Surgical Management of Endocrine Disease

Editors

REBECCA S. SIPPEL
DAVID F. SCHNEIDER

SURGICAL CLINICS OF NORTH AMERICA

www.surgical.theclinics.com

Consulting Editor
RONALD F. MARTIN

August 2019 • Volume 99 • Number 4

ELSEVIER
1600 John F. Kennedy Boulevard • Suite 1800 • Philadelphia, Pennsylvania, 19103-2899
http://www.surgical.theclinics.com

SURGICAL CLINICS OF NORTH AMERICA Volume 99, Number 4
August 2019 ISSN 0039–6109, ISBN-13: 978-0-323-68250-3

Editor: John Vassallo, j.vassallo@elsevier.com
Developmental Editor: Meredith Madeira

Surgical Clinics of North America (ISSN 0039–6109) is published bimonthly by Elsevier Inc., 360 Park Avenue South, New York, NY 10010-1710. Months of publication are February, April, June, August, October, and December. Business and Editorial Offices: 1600 John F. Kennedy Blvd., Suite 1800, Philadelphia, PA 19103-2899. Periodicals postage paid at New York, NY and additional mailing offices. Subscription prices are $417.00 per year for US individuals, $845.00 per year for US institutions, $100.00 per year for US students and residents, $507.00 per year for Canadian individuals, $1071.00 per year for Canadian institutions, $536.00 for international individuals, $1071.00 per year for international institutions and $250.00 per year for Canadian and foreign students/residents. To receive student/resident rate, orders must be accompanied by name of affiliated institution, date of term, and the *signature* of program/residency coordinator on institution letterhead. Orders will be billed at individual rate until proof of status is received. Foreign air speed delivery is included in all *Clinics* subscription prices. All prices are subject to change without notice. POSTMASTER: Send address changes to *Surgical Clinics*, Elsevier Health Sciences Division, Subscription Customer Service, 3251 Riverport Lane, Maryland Heights, MO 63043. **Customer Service (orders, claims, online, change of address): Telephone: 1-800-654-2452 (U.S. and Canada); 314-447-8871 (outside U.S. and Canada). Fax: 314-447-8029. E-mail: journalscustomerservice-usa@elsevier.com (for print support); journalsonline support-usa@elsevier.com (for online support).**

Reprints. For copies of 100 or more, of articles in this publication, please contact the Commercial Reprints Department, Elsevier Inc., 360 Park Avenue South, New York, New York 10010-1710. Tel. 212-633-3874, Fax: 212-633-3820, E-mail: reprints@elsevier.com.

The Surgical Clinics of North America is also published in Spanish by McGraw-Hill Interamericana Editores S.A., P.O. Box 5-237 06500 Mexico D.F. Mexico; and in Portuguese by Interlivros Edicoes Ltda., Rua Comandante Coelho 1085, CEP 21250, Rio de Janeiro, Brazil; and in Greek by Paschalidis Medical Publications, Athens Greece.

The Surgical Clinics of North America is covered in *MEDLINE/PubMed (Index Medicus), EMBASE/Excerpta Medica, Current Contents/Clinical Medicine, Current Contents/Life Sciences, Science Citation Index*, and *ISI/BIOMED*.

Contributors

CONSULTING EDITOR

RONALD F. MARTIN, MD, FACS
Colonel (ret.), United States Army Reserve, Department of Surgery, York Hospital, York, Maine

EDITORS

REBECCA S. SIPPEL, MD
Professor of Surgery, Chief, Division of Endocrine Surgery, Vice Chair of Academic Affairs and Professional Development, University of Wisconsin-Madison School of Medicine and Public Health, Madison, Wisconsin

DAVID F. SCHNEIDER, MS, MD
Assistant Professor, Department of Surgery, Division of Endocrine Surgery, University of Wisconsin-Madison School of Medicine and Public Health, Madison, Wisconsin

AUTHORS

COURTNEY J. BALENTINE, MD, MPH
Assistant Professor, Department of Surgery, The University of Texas Southwestern Medical Center, VA North Texas, Dallas, Texas

KERI DETWEILER, DO
Resident, Department of Surgery, University of California, Irvine, Orange, California

DINA ELARAJ, MD
Associate Professor, Section of Endocrine Surgery, Northwestern University Feinberg School of Medicine, Chicago, Illinois

DAWN M. ELFENBEIN, MD, MPH, FACS
Assistant Professor, Surgical Oncology, Department of Surgery, University of California, Irvine, Orange, California

TONG GAN, MD
General Surgery Resident, Department of Surgery, University of Kentucky, Lexington, Kentucky

RAYMON H. GROGAN, MD, MS, FACS
Associate Professor, Chief of Endocrine Surgery, Baylor St. Luke's Medical Center, Michael E. DeBakey Department of Surgery, Baylor College of Medicine, Houston, Texas

ELIZABETH G. GRUBBS, MD
Associate Professor, Department of Surgical Oncology, The University of Texas MD Anderson Cancer Center, Houston, Texas

JAMES R. HOWE, MD
Department of Surgery, University of Iowa Carver College of Medicine, Division of Surgical Oncology and Endocrine Surgery, University of Iowa Hospitals and Clinics, Iowa City, Iowa

LILY B. HSIEH, MD
Division of Surgical Oncology, Medical College of Wisconsin, Milwaukee, Wisconsin

DYLAN S. JASON, MD
General Surgery Resident, Department of Surgery, The University of Texas Southwestern Medical Center, Dallas, Texas

MAMOONA KHOKHAR, MD
Assistant Professor of Surgery, Division of Endocrine Surgery, University of Arizona College of Medicine–Phoenix, Banner University Medical Center Phoenix, Phoenix, Arizona

COLLEEN M. KIERNAN, MD, MPH
Complex General Surgical Oncology Fellow, Department of Surgical Oncology, The University of Texas MD Anderson Cancer Center, Houston, Texas

FRANCES T. LEE, MD
Surgery Resident, Department of General Surgery, Northwestern University Feinberg School of Medicine, Chicago, Illinois

JAMES A. LEE, MD, FACS
Edwin K. and Anne C. Weiskopf Associate Professor of Surgery, Chief, Endocrine Surgery, Columbia University Irving Medical Center, New York, New York

SAMUEL E. LONG, MD
Clinical Lecturer, Division of Endocrine Surgery, Department of Surgery, University of Michigan, Ann Arbor, Michigan

NIKITA N. MACHADO, MD
Department of General Surgery, University Hospitals Conneaut, Conneaut, Ohio; Assistant Professor, Case Western Reserve University, Cleveland, Ohio

ERIN MACKINNEY, MD
Department of General Surgery, Southern Illinois University School of Medicine, Springfield, Illinois

AMIN MADANI, MD, PhD, FRCSC
Clinical Instructor, Department of Surgery, Columbia University Irving Medical Center, New York, New York

DANIEL MAYERS, DO
Resident, Department of Surgery, University of California, Irvine, Orange, California

ALEXANDRIA D. McDOW, MD
Assistant Professor, Department of Surgery, Section of Endocrine Surgery, Indiana University, Indianapolis, Indiana

MIRA MILAS, MD, FACS
Professor of Surgery, Chief of Endocrine Surgery, Vice Chair for Academic Affairs, Division of Endocrine Surgery, University of Arizona College of Medicine–Phoenix, Banner University Medical Center Phoenix, Phoenix, Arizona

BARBRA S. MILLER, MD
Assistant Professor, Division of Endocrine Surgery, Department of Surgery, University of Michigan, Ann Arbor, Michigan

JANEIL MITCHELL, MD
Fox Valley Surgical Associates, Endocrine Surgery, Appleton, Wisconsin

DALENA T. NGUYEN, MPH
Research Associate, Section of Endocrine Surgery, Department of Surgery, UCLA David Geffen School of Medicine, Los Angeles, California

SARAH C. OLTMANN, MD
Assistant Professor, Department of Surgery, The University of Texas Southwestern Medical Center, Dallas, Texas

SUSAN C. PITT, MD, MPHS
Assistant Professor, Department of Surgery, Division of Endocrine Surgery, University of Wisconsin-Madison, Madison, Wisconsin

REESE W. RANDLE, MD, FACS
Assistant Professor, Section of Endocrine Surgery, Department of Surgery, University of Kentucky, Lexington, Kentucky

AARON T. SCOTT, MD
Department of Surgery, University of Iowa Carver College of Medicine, Iowa City, Iowa

TRACY S. WANG, MD, MPH, FACS
Professor of Surgery, Chief, Section of Endocrine Surgery, Medical College of Wisconsin, Division of Surgical Oncology, Milwaukee, Wisconsin

SCOTT M. WILHELM, MD, FACS
Associate Professor, Department of Surgery, Section Head, Endocrine Surgery, Case Western Reserve University, University Hospitals Cleveland, Cleveland, Ohio

MICHAEL W. YEH, MD
Principal Investigator, Section of Endocrine Surgery, Department of Surgery, UCLA David Geffen School of Medicine, Los Angeles, California

LINWAH YIP, MD, FACS
Department of Surgery, Division of Endocrine Surgery, University of Pittsburgh School of Medicine, Pittsburgh, Pennsylvania

CATHERINE Y. ZHU, MD
Resident Physician, Section of Endocrine Surgery, Department of Surgery, UCLA David Geffen School of Medicine, Los Angeles, California

Contents

Foreword: Endocrine Surgery **xiii**

Ronald F. Martin

Preface: The Art and Science of Endocrine Surgery **xv**

Rebecca S. Sippel and David F. Schneider

Evaluation of Thyroid Nodules **571**

Keri Detweiler, Dawn M. Elfenbein, and Daniel Mayers

This is a brief overview of the initial workup of patients with thyroid nodules. Most nodules are incidentally discovered, benign, and do not require surgery, but the clinician's job is to determine which nodules are concerning and what the appropriate workup should be. Ultrasound examination is the best imaging modality to evaluation thyroid nodules and, when biopsy is indicated, fine needle aspiration is the proper technique to sample thyroid nodules.

Decision Making in Indeterminate Thyroid Nodules and the Role of Molecular Testing **587**

Janeil Mitchell and Linwah Yip

Cytologically indeterminate thyroid nodules are associated with a broad range (5%–75%) of malignant risk and accurately informing definitive management poses a challenge. Advancements in molecular testing of fine-needle aspiration biopsies have improved preoperative diagnostic accuracy and prognostication. For indeterminate nodules, such testing ideally will reduce the need for surgery for benign nodules and potentially guide appropriate extent of initial surgery for malignancy.

Extent of Surgery for Low-Risk Differentiated Thyroid Cancer **599**

Alexandria D. McDow and Susan C. Pitt

Although the incidence of thyroid cancer is increasing, survival remains unchanged. Due to concern for overtreatment, surgical management of thyroid cancer has evolved. Papillary thyroid microcarcinoma measuring 1 cm or smaller are considered very low risk and can be managed with either thyroid lobectomy or active surveillance. Total thyroidectomy is no longer recommended for these cancers unless there is evidence of metastasis, local invasion, or aggressive disease. Recommendations for low-risk differentiated thyroid cancer measuring 1 cm to 4 cm remain controversial. This article explores the controversies over the extent of surgery for patients with very low-risk and low-risk differentiated thyroid cancer.

Management of Nodal Disease in Thyroid Cancer 611

Mamoona Khokhar and Mira Milas

Cervical lymph node metastases are present in a considerable number of patients with differentiated and medullary thyroid cancer. The completeness of surgical resection, including clinically significant lymph node metastases, is an important determinant of outcome, because cervical lymph nodes represent the most common site of persistent and recurrent disease. This article delineates the management of nodal disease in thyroid cancer, focusing on the preoperative evaluation, operative management, and postoperative assessment of cervical lymph nodes.

The Role of Surgery in Autoimmune Conditions of the Thyroid 633

Tong Gan and Reese W. Randle

The two most common autoimmune conditions of the thyroid include chronic lymphocytic (Hashimoto's) thyroiditis and Graves' disease. Both conditions can be treated medically, but surgery plays an important role. Hashimoto's thyroiditis and Graves' disease are mediated by autoantibodies that interact directly with the thyroid, creating inflammation and impacting thyroid function. Patients may develop large goiters with compressive symptoms or malignancy requiring surgical intervention. In addition, there are several surgical indications specific to Hashimoto's and Graves' Disease.

Diagnosis and Evaluation of Primary Hyperparathyroidism 649

Nikita N. Machado and Scott M. Wilhelm

Primary hyperparathyroidism (PHPT) is a common endocrine disorder, resulting from the autonomous production of parathyroid hormone from 1 or more abnormal parathyroid glands. Disease presentation ranges from asymptomatic to multiorgan involvement (skeletal, renal, neurocognitive, and gastrointestinal). This article outlines the epidemiology, clinical presentation, and diagnostic algorithm for PHPT. Key laboratory assessments are discussed, as are imaging studies for preoperative localization. Indications for surgical intervention are detailed, as are potential indications for surveillance. Sporadic and genetic syndromes associated with PHPT are also described.

Who Benefits from Treatment of Primary Hyperparathyroidism? 667

Catherine Y. Zhu, Dalena T. Nguyen, and Michael W. Yeh

Parathyroidectomy (PTx) is the only definitive treatment for primary hyperparathyroidism (PHPT), but is commonly underutilized. Most patients are medically observed, whereas approximately 30% of patients are treated operatively. PTx is a low-risk surgical procedure and the most cost-effective treatment option. An international consensus statement was published in 1990 to guide clinicians in the management of patients with PHPT, particularly those with asymptomatic disease. Most patients with PHPT and low perioperative risk benefit from surgical treatment, regardless of whether they meet consensus criteria, due to fracture risk reduction, health-related quality-of-life improvements, and prevention or mitigation of disease progression.

Intraoperative Decision Making in Parathyroid Surgery **681**

Dylan S. Jason and Courtney J. Balentine

This article reviews intraoperative decision making related to several important aspects of parathyroid surgery. These include how to systematically identify a missing gland, when to perform a unilateral versus bilateral exploration for cure, approaches to secondary hyperparathyroidism, management of familial hyperparathyroidism, and the treatment of parathyroid cancer. The management of intraoperative complications, such as recurrent laryngeal nerve injury and devascularization of parathyroid glands, also is discussed.

Surgical Management of Multiple Endocrine Neoplasia 1 and Multiple Endocrine Neoplasia 2 **693**

Colleen M. Kiernan and Elizabeth G. Grubbs

This article summarizes the surgical management of tumors associated with multiple endocrine neoplasia 1 (MEN1) and multiple endocrine neoplasia 2 (MEN2) and includes discussion of the preoperative planning, the goals, and extent of surgery, as well as the intraoperative considerations and the management of recurrent disease.

The Importance of Family History in the Management of Endocrine Disease **711**

Raymon H. Grogan

Family history is an essential component of the workup of endocrine surgery patients. The family history can change the diagnosis, management, and follow-up of endocrine patients. Here we discuss the importance of family history, review familial endocrine disorders, and develop a list of pertinent questions to ask when taking a family history of patients with endocrine disorders.

Evaluation of an Adrenal Incidentaloma **721**

Dylan S. Jason and Sarah C. Oltmann

Given the frequent use of cross-sectional imaging in medicine, adrenal masses are discovered at an increasing rate. Once detected, it is critical to ensure the patient undergoes the appropriate biochemical/hormonal workup to rule out any aberrant activity and ensure imaging features do not raise suspicion for a malignant neoplasm. Patients with hormonal overactivity, concerning size, and/or imaging characteristics must be referred for surgical consideration. For those not requiring adrenalectomy, it is important to determine which patients mandate follow-up to ensure no further growth or development of hormonal production. It is also critical to understand what is the appropriate follow-up.

Evaluation and Management of Primary Hyperaldosteronism **731**

Frances T. Lee and Dina Elaraj

Primary hyperaldosteronism is an important and increasingly prevalent cause of hypertension that is characterized by unregulated aldosterone excess. More than 90% of primary hyperaldosteronism cases are attributable to either idiopathic adrenal hyperplasia or aldosterone-producing adenomas. The approach to the diagnosis of primary hyperaldosteronism should be step-wise, starting with screening of at-risk populations, confirmatory testing for positively screened patients, and subtype classification in order to direct surgical or medical management. Based on current guidelines, subtype classification of primary hyperaldosteronism should be determined with both imaging and adrenal vein sampling (AVS), reserving deferment of AVS for a selective subset of patients.

When to Intervene for Subclinical Cushing's Syndrome 747

Lily B. Hsieh, Erin Mackinney, and Tracy S. Wang

Without the overt clinical signs and symptoms associated with Cushing's syndrome, the diagnosis of subclinical Cushing's syndrome (SCS) is primarily based on biochemical evaluation. Despite being labeled as "subclinical," SCS is associated with significant morbidity that can be improved with adrenalectomy. Minimally invasive adrenalectomy is associated with low morbidity in the hands of experienced adrenal surgeons and is recommended as the treatment of choice for SCS patients with SCS-associated comorbidities.

Adrenocortical Cancer Treatment 759

Samuel E. Long and Barbra S. Miller

Adrenocortical cancer is a rare disease. Prognosis remains poor but is improving. In this article, initial presentation, biochemical and imaging evaluation, surgical approach to resection, and postoperative care are reviewed. Prognosis, patterns of recurrence, treatment of metastatic disease using medical therapy and other surgical and nonsurgical therapies are discussed.

Surgical Approaches to the Adrenal Gland 773

Amin Madani and James A. Lee

Adrenalectomy can be performed open, endoscopically or robotically, utilizing a transabdominal or retroperitoneal approach. This chapter describes the relevant anatomy, various approaches and surgical techniques, pre-operative work-up and optimization, and post-operative management of patients undergoing an adrenalectomy.

Evaluation and Management of Neuroendocrine Tumors of the Pancreas 793

Aaron T. Scott and James R. Howe

Pancreatic neuroendocrine tumors are a diverse group of neoplasms with a generally favorable prognosis. Although they exhibit indolent growth, metastases are seen in roughly 60% of patients. Pancreatic neuroendocrine tumors may produce a wide variety of hormones, which are associated with dramatic symptoms, but the majority are nonfunctional. The diagnosis and treatment of these tumors is a multidisciplinary effort, and management guidelines continue to evolve. This review provides a concise summary of the presentation, diagnosis, surgical management, and systemic treatment of pancreatic neuroendocrine tumors.

SURGICAL CLINICS OF NORTH AMERICA

FORTHCOMING ISSUES

October 2019
Practicing Primary Palliative Care
Pringl Miller, *Editor*

December 2019
Inflammatory Bowel Disease
Sean J. Langenfeld, *Editor*

February 2020
Melanoma
Rohit Sharma, *Editor*

RECENT ISSUES

June 2019
Management of the Foregut
Sushanth Reddy, *Editor*

April 2019
Diseases of the Biliary Tract
J. Bart Rose, *Editor*

February 2019
Issues in Transplant Surgery
Juan Palma-Vargas, *Editor*

Foreword
Endocrine Surgery

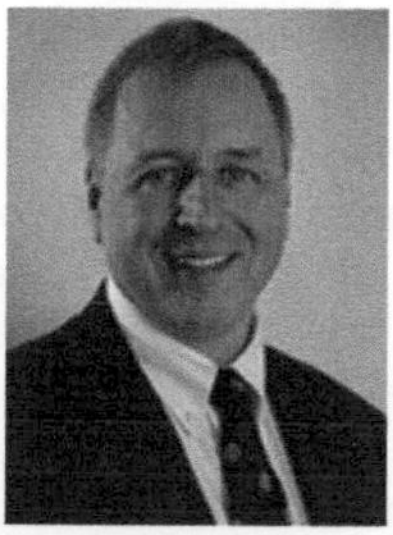

Ronald F. Martin, MD, FACS
Consulting Editor

The current culture in which we live affords us many "instant" opportunities that simply didn't exist even a short while ago. Major online retailers are trying to get delivery times to 1 day or less to their large subscriber base. High-speed Internet capability allows Web-based access at unparalleled speed, and we are on the verge of a 5-G network that will likely bring forth new changes to communications, travel, commerce, and other parts of our lives. On of the derivative effects of this "instant-ality" is the change in the perception of some for the need for humanly stored knowledge (biologically stored in our own brains) as compared with quickly retrievable knowledge by other means (usually electronic), occasionally referred to as JITI (just-in-time information). In theory, one doesn't need to have the information on hand, just the ability to retrieve it quickly by some means when desired. This electronically stored information can be used in much the same way that online retailers use logistical networks to achieve or fulfill rapid delivery of products by prepositioning goods in warehouses close to many different markets.

In some ways, it is completely understandable. Machine-stored facts and other information are usually more easily and accurately retrieved than is information that we rely on memory for. Even some of the best human examples of memory retrieval, *Jeopardy* game-show winners, were outperformed by artificial intelligence machines, such as IBM's *Watson*. While memory and fact retrieval should not be undervalued in any way, excellent recall in and of itself will not likely replace actual mastery of a topic in the near future.

I have suggested in prior issues of the *Surgical Clinics of North America* that the study of gastric surgery from its inception to modern times was probably the best example of surgical thought and discipline that we as surgeons had to offer. From its very humble beginnings as anatomic discipline to its rapid evolution to physiologic observation to a molecular study, it had all of the elements of science that surgeons could want. It also has a long and valued history of identifying limitations and correctly deriving solutions to problems based on an accurate understanding of anatomic structure and

Surg Clin N Am 99 (2019) xiii–xiv
https://doi.org/10.1016/j.suc.2019.05.002
0039-6109/19/© 2019 Published by Elsevier Inc.

physiologic function. I'll admit that my biases as a foregut surgeon affect my judgment here. There are other disciplines that should be in the running as well, such as cardiac surgery and orthopedics, to name just two. I still fall back to gastric surgery as the winner if for no other reason than the advances in gastric surgical thought were made when so little other science was actually available compared with the major advances in the other disciplines coming along more in alignment with the space age.

All the above notwithstanding, it is perhaps time to consider endocrine surgery to be a contender for the intellectual crown. The reasons for this are many, but chief among them are that endocrine surgery has perhaps more than any other surgical discipline incorporated anatomic structure, physiologic understanding, rigorous structural- and physiologic-based imaging, and genetic understanding both on the individual patient level and on the epidemiologic level. Our endocrine colleagues are probably as far if not farther along to functioning on the truly "precision" level of surgery and medicine than any of our other surgical colleagues.

The advances in the molecular-level understanding of endocrine diseases and endocrine neoplastic disease have largely rendered many of the concepts that surgical residents were forced to commit to memory even two decades ago less relevant. What used to be a wide list of memorized associations is now largely replaced with understanding how processes are related at the level of genetic markers or miRNA panels.

Despite all these advances in genetic and chemical markers, testing panels, and imaging or even the advances in operative approaches to removing endocrine tissue, one still has to develop mastery of the underlying processes in order to best care for patients. To that end, we are deeply indebted to Drs Sippel and Schneider, who have assembled an outstanding group of contributors to help us all improve our mastery of a wide array of topics. As a former general surgery training program director, I would encourage any resident (or any of the rest of us) to start with this collection of articles if one wants to know what one needs to know to comfortably do well on the ABSITE, pass the ABS Qualifying Exam or Certifying Exam, or most importantly, be more comfortable caring for patients.

To go back to the online retail analogy, just because one can rapidly acquire some good or tool from an Internet retailer quicker than quick, it still doesn't mean that one needed the good or one knows how to use the tool. To understand what goods are needed and how tools are used, one needs something more than a credit card and an online account: one needs knowledge. Being able to recall facts or data is good. Being able to remember treatment algorithms also is good. They are both good examples of coming up with answers. Understanding the questions, though, is better, for that allows us to go beyond the answers we have today. One must first acquire knowledge, and over time, with practice and reflection, one can develop mastery, at which time the questions will become clearer.

We hope you enjoy this issue of the *Surgical Clinics of North America*. As always, we welcome your feedback and observations.

Ronald F. Martin, MD, FACS
Colonel (retired), United States Army Reserve
Department of Surgery
York Hospital
16 Hospital Drive, Suite A
York, ME 03909, USA

E-mail address:
rmartin@yorkhospital.com

Preface
The Art and Science of Endocrine Surgery

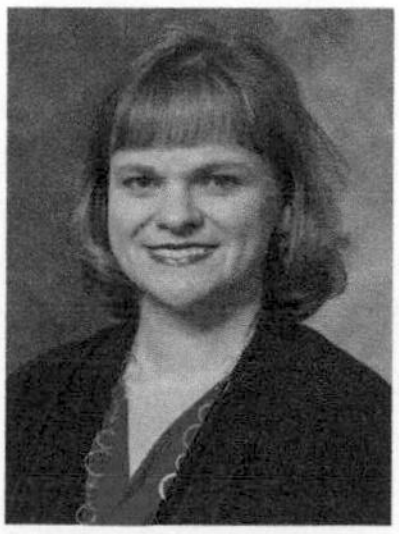

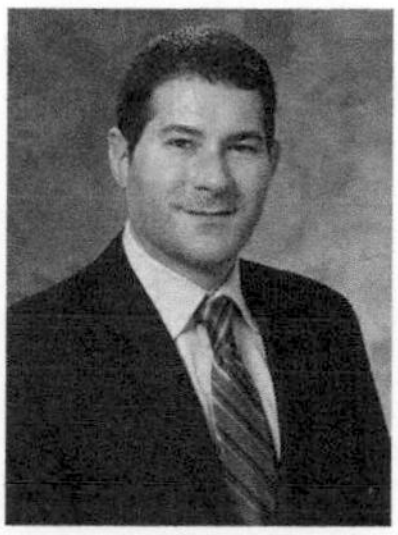

Rebecca S. Sippel, MD   David F. Schneider, MS, MD
Editors

> *The concept of medicine as art, the physician as artist, or the artist as scientist is not as contradictory as it would seem.*
>
> —*Carol Z. Clark and Orlo H. Clark, MD*
>
> The Remarkables:
> Endocrine Abnormalities in Art

As Endocrine Surgeons, we celebrate the long-held belief that the practice of surgery is both art and science. In this issue of *Surgical Clinics of North America*, "Surgical Management of Endocrine Disease," we emphasize the latest developments in our field. Certainly, the science has advanced, with newer, molecular-based diagnostics for thyroid nodules, state-of-the-art imaging techniques for neuroendocrine tumors, and intraoperative techniques for parathyroid localization. Yet, the reader will still find evidence of artistry in these pages. We have assembled a prestigious group of authors, all experts in the field of Endocrine Surgery. They share the latest science, but they also provide their guides for preoperative workup, intraoperative decision making, and postoperative patient management. While we always strive to base these tasks on evidence or science, these decisions also reflect an artistry. The intangible value added when an experienced surgeon combines the latest science with his or her experience and unique touch is truly an art. It is an artistry informed by the authors' experience and training as well as the latest science. We hope you will enjoy both the science and the art as you read these articles.

Like many in our field, we have always treasured the *Surgical Clinics of North America* issues dedicated to Endocrine Surgery. Each new issue serves as both review and an update on the current thinking in our field. This issue is no exception. While many readers have certainly attended meetings and read the literature, we feel that

Surg Clin N Am 99 (2019) xv–xvi
https://doi.org/10.1016/j.suc.2019.05.001
0039-6109/19/© 2019 Published by Elsevier Inc.

this issue of *Surgical Clinics of North America* compiles and summarizes the current science and controversies, something that is particularly useful with the rapid pace of new information. A lot has changed since the last issue. Guidelines have evolved. An ever-increasing number of molecular diagnostics continue to guide treatment decisions. In addition, more research has changed our thinking on the long-term management of differentiated thyroid cancer and parathyroid disease. We hope that this issue serves as a useful summary for all the latest progress in Endocrine Surgery.

Last, we wish to thank all the contributing authors. They are truly leaders in our field, and we thank them for their time, diligence, and writing skills in producing this collection. We truly appreciate them sharing their knowledge, expertise, and, yes, artistry, for this issue.

Rebecca S. Sippel, MD
Division of Endocrine Surgery
Department of Surgery
University of Wisconsin
School of Medicine and Public Health
H4/722 CSC
600 Highland Avenue
Madison, WI 53792-7375, USA

David F. Schneider, MS, MD
Division of Endocrine Surgery
Department of Surgery
University of Wisconsin
School of Medicine and Public Health
K4/738 CSC
600 Highland Avenue
Madison, WI 53792-7375, USA

E-mail addresses:
sippel@surgery.wisc.edu (R.S. Sippel)
schneiderd@surgery.wisc.edu (D.F. Schneider)

Evaluation of Thyroid Nodules

Keri Detweiler, DO[a], Dawn M. Elfenbein, MD, MPH[b,*], Daniel Mayers, DO[a]

KEYWORDS

- Thyroid nodule • Thyroid ultrasound • Fine needle aspiration • Bethesda criteria

KEY POINTS

- Most thyroid nodules are asymptomatic and benign, but nodules that cause compression symptoms or are concerning for cancer should be referred for surgery.
- Ultrasound examination is the best imaging modality to evaluation thyroid nodules.
- Various organizations have published guidelines to help decide how to manage various types of nodules.
- For nodules that require biopsy, fine needle aspiration biopsy is the best technique for sampling thyroid nodules.

INTRODUCTION

Thyroid nodules are incredibly common: more than one-half of everyone living will develop a thyroid nodule at some point in their life. Women are more likely than men to have nodules, and nodules seem to grow with age, because older individuals have more nodules than younger ones.[1] As imaging techniques become more sensitive at finding smaller lesions, the incidence will continue to increase. When the only way to detect thyroid nodules was by palpation, 5% to 10% of the population had them.[2,3] Now with high-resolution ultrasound imaging, nearly 70% of people are found to have at least 1 small nodule.[4] The presence of small nodules is not a new phenomenon; a classic study from the 1930s found that 57% of people who died of other causes had thyroid nodules discovered on autopsy[5]; we now are finding them while people are living.

The vast majority of nodules are benign (>90%),[6] and small cancers may not ever cause problems for an individual patient.[7] However, the discovery of a mass is one of the most anxiety-producing events for an individual patient; cancer is the most feared diagnosis for Americans and often this fear triggers an emotional desire for aggressive

Disclosure statement: The authors have nothing to disclose.
[a] Department of Surgery, University of California, Irvine, 333 City Boulevard West, Suite 1600, Orange, CA 92868, USA; [b] Surgical Oncology, Department of Surgery, University of California, Irvine, 333 City Boulevard West, Suite 1600, Orange, CA 92868, USA
* Corresponding author.
E-mail address: delfenbe@uci.edu

Surg Clin N Am 99 (2019) 571–586
https://doi.org/10.1016/j.suc.2019.04.001

treatment.[8] Our role as clinicians is to understand when thyroid nodules are problematic, which nodules are at risk to be clinically significant (either cancer or risk of causing significant compression symptoms), and finally what to do about them.

RELEVANT ANATOMY AND PATHOPHYSIOLOGY

The thyroid is a butterfly-shaped gland in the neck composed of follicular cells that secrete thyroid hormone, and parafollicular cells (or C cells) that secrete calcitonin. The follicular cells are arranged in small spherical groupings of cells around a core of colloid that contains thyroid hormone precursor proteins (**Fig. 1**). The thyroid also contains endothelial cells, blood vessels, nerves, and lymphatic vessels. The gross appearance of a normal thyroid gland is smooth and homogeneous. Nodule is a term that refers to a lump within the thyroid parenchyma and is distinguished from a simple cyst in that it is composed of at least some cellular material, not simply filled with fluid.

The thyroid lies around the trachea below the thyroid cartilage (**Fig. 2**). It is attached to the anterior surface of the trachea with its thin fibrous capsule that thickens posterolaterally to form the ligaments of Berry. The gland is in close proximity to several structures including the esophagus, typically posterior to the trachea on the left side of the neck, the carotid arteries, and the larynx. The recurrent laryngeal nerves, which innervate the intrinsic muscles of the larynx, pass behind the gland. Enlargement of the thyroid, particularly caused by a nodule, that is more dense or firm than a normal thyroid, can therefore cause symptoms of impingement on any of these nearby structures.

Because not all thyroid nodules are biopsied or surgically removed, we can never know the true breakdown of the types of nodules. However, surgical series have shown that of thyroids that have been surgically removed for nodular disease, 44% to 77% of nodules are benign colloid nodules, 15% to 40% of nodules are benign follicular adenomas, and 8% to 17% are differentiated thyroid cancer.[9–11] Very small percentages of thyroid nodules turn out to be more aggressive forms of thyroid cancer, such as medullary, anaplastic, or primary thyroid lymphoma.

CLINICAL PRESENTATION AND EXAMINATION

Risk Factors

Although nodules are common and seen all over the world, there are some risk factors associated with the development of thyroid nodules. Although we have known for a

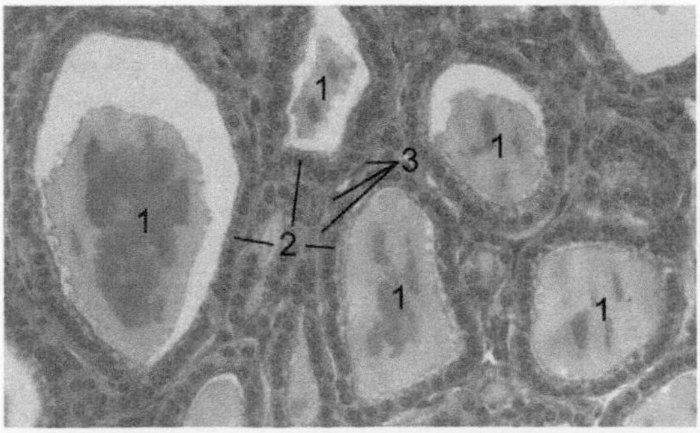

Fig. 1. Thyroid histology. (1) Colloid-containing follicle, (2) Follicular cells, (3) Endothelial cells. (*From* Wikimedia Commons, https://en.wikipedia.org/wiki/Thyroid#/media/File:Thyroid-histology.jpg, with permission.)

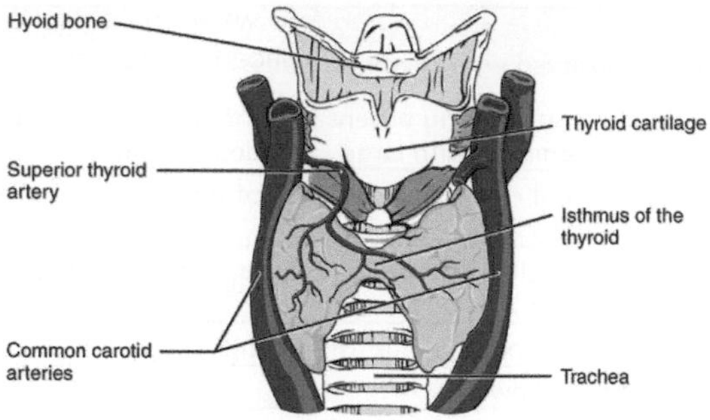

Fig. 2. Thyroid anatomy. The thyroid lies in close proximity to the trachea, carotid arteries, esophagus (not shown, posterior and to the left of the trachea), and larynx (posterior to the thyroid cartilage). (*From* Wikimedia Commons, https://commons.wikimedia.org/wiki/File:Anterior_thyroid.jpg, with permission.)

long time that nodules are more common in women, older individuals, people with decreased iodine intake, and a history of radiation exposure,[2,12] recently a few more specific risk factors have been identified. Smoking,[13] obesity,[14] alcohol consumption,[15] uterine fibroids,[16] and higher insulin-like growth factor-1 levels[17] have been found to be associated with thyroid nodule presence. Interestingly, use of oral contraceptive pills[18] and 3-hydroxy-3-methyl-glutaryl-coenzyme A reductase (statin) medications[19] have been found to have a negative correlation with the presence of thyroid nodules, but whether these medications confer a protective effect is not yet clear.

A family history of thyroid disease, thyroid cancer, and other endocrine conditions should be elucidated during a thorough history of anyone who presents with a thyroid nodule. The multiple endocrine neoplasia syndromes, specifically multiple endocrine neoplasia types 2a and 2b, are associated with a high risk of medullary thyroid cancer. Although familial nonmedullary thyroid cancer is fairly rare and not well-defined, there are several syndromes to be aware of that confer increased risk, including Cowden syndrome, familiar adenomatous polyposis, Gardner syndrome, Carney complex type 1, Werner syndrome, and DICER1 syndrome.[20]

Signs and Symptoms

The most common presentation of a thyroid nodule is an incidental finding from an imaging study done for another reason (ie, trauma scans, chest computed tomography scan for pulmonary complaints, carotid artery ultrasound examination for stroke workup).[21] Some patients present having felt a neck mass, either on their own or on routine physical examination. Other than being able to feel the mass, palpable masses may not cause localized compression. In any person who presents with either a palpable or nonpalpable mass, it is important to inquire about possible related symptoms. As nodules get to be 2 to 3 cm or if they are peripherally located where they can compress other structures,[22–25] they may start to cause symptoms. It is important to inquire specifically about the symptoms listed on **Table 1** when taking a history of anyone with a thyroid nodule.

Thyroid Function and Nodules

Although most thyroid nodules do not interfere with thyroid function, it is important to inquire about any hypothyroid or hyperthyroid symptoms. A small number of thyroid nodules are made up of autonomously functioning follicular cells and overproduce

Table 1 Compressive symptoms associated with thyroid nodules	
Dysphagia	Difficulty swallowing or sensation of food getting "caught" in throat, more common with large left-sided nodules
Neck fullness	Sensation of excess tissue at base of throat, some patient describe a "tightness"
Choking	Related to fullness, patients feel a squeezing sensation around the region of their thyroid gland
Dyspnea	Shortness of breath, most often while supine
Odynophagia	Painful swallowing
Globus sensation	Sensation of a lump or foreign body in the throat that does not go away when a person swallows
Voice changes	True voice changes are concerning for malignant invasion of nerves, but some patients with large compressive nodules may complain of subtle voice fatigue or weakness

thyroid hormone. Additionally, thyroid nodules can exist in a background of hyperthyroidism (ie, nodular Graves' disease) or hypothyroidism (ie, Hashimoto's thyroiditis). In an individual who is hyperthyroid with nodules, it is important to perform thyroid scintigraphy to determine whether the nodule itself is producing excess hormone or whether the surrounding thyroid is hyperactive—the workup and treatment of these conditions is quite different. **Table 2** lists common hyperthyroid and hypothyroid symptoms that one should elicit while taking a history of anyone with thyroid nodules.

Table 2
Functional thyroid symptoms by body system

Hyperthyroidism	Hypothyroidism
General	General
Feeling warm	Feeling cold
Weight loss with high appetite	Weight gain with poor appetite
Increased sweating	Fatigue/sluggishness
Insomnia/fatigue	Need for sleep during the day
Psychological	Psychological
Irritability	Poor memory
Nervousness	Difficulty concentrating
Anxiety	Depression
Cardiovascular	Cardiovascular
Fast heart rate/palpitations	Slow heart rate
Muscular	Muscular
Weakness, upper arms and thighs	Delayed reflexes
Gastrointestinal	Gastrointestinal
Frequent bowel movements	Constipation
Genitourinary	Genitourinary
Amenorrhea	Menorrhagia
Skin	Skin
Thinning of skin	Myxedema, dry skin
Fine, brittle hair	Hair loss
	Brittle nails

Thyroid Nodule Physical Examination

Characteristics to note on physical examination of the thyroid should include size, consistency, location, and movement with deglutition (swallowing). Nodules that are very firm—like a pebble or rock instead of a rubbery, compressible mass—or nodules that are fixed in place when the patient swallows are more concerning for malignancy. Careful palpation of the jugular lymph node chain in levels 2 through 4 should be performed, and any palpable nodes investigated further with imaging. Although palpable nodes can be concerning for malignancy, they are not uncommon in inflammatory thyroid conditions such as Hashimoto's thyroiditis. In any patient with a large (>4 cm) nodule or compressive symptoms at rest, the patient should be instructed to lift their arms above their head and the examiner looks for facial plethora, distension of the jugular veins, or symptoms of dyspnea. This sign is referred to as Pemberton sign and is a concerning finding for severe compression symptoms from a retrosternal goiter.[26]

DIAGNOSTIC PROCEDURES

Regardless of how the nodule was discovered initially, and irrespective of any symptoms or examination findings, it is appropriate for every patient who has a thyroid nodule to undergo an ultrasound examination of the thyroid and any suspicious lymphadenopathy, and to have measurements of thyroid function by checking a serum thyroid-stimulating hormone (TSH) level. This is the most appropriate initial workup of every thyroid nodule. Depending on the results of these 2 initial studies, the workup either concludes or proceeds in a stepwise fashion. **Fig. 3** shows a suggested algorithm for the initial workup of a thyroid nodule.

Hyperthyroid with Nodules

For patients who have a suppressed TSH and thyroid nodules, radioiodine scintigraphy can distinguish whether nodules themselves are hyperactive ("hot" nodule), isoactive ("warm" nodule), or hypoactive ("cold" nodule). Although there are case reports of "hot" nodules harboring differentiated thyroid cancer,[27] because the rate of malignancy is so low, no cytologic evaluation is necessary (latest American Thyroid Association [ATA] guidelines). If nodules show similar or decreased uptake ("warm" or "cold" nodules), the algorithm is similar to that of a patient with nodules and normal or low thyroid function.

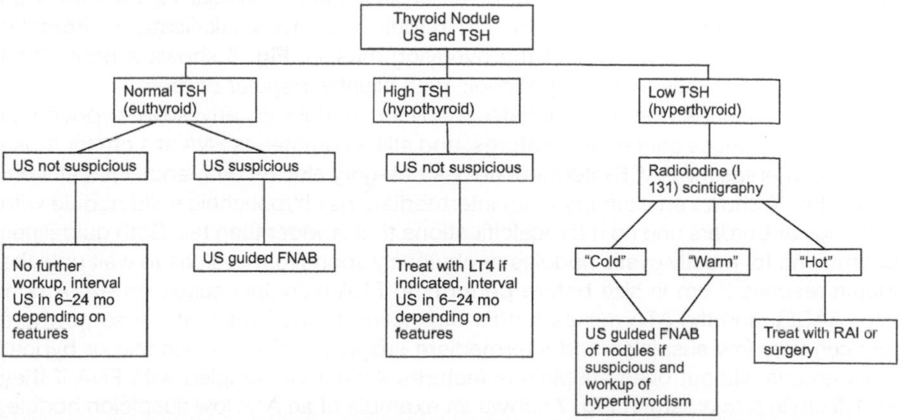

Fig. 3. Initial evaluation of a thyroid nodule. FNAB, fine needle aspiration biopsy; RAI, radioactive iodine ablation; US, ultrasound.

Treatment options for hyperfunctioning nodules are stabilization with antithyroid medications followed by treatment with either surgery or radioactive iodine, unless there are major contraindications for these definitive options. Hemithyroidectomy can be performed if the disease is unilateral and the success rate of this surgery at curing hyperthyroidism is very high (>99%). Hypothyroidism is rare after hemithyroidectomy for a single toxic nodule, occurring 2% to 3% of the time. A total thyroidectomy may be necessary in a patient with multiple toxic nodules. Radioactive iodine carries a 6% to 18% risk of recurrence of hyperthyroidism when used for single toxic nodules and also carries a risk of subclinical or overt hypothyroidism developing in the years after treatment, and as many as 46% of patients may develop hypothyroidism after 10 years owing to unavoidable damage to the normal thyroid parenchyma.[28]

Euthyroid or Hypothyroid with Nodules

For patients with decreased or normal thyroid function and nodules, the decision about whether cytologic sampling is recommended is based on the ultrasound features such as size, composition (solid vs cystic), high-risk features (microcalcifications, shape, borders, etc), and rate of growth (if known). Although historically there has been a recommendation to perform fine needle aspiration biopsy (FNAB) of any nodule greater than 1 cm in the largest dimension, more recent guidelines take into account the slow growth pattern of most thyroid cancers and the concern that diagnosing small and clinically insignificant thyroid cancers leads to overtreatment.[29] There are 3 organizations that have published recent guidelines about the ultrasound features of thyroid nodules and at what size one should consider performing FNAB: the ATA, the American Association of Clinical Endocrinologists (AACE), and the American College of Radiology (TI-RADS).

The ATA guidelines[3] describe 5 categories of thyroid nodules (high suspicion, intermediate suspicion, low suspicion, very low suspicion, and benign), whereas the AACE guidelines[30] describe 3 categories (high risk, intermediate risk, and low risk). Each of these categories have ultrasound features associated with them, and the recommended size at which to offer FNA. Both organizations describe nodules that are irregularly shaped or obviously invasive, microcalcifications, and taller-than-wide shape as very concerning for malignancy and recommend FNA for any nodule larger than 1 cm with these features. The AACE guidelines contain a caveat to consider biopsy for these high-risk lesions 5 to 9 mm in size if a person has a personal or family history of thyroid cancer, high-risk radiation exposure, or other suspicious findings. **Fig. 4** shows an example of a left-sided high-risk thyroid nodule with microcalcifications, irregular shape, and possible invasion into the overlying muscle. **Fig. 5** shows a right-sided taller-than-wide nodule that is hypoechoic with slightly irregular borders.

The ATA describes an intermediate suspicion nodule as any solid hypoechoic nodule without those concerning features, and still recommends FNA at 1 cm for those nodules, whereas the AACE intermediate risk category also recommends FNA at 1 cm in size. **Fig. 6** shows an example of an intermediate risk hypoechoic solid nodule with fairly regular borders and no microcalcifications that is wider than tall. Both guidelines recommend for mostly cystic nodules or obviously spongiform lesions to wait until the nodule reaches 2 cm in size before performing FNA (very low suspicion—ATA, low risk—AACE), and the ATA makes further distinction for nodules that are somewhere between very low suspicion and intermediate suspicion. These isoechoic or hypoechoic lesions without overt suspicious features should be sampled with FNA if they are 1.5 cm in size or larger. **Fig. 7** shows an example of an ATA low suspicion nodule. Finally, the ATA describes purely cystic nodules as benign with no risk of cancer so FNA is not necessary for diagnosis. Sometimes simple cysts can be quite large and

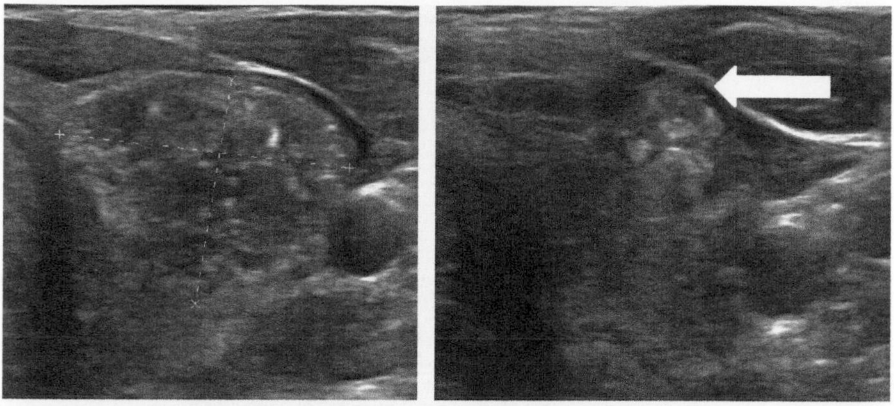

Fig. 4. Ultrasound image of a highly suspicious thyroid nodule. Note microcalcifications, irregular shape, and in the second panel (*white arrow*) there is possible invasion into overlying strap muscles. (*Courtesy of* Dawn M. Elfenbein, MD, MPH, FACS, Department of Surgery, University of California Irvine, Orange, CA)

the aspiration of the cyst fluid may provide symptom relief, but cytologic sampling to rule out cancer is not recommended.

Although the ATA and AACE guidelines are descriptive and leave more room for clinical interpretation, the TI-RADS[31] system is designed to standardize the language radiologists use to communicate findings to the ordering physician of a thyroid ultrasound examination. Instead of describing the features of a high-risk nodule and leaving it to an individual to interpret as they will if a nodule only has 3 out of 4 of those features, TI-RADS describes 5 categories of ultrasound features and assigns point values for each feature a nodule has (**Table 3**). This system is based off the success of other similar cancer imaging reporting systems, such as used in breast and lung cancer

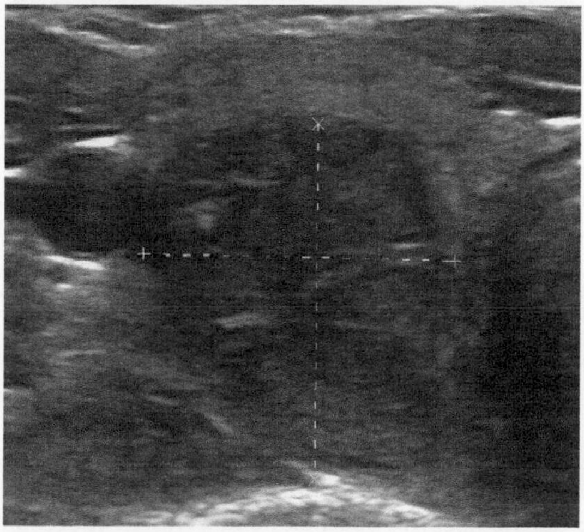

Fig. 5. Ultrasound image of a highly suspicious thyroid nodule. This hypoechoic, irregularly shaped nodule is taller than wide. (*Courtesy of* Dawn M. Elfenbein, MD, MPH, FACS, Department of Surgery, University of California Irvine, Orange, CA)

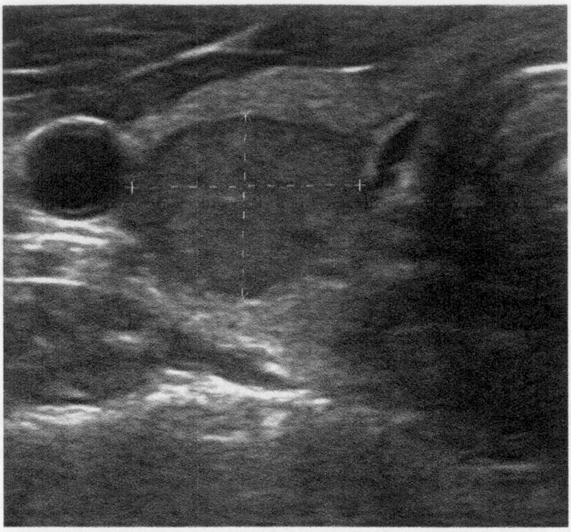

Fig. 6. Ultrasound image of an intermediate risk thyroid nodule. This hypoechoic, regularly shaped nodule is wider than tall and lacks microcalcifications or obvious invasion. (*Courtesy of* Dawn M. Elfenbein, MD, MPH, FACS, Department of Surgery, University of California Irvine, Orange, CA.)

(https://www.acr.org/Clinical-Resources/Reporting-and-Data-Systems). Because the size cutoffs are on average a bit larger than the other 2 systems, the implementation of this system will result in fewer biopsies of benign nodules, but will also result in fewer biopsies of malignant nodules.[32] Although all 3 guidelines are roughly the same, many clinicians are reluctant to adhere strictly to 1 system all the time. Clinical judgment, shared decision making, and individual risk assessment still play a critical role in

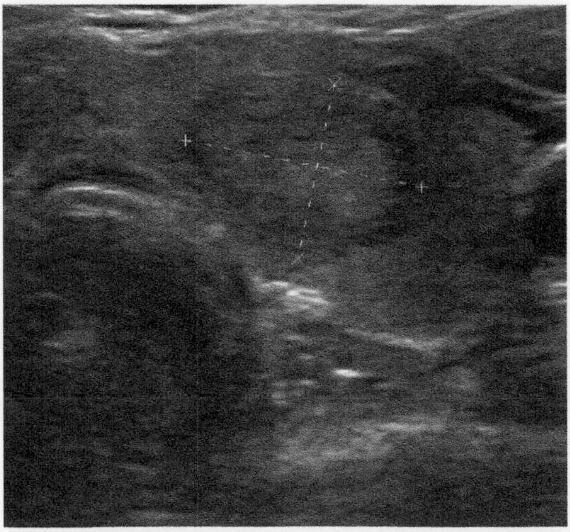

Fig. 7. ATA low suspicion nodule. This isoechoic nodule with a hypoechoic rim without overt suspicious features in an example of an ATA low-risk nodule. The AACE would consider this an intermediate risk nodule. (*Courtesy of* Dawn M. Elfenbein, MD, MPH, FACS, Department of Surgery, University of California Irvine, Orange, CA.)

Table 3
TI-RADS system of classification of thyroid nodules

TI-RADS Categories	Ultrasound Features
Composition	Cystic, or completely cystic - 0 points Spongiform - 0 points Mixed cystic/solid - 1 point Solid, or almost completely solid - 2 points
Echogenicity	Anechoic - 0 points Hyperechoic or isoechoic - 1 point Hypoechoic - 2 points Very hypoechoic - 3 points
Shape (in transverse plane)	Wider than tall - 0 points Taller than wide - 3 points
Margin	Smooth - 0 points Ill defined - 0 points Lobulated or irregular - 2 points Extrathyroidal extension - 3 points
Echogenic foci	None - 0 points Comet tail artifact - 0 points Macrocalcifications - 1 point Peripheral or rim calcifications - 2 points Punctate echogenic foci - 3 points

For each nodule, add up score from each of the 5 categories. **Table 4** provides FNA recommendations and/or follow up ultrasound suggestions for each nodule.

Adapted from Grant EG, Tessler FN, Hoang JK, et al. Thyroid Ultrasound Reporting Lexicon: White Paper of the ACR Thyroid Imaging, Reporting and Data System (TIRADS) Committee. Journal of the American College of Radiology 2015;12(12):1272–9; with permission.

deciding when to perform FNA biopsy of thyroid nodules, but the guidelines are a useful tool in decision making.

In addition to ultrasound characteristics, two other features are associated with increased risk for malignancy. Interestingly, for euthyroid patients, the actual value of TSH within the normal range is correlated with malignancy rates. Patients with values closer to the higher limit of normal (1.7 mU/L) have a 2.7 times increased adjusted odds ratio of malignancy versus those who have TSH closer to the lower limit of normal (0.4 mU/L).[33] Additionally, those thyroid nodules found incidentally on a PET-computed tomography scan have a higher risk of being malignant than those found incidentally on other imaging modalities, such as a plain computed tomography scan or MRI. Nearly 1 in 3 nodules that are PET with fludeoxyglucose F 18 avid turn out to be malignant, which is a much higher rate than the 5% to 10% overall rate of thyroid cancer.[34]

Fine Needle Aspiration Biopsy

For patients in whom it is determined based on history, physical examination, imaging and laboratory results that an FNA biopsy is indicated of their thyroid nodule, this procedure should be done expeditiously and under ultrasound guidance. Ultrasound-guided FNA is a minor, office-based procedure that can be performed without general anesthesia. Typically, small gauge (25–27 gauge) needles are inserted into the nodule and the liquid obtained is smeared onto glass slides. The follicular cells and presence of colloid are analyzed and reported based on the Bethesda System for Reporting Thyroid Cytopathology.[35] This system was recently updated in 2017 after new

Table 4
TI-RADS Score and FNA or follow-up ultrasound recommendations based on size of nodule

	FNA Cutoff (Largest Dimension)
TR5—highly suspicious (>7 points)	FNA recommended at 1 cm 0.5–1.0 cm—follow-up ultrasound examination annually for ≥5 y
TR4—moderately suspicious (4–6 points)	FNA recommended at 1.5 cm 1–1.5 cm—follow-up ultrasound examination at 1, 3, and 5 y
TR3—mildly suspicious (3 points)	FNA recommended at 2.5 cm 1.5–2.5 cm—follow-up ultrasound examination at 1, 3, and 5 y
TR2—not suspicious (1–2 points)	FNA not recommended
TR1—benign (0 points)	FNA not recommended

Adapted from Grant EG, Tessler FN, Hoang JK, et al. Thyroid Ultrasound Reporting Lexicon: White Paper of the ACR Thyroid Imaging, Reporting and Data System (TIRADS) Committee. Journal of the American College of Radiology 2015;12(12):1272–9; with permission.

information about the noninvasive follicular variant papillary thyroid carcinoma altered the way we think about some cancers, as well as the introduction of various molecular testing techniques for indeterminate nodules.[36]

The Bethesda system provides 6 distinct categories with specific features associated with each. Bethesda I lesions are nondiagnostic, and means not enough cells were obtained to provide a diagnosis. The risk of malignancy for these nodules is the same as it is for a nodule that had never been biopsied, and that is somewhere between 5% and 10%. Bethesda II lesions are benign and although no test is absolutely perfect at ruling out malignancy, the false-negative rate in this category is low, between 0% and 3%. Bethesda III, IV, and IV lesions are the "indeterminate nodule" categories, and with the introduction of molecular testing, the usual management has changed in recent years, but the risk of malignancy for these categories ranges from 6% to 75%. Bethesda VI or malignant lesions are cancer almost all of the time, with a false-positive rate of 1% to 6%.

Janeil Mitchell and Linwah Yip's article, "Decision-Making in Indeterminate Thyroid Nodules and the Role of Molecular Testing," in this issue discusses in detail the role of molecular testing for Bethesda III, IV, and V lesions, and Alexandria D. McDow and Susan C. Pitt's article, "Extent of Surgery for Low-Risk Differentiated Thyroid Cancer," and Mamoona Khokhar and Mira Milas' article, "Management of Nodal Disease in Thyroid Cancer," in this issue, discusses the extent of surgery for Bethesda VI malignant thyroid lesions and nodal involvement, so the remainder of this article focuses mostly on Bethesda I and II lesions.

Bethesda I: Nondiagnostic

Nondiagnostic cytology samples are FNA samples that fail to yield at least 6 clusters of well-visualized follicular cells, each group containing at least 10 follicular cells. The ATA recommends repeating the FNA with on-site cytologic evaluation (where the slides are immediately evaluated for the presence of follicular cells and repeat samples are taken until adequate amounts are obtained). Nodules that have a large cystic component are often more difficult to sample because the cyst fluid preferentially fills the needle and the larger, more dense follicular cells are not sampled, and in some cases enough follicular cells will never be obtained. In these cases, clinical judgment must be used to determine how concerning the nodule is for cancer and choosing between diagnostic lobectomy versus close observation measuring for interval growth.

In most nodules, however, a repeat FNA will yield enough cells to make a diagnosis, and most clinicians recommend a waiting period of around 3 months to allow any inflammation from the first FNA to subside. Recent studies have questioned whether this 3-month waiting period is necessary, and in some nodules with highly suspicious ultrasound features, it is probably appropriate to repeat the sample sooner.[3]

Bethesda II: Benign

Because the most common type of thyroid nodule by far is a benign colloid nodule, the vast majority of thyroid nodule FNA biopsy samples will show benign appearing follicular cells and abundant colloid (**Fig. 8**). Patients and physicians who receive this report of an FNA of a thyroid nodule should be very reassured that the nodule is not an aggressive cancer. As with any diagnostic test, however, the false-negative rate is not absolutely zero, and anyone who has had a thyroid FNAB of a nodule should be followed at least for a short time with interval ultrasound examinations. Although there is no widely accepted surveillance strategy for benign thyroid nodules, the ATA and American College of Radiology have similar recommendations for repeat ultrasound in 1 to 2 years.[3,31] For patients with highly suspicious ultrasound characteristics but benign FNA, a repeat ultrasound examination should be done within 12 months of the FNA biopsy, sooner if clinically indicated (growth by physical examination, new compressive symptoms, new neck mass in a different location, etc). For those with ultrasound characteristics that are low suspicion and benign FNA result, the ultrasound examination should be repeated 12 to 24 months after the FNA. At the repeat ultrasound examination, the nodule should be measured and growth reported as precisely as possible. True growth is defined as a 20% increase in at least 2 dimensions or more than a 50% increase in overall volume of the nodule. If there is true growth of the nodule, or new concerning ultrasound features, repeat FNA should be strongly considered.

If there is no growth of the nodule at this first repeat ultrasound examination, the next ultrasound examination can be recommended at an even longer interval, probably 2 or more years, although there is no widely accepted time interval. If the repeat ultrasound examination does show growth and a repeat FNA again finds a second benign cytology specimen, the risk of malignancy in this thyroid nodule is virtually zero, despite interval growth. Benign thyroid nodules also can grow, so as long as

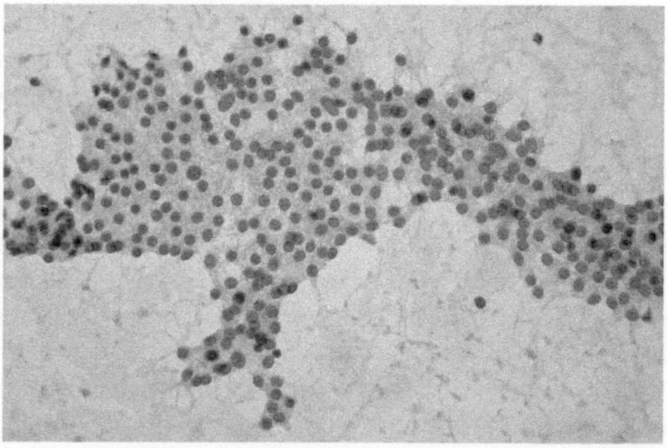

Fig. 8. Cytology of a benign thyroid FNA (papanicoloau). Note the follicular cells with homogeneous small, dark, round nuclei with a background of colloid. (*From* Wikimedia Commons, https://commons.wikimedia.org/wiki/File:Thyroid_FNA,_Benign,_Consistent_with_Adenomatoid_Nodule_(8116075837).jpg, with permission.)

the nodule remains asymptomatic without compressive symptoms, routine surveillance with ultrasound examination is no longer indicated,[3] although in practice patients often end up being followed for years with annual ultrasound examination and multiple FNA biopsies.

There are reasons to surgically remove thyroid nodules other than risk of malignancy, however, and patients with compressive or globus symptoms may benefit from thyroid surgery for relief of those symptoms. A conversation about the risks of thyroid surgery, including the risk of recurrent nerve injury causing temporary or permanent voice changes, subjective more subtle voice and swallow issues, and the risk for thyroid hormone insufficiency after surgery must be had with the patient and it is essential to involve the patient in this decision. The patient has to decide how symptomatic they are and whether the immediate risks of surgery is worth it to them. For those patients who have occasional dysphagia that does not seem to be worsening over time and benign thyroid nodules, surgery may not be worth it. But for another patient with a constant globus sensation that is causing significant anxiety and poor quality of life, surgery may be very much worth it. As with any symptoms, individuals have varying tolerance for certain sensations, and the size of the nodule may not directly correlate with the severity of symptoms. Some patients with large growing nodules that have been followed for some time and have established a pattern of growth, one may consider removing large nodules before they cause severe symptoms. It can be a less complicated surgery to remove a 4-cm nodule in a relatively healthy 65-year-old person than it might be to remove a 6-cm nodule 5 years down the road in the same person who may have other medical diagnoses occur in the interval. It is up to the physician and the patient to come to an agreement about when the benefits outweigh the risks of surgery for an individual patient in the case of compressive symptoms from benign nodules.

Bethesda III: Atypia or Follicular Lesion of Undetermined Significance

Perhaps the most diagnostic dilemmas arise from nodules that result in this atypia or follicular lesion of undetermined significance category. The true rate of malignancy in this category is difficult to determine, because unless there are obvious concerning features or compressive symptoms, many of these do not get surgically removed and the true rate of cancer is not known. This is also a bit of a "catch all" category where nodules that have some minor abnormalities that make it so that a cytologist cannot definitively call a nodule benign, but not so abnormal that there is a real concern for cancer, are called atypical. The true rate of malignancy likely varies by institution, and it is important for clinicians to have a general sense in their institution how high the rate of cancer is in this category to make the best recommendation for further treatment.

The appropriate next step in management, therefore, should be tailored to the specific circumstances of an individual patient, and with the introduction of molecular testing techniques described in detail in Janeil Mitchell and Linwah Yip's article, "Decision-Making in Indeterminate Thyroid Nodules and the Role of Molecular Testing," in this issue, the rate of diagnostic lobectomy will probably continue to decrease for atypia or follicular lesion of undetermined significance. Before the era of molecular testing, the general recommendation was to repeat the FNA and if the second sample also showed atypia or follicular lesion of undetermined significance, a diagnostic lobectomy was recommended. This process resulted in many surgeries for what turned out to be a benign nodule around 70% of the time. Today, there are options for repeating the FNA and obtaining a risk profile based on the genetic and molecular profile of a particular tumor to determine if there is a high or low likelihood of cancer for an individual patient. If molecular testing is available, it should be strongly considered for patients with a Bethesda III lesion, and some sites are now obtaining an additional FNA sample at the time of original biopsy to send for molecular testing in case the cytologic result shows a Bethesda III, IV, or V lesion. If molecular testing is not available or is cost prohibitive for an individual patient, the options remain to repeat FNA or perform a lobectomy. If the nodule is large, has any suspicious ultrasound features, or is causing even mild compression symptoms in a patient who is a surgical candidate, it is probably appropriate to proceed to surgery. If the nodule is small, benign appearing on ultrasound examination, has been followed for some time and is stable in size, it is appropriate to repeat the FNA.

Bethesda IV: Follicular Neoplasm

Like with Bethesda III lesions, the majority of nodules with this cytologic pattern of sheets of follicular cells with relative lack of colloid turn out to be benign follicular adenomas. However, because FNA does not preserve the microscopic architecture of the nodule, it is impossible to tell an invasive follicular cancer from a benign follicular adenoma by looking at cells alone. These lesions are managed much like Bethesda III lesions, as described in Bethesda III: Atypia or Follicular Lesion of Undetermined Significance.

Bethesda V: Suspicious for Malignancy

Unlike Bethesda III and IV lesions, most of the nodules in this category do turn out to be malignant, and most of these patients will ultimately be recommended for surgical resection. Although molecular testing may be helpful in this category to determine if there are any high-risk features that would require total thyroidectomy, it is unlikely molecular testing will be reassuring enough to not recommend at least a lobectomy for most of these patients. The extent of surgery for thyroid cancer has changed with the newest ATA guidelines, and cancers that are unilateral, less than 4 cm in size with no high-risk features such as lymph node metastases or high-grade pathologic features, can be managed with lobectomy alone. Alexandria D. McDow and Susan C. Pitt's article, "Extent of Surgery for Low-Risk Differentiated Thyroid Cancer," in this issue describes in detail the decision making that goes into deciding how much surgery to perform for differentiated thyroid cancers.

CLINICAL OUTCOMES IN THE LITERATURE

For patients with benign thyroid nodules that do not undergo surgery, often they get into a pattern of frequent ultrasound examinations and repeat biopsies, because the published guidelines are fairly vague about how often to repeat imaging and cytologic sampling. If a patient has a repeat ultrasound examination 1 year after a benign biopsy and the nodule has grown significantly, a second FNA is indicated. If that repeat biopsy is also benign, the chances of a false-negative result are exceedingly low, although often these patients are reimaged in a year, and potentially rebiopsied. The answer to the question, "At what point can we stop imaging and sampling benign nodules?" is not well-studied, and probably leads to excessive cost and anxiety for patients. One recent study found that, among patients who have had multiple biopsies of the same benign nodule, 72% ultimately underwent surgery for symptoms, but 18.5% elected to have the nodule removed despite being asymptomatic.[37] One can assume that the stress of being subjected to repeated tests contributed to this decision. Another study suggests that, after 3 years of follow-up, patients should be followed clinically for development of symptoms, but routine ultrasound examinations and FNA are unlikely to reveal a future problem.[38]

SUMMARY

Most patients with thyroid nodules have small and asymptomatic benign nodules. Nodules that are large enough to cause compression symptoms or have concerning features for cancer should be worked up with ultrasound and FNA. Among nodules that are subjected to FNAB, most are benign, and indeterminate nodules that traditionally were managed with a diagnostic lobectomy now may benefit from molecular testing to stratify malignancy risk. Benign thyroid nodules should be followed for a period of a few years, but there is no widely accepted strategy for long-term follow-up.

REFERENCES

1. Brander A, Viikinkoski P, Nickels J, et al. Thyroid gland: US screening in a random adult population. Radiology 1991;181(3):683–7.
2. Vander JB, Gaston EA, Dawber TR. The significance of nontoxic thyroid nodules. Final report of a 15-year study of the incidence of thyroid malignancy. Ann Intern Med 1968;69(3):537–40.
3. Haugen BR, Alexander EK, Bible KC, et al. 2015 American Thyroid Association Management guidelines for adult patients with thyroid nodules and differentiated thyroid cancer: the American Thyroid Association guidelines task force on thyroid nodules and differentiated thyroid cancer. Thyroid 2016;26(1):1–133.
4. Guth S, Theune U, Aberle J, et al. Very high prevalence of thyroid nodules detected by high frequency (13 MHz) ultrasound examination. Eur J Clin Invest 2009;39(8):699–706.
5. Rice CO. Incidence of nodules in the thyroid: a comparative study of symptomless thyroid glands removed at autopsy and hyperfunctioning goiters operatively removed. Arch Surg 1932;24(3):505–15.
6. Hegedus L. Clinical practice. The thyroid nodule. N Engl J Med 2004;351(17): 1764–71.
7. Ito Y, Miyauchi A, Kudo T, et al. Trends in the implementation of active surveillance for low-risk papillary thyroid microcarcinomas at Kuma Hospital: gradual increase and heterogeneity in the acceptance of this new management option. Thyroid 2018;28(4):488–95.
8. Vrinten C, McGregor LM, Heinrich M, et al. What do people fear about cancer? A systematic review and meta-synthesis of cancer fears in the general population. Psychooncology 2017;26(8):1070–9.
9. Christensen SB, Bondeson L, Ericsson UB, et al. Prediction of malignancy in the solitary thyroid nodule by physical examination, thyroid scan, fine-needle biopsy and serum thyroglobulin. A prospective study of 100 surgically treated patients. Acta Chir Scand 1984;150(6):433–9.
10. Mazzaferri EL. Management of a solitary thyroid nodule. N Engl J Med 1993; 328(8):553–9.
11. Walsh RM, Watkinson JC, Franklyn J. The management of the solitary thyroid nodule: a review. Clin Otolaryngol Allied Sci 1999;24(5):388–97.
12. Burch HB. Evaluation and management of the solid thyroid nodule. Endocrinol Metab Clin North Am 1995;24(4):663–710.
13. Knudsen N, Bulow I, Laurberg P, et al. Association of tobacco smoking with goiter in a low-iodine-intake area. Arch Intern Med 2002;162(4):439–43.
14. Sousa PA, Vaisman M, Carneiro JR, et al. Prevalence of goiter and thyroid nodular disease in patients with class III obesity. Arq Bras Endocrinol Metabol 2013;57(2): 120–5.

15. Valeix P, Faure P, Bertrais S, et al. Effects of light to moderate alcohol consumption on thyroid volume and thyroid function. Clin Endocrinol 2008;68(6):988–95.
16. Spinos N, Terzis G, Crysanthopoulou A, et al. Increased frequency of thyroid nodules and breast fibroadenomas in women with uterine fibroids. Thyroid 2007; 17(12):1257–9.
17. Volzke H, Friedrich N, Schipf S, et al. Association between serum insulin-like growth factor-I levels and thyroid disorders in a population-based study. J Clin Endocrinol Metab 2007;92(10):4039–45.
18. Knudsen N, Bulow I, Laurberg P, et al. Low goitre prevalence among users of oral contraceptives in a population sample of 3712 women. Clin Endocrinol 2002; 57(1):71–6.
19. Cappelli C, Castellano M, Pirola I, et al. Reduced thyroid volume and nodularity in dyslipidaemic patients on statin treatment. Clin Endocrinol 2008;68(1):16–21.
20. Peiling Yang S, Ngeow J. Familial non-medullary thyroid cancer: unraveling the genetic maze. Endocr Relat Cancer 2016;23(12):R577–95.
21. Hoang JK, Langer JE, Middleton WD, et al. Managing incidental thyroid nodules detected on imaging: white paper of the ACR Incidental Thyroid Findings Committee. J Am Coll Radiol 2015;12(2):143–50.
22. Alfonso A, Christoudias G, Amaruddin Q, et al. Tracheal or esophageal compression due to benign thyroid disease. Am J Surg 1981;142(3):350–4.
23. Banks CA, Ayers CM, Hornig JD, et al. Thyroid disease and compressive symptoms. Laryngoscope 2012;122(1):13–6.
24. Eng OS, Potdevin L, Davidov T, et al. Does nodule size predict compressive symptoms in patients with thyroid nodules? Gland Surg 2014;3(4):232–6.
25. Nam IC, Choi H, Kim ES, et al. Characteristics of thyroid nodules causing globus symptoms. Eur Arch Otorhinolaryngol 2015;272(5):1181–8.
26. Antonarakis ES. Pemberton sign. Mayo Clin Proc 2007;82(7):859.
27. Mirfakhraee S, Mathews D, Peng L, et al. A solitary hyperfunctioning thyroid nodule harboring thyroid carcinoma: review of the literature. Thyroid Res 2013; 6(1):7.
28. Ross DS, Burch HB, Cooper DS, et al. 2016 American Thyroid Association guidelines for diagnosis and management of hyperthyroidism and other causes of thyrotoxicosis. Thyroid 2016;26(10):1343–421.
29. Ahn HS, Kim HJ, Welch HG. Korea's thyroid-cancer "epidemic"–screening and overdiagnosis. N Engl J Med 2014;371(19):1765–7.
30. Gharib H, Papini E, Garber JR, et al. American Association of Clinical Endocrinologists, American college of endocrinology, AND Associazione Medici Endocrinologi Medical guidelines for clinical practice for the diagnosis and management of thyroid nodules–2016 update. Endocr Pract 2016;22(5):622–39.
31. Grant EG, Tessler FN, Hoang JK, et al. Thyroid ultrasound reporting lexicon: white paper of the ACR thyroid imaging, reporting and data system (TIRADS) committee. J Am Coll Radiol 2015;12(12 Pt A):1272–9.
32. Tessler FN, Middleton WD, Grant EG. Thyroid imaging reporting and data system (TI-RADS): a user's guide. Radiology 2018;287(3):1082.
33. Boelaert K, Horacek J, Holder RL, et al. Serum thyrotropin concentration as a novel predictor of malignancy in thyroid nodules investigated by fine-needle aspiration. J Clin Endocrinol Metab 2006;91(11):4295–301.
34. Soelberg KK, Bonnema SJ, Brix TH, et al. Risk of malignancy in thyroid incidentalomas detected by 18F-fluorodeoxyglucose positron emission tomography: a systematic review. Thyroid 2012;22(9):918–25.

35. Crippa S, Mazzucchelli L, Cibas ES, et al. The Bethesda System for reporting thyroid fine-needle aspiration specimens. Am J Clin Pathol 2010;134(2):343–4 [author reply: 345].
36. Cibas ES, Ali SZ. The 2017 Bethesda system for reporting thyroid cytopathology. Thyroid 2017;27(11):1341–6.
37. Ajmal S, Rapoport S, Ramirez Batlle H, et al. The natural history of the benign thyroid nodule: what is the appropriate follow-up strategy? J Am Coll Surg 2015; 220(6):987–92.
38. Lee S, Skelton TS, Zheng F, et al. The biopsy-proven benign thyroid nodule: is long-term follow-up necessary? J Am Coll Surg 2013;217(1):81–8 [discussion: 88–9].

Decision Making in Indeterminate Thyroid Nodules and the Role of Molecular Testing

Janeil Mitchell, MD[a], Linwah Yip, MD[b,*]

KEYWORDS

• Indeterminate thyroid nodule • Gene mutations • Molecular testing
• Mutational analysis • Gene expression classifier • Gene sequencing
• microRNA classifier

KEY POINTS

- Indeterminate thyroid nodules (Bethesda System for Reporting Thyroid Cytopathology categories III–V) are a common cytologic entity, occurring in 25% of fine-needle aspirations and representing a risk of malignancy ranging from 5% to 75%.
- Tumor profiling and risk stratification of indeterminate thyroid nodules using adjunct DNA, mRNA, or microRNA molecular genetic testing may reduce the need for diagnostic surgery.
- Clinical algorithms incorporating molecular testing exist and may aid decision making in the initial management of indeterminate thyroid nodules, further providing precise treatment options of both nodules and thyroid cancer.

INTRODUCTION

Differentiated thyroid cancer (DTC) is increasing in incidence in the United States[1] although 5-year survival rates for the most common subtype of thyroid cancer, papillary thyroid cancer (PTC), have been greater than 95% over the past 20 years.[2] Optimizing survivorship and reducing long-term health care costs associated with diagnosis, treatment, and surveillance have been important aspects of thyroid cancer and indeterminate thyroid nodule management. Thus, current algorithms include

Disclosures: The authors have no conflicts of interest or financial disclosures to declare. No financial support was received for the completion of this work.
[a] Fox Valley Surgical Associates, Endocrine Surgery, 1818 North Meade Street, Appleton, WI 54911, USA; [b] Department of Surgery, Division of Endocrine Surgery, University of Pittsburgh School of Medicine, Kaufman Medical Building, 3471 Fifth Avenue, Suite 101, Pittsburgh, PA 15213, USA
* Corresponding author.
E-mail address: yipl@upmc.edu

Surg Clin N Am 99 (2019) 587–598
https://doi.org/10.1016/j.suc.2019.04.002

options for utilization of molecular tests to improve prediction of malignancy for indeterminate thyroid nodules.[3–5]

During the initial assessment of a thyroid nodule, the 2015 American Thyroid Association (ATA) guidelines recommend classifying nodules based on sonographic features which may be concerning for malignancy.[3] Whether additional assessment with fine-needle aspiration biopsy (FNAB) is needed also may depend on nodule size and other clinical factors that can affect the likelihood of malignancy.[3,6] Nodule cytology results are standardized according to the 6 categories in the Bethesda System for Reporting Thyroid Cytopathology: BI, nondiagnostic; BII, benign; BIII, atypia of undetermined significance/follicular lesion of undetermined significance; BIV, follicular neoplasm/suspicious for follicular neoplasm; BV, suspicious for malignancy; and BVI, malignant.[7,8] The benign and malignant Bethesda diagnoses are accurate, and in meta-analysis of histologically evaluated nodules the rate of malignancy is at less than 4% and 99%, respectively.[9]

Approximately 20% to 25% of FNAB results, however, fall into 1 of the BIII, BIV, or BV categories, which are associated with a range of malignancy that varies from 5% to 75%. BV is the least common cytology category, occurring in 5% to 7% of biopsies, and, due to the relatively high risk of cancer (up to 75%), diagnostic surgery typically is recommended.[3,8,9] For BIII/BIV biopsy results, often additional factors need to be incorporated into deciding whether the nodule requires diagnostic surgery or if surveillance is appropriate. The 2015 ATA guidelines recommend pursuing either repeat FNAB, thyroid surgery, or consideration of molecular testing[3] (**Fig. 1**). There is significant interobserver variability in the indeterminate category of thyroid FNAB, further complicating initial cytologic diagnosis.[10]

In the United States, more than a half million FNABs are estimated to be performed each year and, of these, approximately 100,000 are indeterminate, and this subset of thyroid nodules represents a target for improved diagnostic accuracy and potentially effective use of prognostic testing to aid in the delivery of risk-stratified appropriate care.[1,11] Molecular testing has emerged as an adjunct for cytologically indeterminate

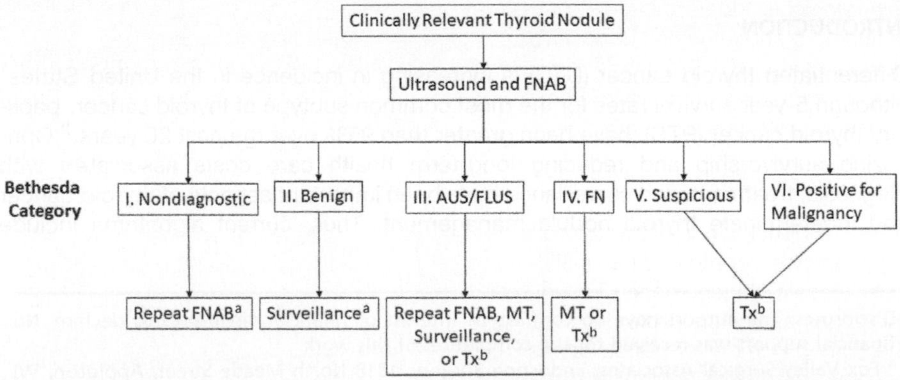

Fig. 1. Algorithm of thyroid nodule management, including molecular testing adapted from 2015 ATA Management Guidelines for Adult Patients with Thyroid Nodules and Differentiated Thyroid Cancer. AUS/FLUS, atypia or follicular lesion of undetermined significance; FN, follicular neoplasm; MT, molecular testing; Tx, thyroidectomy. [a] If clinical or sonographic features are concerning for malignancy, then thyroidectomy (either lobectomy or total thyroidectomy) can be considered. [b] When thyroidectomy is considered, either lobectomy or total thyroidectomy is an acceptable option, depending on concern for ATA intermediate-risk or high-risk malignancy, patient-specific factors and preferences.

nodules, allowing for more precise estimation of the probability of malignancy and preoperative prediction of either an aggressive or indolent malignancy.

THYROID CANCER–RELATED GENETIC MUTATIONS AND ONCOLOGIC RISK

The basis of molecular testing arises from the identification of genetic alterations involved in thyroid cancer tumorigenesis. A majority of thyroid cancer–related gene mutations are drivers of the mitogen-activated protein kinase (MAPK) and phosphatidylinositol-3 kinase-Akt (PI3K-AKT) pathways involving tyrosine kinase cell membrane receptors, intracellular signaling proteins, and nuclear receptors encoded by *BRAF, RAS, RET,* and *PPARG* genes as well as regulatory genes, such as *PTEN* and *PAX8.*[12]

One of the frequently studied molecular markers in thyroid cancer is an activating point mutation of the *BRAF* gene, V600E. *BRAF* V600E is the most commonly identified genetic alterations in PTC and is seen in 40% to 80% of PTC tumors, which varies depending on geographic region.[13–15] *BRAF* V600E is a specific marker for PTC, often classic or tall cell variant, and, although the majority of *BRAF* V600E–positive PTCs do not have aggressive tumor characteristics, the mutation is associated with a well-documented increased risk of locally advanced presentation, disease recurrence, and regional lymph node metastasis.[16–20] Conventional PTCs with a risk of lymph node metastasis also are seen when *RET/PTC* and *NTRK* fusions are detected.[18,21,22] *TERT* promoter mutations also are strongly associated with aggressive DTC as well as poorly differentiated thyroid cancer and anaplastic cancer.[23,24] *TERT*-positive tumors have an increased risk of disease-related mortality, which is even further elevated by the presence of a concurrent *BRAF* V600E mutation.[25–27]

The other commonly affected gene in thyroid malignancy is *RAS*. Mutations causing constitutive activation of the MAPK pathway can be found in 1 of the *K-RAS*, *H-RAS*, and *N-RAS* isoforms but affects *N-RAS* most frequently.[28–30] *RAS*-associated tumors can be seen across the spectrum of follicular-patterned lesions from benign follicular adenomas to poorly differentiated cancers, although it is rare to have an aggressive cancer with an isolated *RAS* mutation. *H-RAS* and *K-RAS* mutations also have been identified in medullary thyroid cancers.[29,31] When *RAS* is detected preoperatively in a cytologically indeterminate nodule, follicular variant PTC is the most likely histology, including a subset which is noninvasive follicular thyroid neoplasm with papillary-like nuclear features (NIFTP).[32,33] Similar to *RAS*, *BRAF* K601E and *PAX8/PPARG* rearrangements have demonstrated more favorable long-term tumor behavior and rarely cause disease-related death.[18,34,35]

MOLECULAR GENE TESTING

After the identification of thyroid cancer–related genes, single-gene arrays were developed and then combined into initial multigene panels, which were available for clinical use. These multigene panels included testing for *BRAF* V600E, *BRAF* K601E, and *RAS* mutations as well as *PAX8/PPARG, RET/PTC1* and *RET/PTC3* fusions.[36] Because of the limited number of tested genes, the initial gene panel tests did not have strong negative predictive value (NPV); thus, BIII/BIV nodules still required diagnostic surgery. But the panel did provide increased diagnostic specificity and could be used cost effectively to guide the extent of initial surgery particularly under prior ATA guidelines, wherein initial total thyroidectomy was recommended for DTC greater than 1 cm.[37–39]

Historically, Afirma (Veracyte, South San Francisco, California) was a primarily mRNA-based gene expression panel, which was optimized to identify benign nodules.[40] Using microarray analysis, the expression profile of benign nodules was characterized and subsequently utilized in a commercially available assay. A multicenter study demonstrated high sensitivity and NPV but low specificity.[41] The introduction and accessibility of next-generation sequencing technology allowed for simultaneous detection of multiple genetic alterations and is the methodology utilized in ThyroSeq (TS) testing (CBLPath, Rye Brook, New York).[42] TSv2 was the initial commercially available next-generation thyroid-specific test, and detected 72 variations, including point mutations, fusions, and expression levels of tumor markers, such as calcitonin.[43,44] The first microRNA (miRNA)-based test, ThyGenX/ThyraMIR (Interpace Diagnostics, Parsippany, New Jersey) was offered as a combined 7-gene panel and 10-miRNA test and is now available as an expanded gene and miRNA panel, ThyGeNEXT/ThyraMIR[45] (**Table 1**). Until recently, Rosetta GX Reveal (Rosetta Genomics, Princeton, New Jersey) was another commercially available miRNA panel with 24 tumor markers.[46]

Since the first molecular tests were made available for clinical use, significant advancements have been made in understanding the drivers of tumorigenesis in DTC. To date, more than 10,000 DNA, mRNA, and miRNA gene mutations have been implicated in the development of papillary, follicular, medullary, and anaplastic thyroid cancer, accounting for approximately 90% of genetic aberrations believed involved in thyroid oncogenesis.[12] Current management guidelines from the ATA and National Comprehensive Cancer Network (NCCN) suggest algorithms that incorporate the use of molecular testing for cytologically indeterminate nodules and, at present, there are 2 commercially available multigene molecular tests for clinical use[3,47] (see **Table 1**).

AFIRMA GENOMIC SEQUENCING CLASSIFIER/XPRESSION ATLAS

The Afirma Genomic Sequencing Classifier (GSC) is the latest mRNA gene mutation study featuring 511 genes, representing an expanded version of the preceding Gene Expression Classifier (GEC), which consisted of a 167-gene microarray panel and 6-gene malignancy classifier panel.[48] Tested genes are proprietary, and test results are reported as benign or suspicious. *TERT* analysis is not offered in the current test whereas *BRAF V600E*, *RET/PTC1*, and *RET/PTC3* mutations are described when present. In initial study, GEC testing was found to have an overall high sensitivity (92%) and NPV (93%) for BIII/BIV nodules at a prevalence of malignancy ranging from 15% to 21% but low specificity and reported positive predictive values (PPVs) of only 14% to 57%.[41,49,50] GSC added additional expression markers and, except for 9% of samples that had insufficient mRNA for testing, used the same data samples initially collected for the GEC validation study. The cancer prevalence was 24.1% and among BIII/BIV nodules, the test demonstrated a sensitivity similar to GEC (91%) but had higher specificity (68%).[48] Furthermore, 54% of patients with indeterminate nodules had negative or benign test results, representing a population that could potentially avoid unneeded surgery.[48]

GSC added expression panels for Hürthle cell lesions, which were poorly risk stratified using GEC.[48,51] The molecular changes associated with Hürthle cell cancers are different compared with the changes associated with follicular-patterned malignancies and, until recently, have not been well characterized. In a comprehensive molecular analysis of a Hürthle cell cancer cohort, activation of the PI3K-AKT-mTOR and Wnt/β-catenin pathways were seen in addition to increased chromosomal instability.[52] A total of 26 Hürthle cell adenomas/carcinomas were analyzed in the recent GSC assessment, and sensitivity for this subset was 89% with specificity of 59% which is improved compared with GEC specificity of 11% for these lesions.[48] Although it

Table 1
Comparison of characteristics and performance of available molecular tests for thyroid nodules with Bethesda III/IV cytology

	Gene Sequencing Classifier[48]	Thyroseq v3[53]	ThyGenX/ThyraMIR[45]
Methodology	mRNA gene sequencing and gene expression	DNA and mRNA gene sequencing and expression	DNA and mRNA gene sequencing, quantitative polymerase chain reaction miRNA expression
Tested genetic alterations	511 mRNA panel (761 variants and 130 fusions), gene expression	112 DNA and mRNA panel (>12,000 variants and 150 gene fusions), copy number alterations, gene expression	10 DNA and mRNA panel (17 variants), 10 miRNA expression
Specimen requirements	Dedicated fine-needle aspiration pass	Dedicated fine-needle aspiration pass, direct smears, or paraffin-embedded cell block sections	Dedicated fine-needle aspiration pass, direct smears, or ThinPrep slides
Multicenter study validation	Y (n = 190 nodules, 24% cancer)	Y (n = 247 nodules, 28% cancer)	Y (n = 109 nodules, 32% cancer)
Sensitivity (95% CI)	91% (79–98)	94% (85–100)	89% (73–97)
Specificity (95% CI)	68% (60–76)	82% (63–84)	85% (75–92)
NPV (95% CI)	96% (90–99)	97% (93–99)	94% (85–98)
PPV (95% CI)	47% (36–58)	66% (56–75)	74% (58–86)
Reported results	Benign or suspicious *BRAF* V600E, *RET/PTC* mutations specified when present.	Cancer association: none, low, or high Specific gene mutation, fusion, and/or translocation reported	Negative or positive *BRAF* V600E, *TERT*, *RET/PTC* mutations specified when present
Additional factors	Xpression Atlas can provide DNA and fusion data, but validation and added cost data not available	Risk of cancer variable and dependent on detected genetic alterations	Current version is ThyGeNEXT/ThyraMIR with no available performance data

is not known what added changes to GSC contributed to the overall higher specificity, better discrimination of oncocytic lesions was likely 1 contributing factor. The Xpression Atlas is a supplemental component of GSC and is described as additional DNA and fusion data; however, studies validating the clinical utility of the detected gene variants are to date not yet available.

THYROSEQ V3 GENOMIC CLASSIFIER

TSv3 is the most recent thyroid molecular panel test using next-generation sequencing. The current version is composed of a 112-gene panel evaluating mutations, gene fusions, expression alterations, and copy number alterations.[53] A prospective, multi-institutional study with cytologists and pathologists blinded to molecular results recently was completed. Recommendations for thyroidectomy were not led by molecular results, and, among 247 nodules with BIII/BIV cytology and histologic correlation, the cancer prevalence was 28%. Benign or negative test results were obtained in 61%, and sensitivity and specificity were high at 94% and 82%, respectively.[53]

Similar to GSC, better discrimination of malignant from benign Hürthle cell neoplasms likely contributed to the improved test performance. A total of 44 Hürthle cell lesions were assessed with TSv3, and sensitivity was 100% with specificity of 62%. Negative TSv3 results were seen in 5 (3%) of histologic cancers ranging in size from 1.1 cm to 4 cm; 1 was a minimally invasive FTC and 4 were PTCs without extrathyroidal extension (American Joint Committee on Cancer staging categories T1–T2).[53]

ThyGeNEXT/ThyraMIR

ThyraMIR was initially a 10-miRNA expression analysis to be used in conjunction with next-generation DNA/mRNA testing for a concise panel of 7 genes associated with thyroid cancer, called ThyGenX. In a cost-reducing testing algorithm, if ThyGenX was negative, then reflex ThyraMIR analysis was performed. The cumulative test has reported sensitivity and specificity of 85% and 89%, respectively.[45] ThyGeNEXT has recently replaced ThyGenX with an expanded DNA and mRNA panel.[54] Test performance after this change has not been published and prospective large multicenter studies are lacking for both versions. The test is unique in that specimen refrigeration is not required and samples for analysis may be procured from several smear preparation types or directly from thin prep slides instead of requiring an additional biopsy.

CLINICAL UTILITY OF MOLECULAR TESTING IN INDETERMINATE NODULES OF MOLECULAR ANALYSIS

A recent meta-analysis of GEC, TSv2, ThyGenX/ThyraMIR, and RosettaGx (which is no longer available) estimated that when cancer prevalence was 25%, surgery for 27%, 79%, 85%, and 74%, respectively, of indeterminate nodules could be avoided with negative molecular testing results.[55] After a 6-month implementation period of GEC, a multicenter cross-sectional cohort survey study found a decline in surgical resection rates from 74% for cytologically indeterminate nodules to 7.6%, although long-term follow-up for the GEC-benign nodules was not described.[56]

Preoperative testing for thyroid-related mutations may contribute to observed reductions in effectiveness of intraoperative pathologic examination during diagnostic lobectomy.[57] Another study on molecular genotyping of 471 BIII/BIV nodules found that per the 2009 ATA guidelines, molecular testing reduced the need for 2-stage thyroidectomy by 2.5-fold.[39] Other studies of GEC suggest, however, that reductions in diagnostic lobectomies are lower than expected[58] and only rarely may change extent of planned surgery.[59]

Direct comparison of different molecular tests on the same nodule cohort is lacking. The exception is a recent study of 129 BIII/BIV nodules, which were randomized to have either GEC or TSv2 testing. The benign call rate was higher for TSv2 (77%), vs GEC 43%, and although histology was not available for all mutation-negative nodules, the specificity of TSv2 also was higher compared with GEC.[60] Use of more than 1 test clinically has not been studied and is unlikely cost effective. A proposed algorithm for management of indeterminate nodules utilizing molecular test and potential results is presented in **Fig. 1**. Although some specific mutations can have prognostic implications if cancer is confirmed on histology, it is not yet clear whether use of the preoperative molecular signature to guide treatment (including extent of surgery or need for radioactive iodine ablation) has a beneficial impact on disease-related outcomes.

LIMITATIONS OF MUTATIONAL TESTING

Despite advancements, there are still undetected genetic abnormalities underlying some thyroid cancers. Prior to the recent GSC and TSv3 reports, an estimated 5% of papillary, 50% of medullary, and 10% of anaplastic thyroid cancers had a genetic aberration that was not identifiable by available molecular panels.[61] Thus, mutation-negative indeterminate thyroid nodules still require surveillance. The natural history of mutation-negative yet cytologically indeterminate nodules has not yet been characterized. Positive molecular test results also need to be appropriately interpreted. Results often are reported dichotomously (see **Table 1**) and when all DTC greater than 1 cm was recommended for total thyroidectomy, the prognostic implications of thyroid cancer subtype was less of a preoperative concern. In reality, however, associated malignancies have a variable range of aggressiveness that may depend on more specific assessment of the exact molecular profile. Although these additional prognostic data are provided by some molecular tests, they are not available for all. Finally, even with positive molecular test results, not all nodules are malignant. Studies have suggested that misinterpretation of positive results may lead to overuse of total thyroidectomy when molecular marker testing is used, particularly in the era of the 2009 ATA guideline recommendations.[62]

The NPV and PPV of diagnostic testing vary with prevalence of malignancy which is geographically and institutionally variable.[50] Histologic classification of follicular-patterned lesions is associated with an approximately 70% interobserver and intraobserver variability, even among experienced thyroid pathologists, contributing to some of the prevalence variability.[63,64] NIFTP tumors are a subset of encapsulated follicular-variant PTC, meet specific histologic criteria consistent with nonaggressive lesions, and thus likely have minimal invasive potential.[64] Since the nomenclature revision describing NIFTP, studies have demonstrated lower rates of malignancy for BIII, BIV, and BV cytology categories.[65,66] The accuracy of all molecular tests likely will be altered depending on whether NIFTP is considered malignant or benign. Currently, NIFTP require pathologic evaluation for diagnosis; however, NIFTP is more likely with *RAS*-like mutations (*RAS*, *EIF1AX*, *BRAF* K601E, *PTEN*) and likely not seen with high-risk (*TERT*) or *BRAF*-like mutations (*BRAF* V600E, *RET* fusions).[53,67]

Appropriately, the NCCN Clinical Practice Guidelines and ATA guidelines advise careful interpretation of test results within clinical context as well as restricting their use to scenarios whereby test findings would change management.[3,47] For example, if surgery is indicated for compressive symptoms, large nodule size, concerning imaging and/or clinical features, then molecular testing likely will not provide additional information. TSv3 and ThyGeNEXT/ThyroMIR include prognostic markers, such as *TERT*, but it is not yet known if the preoperative detection of such markers should alter the initial extent of surgery. Always in considering molecular testing in cytologically indeterminate nodules, other factors beyond molecular test findings should be incorporated into clinical decision making prior to developing an operative or nonoperative management plan, including ultrasound appearance, nodule size, existing risk factors for malignancy, and patient preference.

Cost of care is a consideration including the costs of molecular testing, diagnostic surgery, and surveillance if molecular testing is negative. Cost-efficacy analyses have shown that in hypothetical modeling, cost-savings seem proportional to the number of diagnostic surgeries avoided and cancer prevalence and also are dependent on test costs.[68–70] One study recently suggested, however, superiority of thyroidectomy over GEC testing of BIII/BIV nodules, when long-term cost of surveillance is included in cost-effectiveness modeling.[71] Published costs of testing can range from $1675 for ThyGenX alone to greater than $3500 for the more comprehensive panels.[72] Furthermore, unless obtained during the initial biopsy, an additional FNAB may be required to obtain specimen for the test, which incurs cost and risk.

FUTURE OF MOLECULAR TESTING AND SUMMARY

The technical advances in detection of molecular signatures combined with a better understanding of the genetic changes that lead to thyroid carcinogenesis have contributed to the development of available molecular tests that can now be used to direct decision making for optimal management of cytologically indeterminate nodules. Utilization of diagnostic surgery should be reserved only for nodules that have clinical, imaging, and molecular features guiding the need for intervention. Furthermore, as understanding of the prognostic significance of different molecular signatures continues to expand, molecular-based treatment algorithms may become more standardized mirroring other cancer pathways.

REFERENCES

1. Rahib L, Smith BD, Aizenberg R, et al. Projecting cancer incidence and deaths to 2030: the unexpected burden of thyroid, liver, and pancreas cancers in the United States. Cancer Res 2014;74(11):2913–21.
2. SEER*Explorer: an interactive website for SEER cancer statistics [Internet]. Surveillance Research Program, National Cancer Institute. Available at: https://seer.cancer.gov/explorer/. Accessed April 28, 2019.
3. Haugen BR, Alexander EK, Bible KC, et al. 2015 American Thyroid Association management guidelines for adult patients with thyroid nodules and differentiated thyroid cancer: the American Thyroid Association guidelines task force on thyroid nodules and differentiated thyroid cancer. Thyroid 2016;26(1):1–133.
4. Sawka AM, Ghai S, Tomlinson G, et al. A protocol for a Canadian prospective observational study of decision-making on active surveillance or surgery for low-risk papillary thyroid cancer. BMJ Open 2018;8(4):e020298.
5. Tuttle RM, Zhang L, Shaha A. A clinical framework to facilitate selection of patients with differentiated thyroid cancer for active surveillance or less aggressive initial surgical management. Expert Rev Endocrinol Metab 2018;13(2):77–85.
6. Tessler FN, Middleton WD, Grant EG, et al. ACR thyroid imaging, reporting and data system (TI-RADS): white paper of the ACR TI-RADS committee. J Am Coll Radiol 2017;14(5):587–95.

7. Cibas ES, Ali SZ. The Bethesda system for reporting thyroid cytopathology. Thyroid 2009;19(11):1159–65.
8. Cibas ES, Ali SZ. The 2017 Bethesda system for reporting thyroid cytopathology. Thyroid 2017;27(11):1341–6.
9. Bongiovanni M, Spitale A, Faquin WC, et al. The Bethesda system for reporting thyroid cytopathology: a meta-analysis. Acta Cytol 2012;56(4):333–9.
10. Olson MT, Boonyaarunnate T, Aragon Han P, et al. A tertiary center's experience with second review of 3885 thyroid cytopathology specimens. J Clin Endocrinol Metab 2013;98(4):1450–7.
11. Nikiforov YE. Role of molecular markers in thyroid nodule management: then and now. Endocr Pract 2017;23(8):979–88.
12. Cancer Genome Atlas Research Network. Integrated genomic characterization of papillary thyroid carcinoma. Cell 2014;159(3):676–90.
13. Xing M, Westra WH, Tufano RP, et al. BRAF mutation predicts a poorer clinical prognosis for papillary thyroid cancer. J Clin Endocrinol Metab 2005;90(12): 6373–9.
14. Xing M. BRAF mutation in thyroid cancer. Endocr Relat Cancer 2005;12(2): 245–62.
15. Kim TH, Park YJ, Lim JA, et al. The association of the BRAF(V600E) mutation with prognostic factors and poor clinical outcome in papillary thyroid cancer: a meta-analysis. Cancer 2012;118(7):1764–73.
16. Kim SJ, Lee KE, Myong JP, et al. BRAF V600E mutation is associated with tumor aggressiveness in papillary thyroid cancer. World J Surg 2012;36(2):310–7.
17. Li C, Lee KC, Schneider EB, et al. BRAF V600E mutation and its association with clinicopathological features of papillary thyroid cancer: a meta-analysis. J Clin Endocrinol Metab 2012;97(12):4559–70.
18. Yip L, Nikiforova MN, Yoo JY, et al. Tumor genotype determines phenotype and disease-related outcomes in thyroid cancer: a study of 1510 patients. Ann Surg 2015;262(3):519–25 [discussion: 524–5].
19. Xing M, Alzahrani AS, Carson KA, et al. Association between BRAF V600E mutation and recurrence of papillary thyroid cancer. J Clin Oncol 2015;33(1):42–50.
20. Xing M, Alzahrani AS, Carson KA, et al. Association between BRAF V600E mutation and mortality in patients with papillary thyroid cancer. JAMA 2013;309(14): 1493–501.
21. Elisei R, Romei C, Vorontsova T, et al. RET/PTC rearrangements in thyroid nodules: studies in irradiated and not irradiated, malignant and benign thyroid lesions in children and adults. J Clin Endocrinol Metab 2001;86(7):3211–6.
22. Prasad ML, Vyas M, Horne MJ, et al. NTRK fusion oncogenes in pediatric papillary thyroid carcinoma in northeast United States. Cancer 2016;122(7):1097–107.
23. Liu X, Bishop J, Shan Y, et al. Highly prevalent TERT promoter mutations in aggressive thyroid cancers. Endocr Relat Cancer 2013;20(4):603–10.
24. Bullock M, Ren Y, O'Neill C, et al. TERT promoter mutations are a major indicator of recurrence and death due to papillary thyroid carcinomas. Clin Endocrinol 2016;85(2):283–90.
25. Landa I, Ganly I, Chan TA, et al. Frequent somatic TERT promoter mutations in thyroid cancer: higher prevalence in advanced forms of the disease. J Clin Endocrinol Metab 2013;98(9):E1562–6.
26. Melo M, da Rocha AG, Vinagre J, et al. TERT promoter mutations are a major indicator of poor outcome in differentiated thyroid carcinomas. J Clin Endocrinol Metab 2014;99(5):E754–65.

27. Liu X, Qu S, Liu R, et al. TERT promoter mutations and their association with BRAF V600E mutation and aggressive clinicopathological characteristics of thyroid cancer. J Clin Endocrinol Metab 2014;99(6):E1130–6.
28. Rossi M, Buratto M, Tagliati F, et al. Relevance of BRAF(V600E) mutation testing versus RAS point mutations and RET/PTC rearrangements evaluation in the diagnosis of thyroid cancer. Thyroid 2015;25(2):221–8.
29. Patel SG, Carty SE, McCoy KL, et al. Preoperative detection of RAS mutation may guide extent of thyroidectomy. Surgery 2017;161(1):168–75.
30. Radkay LA, Chiosea SI, Seethala RR, et al. Thyroid nodules with KRAS mutations are different from nodules with NRAS and HRAS mutations with regard to cytopathologic and histopathologic outcome characteristics. Cancer Cytopathol 2014; 122(12):873–82.
31. Vasko V, Ferrand M, Di Cristofaro J, et al. Specific pattern of RAS oncogene mutations in follicular thyroid tumors. J Clin Endocrinol Metab 2003;88(6):2745–52.
32. Bae JS, Choi SK, Jeon S, et al. Impact of NRAS mutations on the diagnosis of follicular neoplasm of the thyroid. Int J Endocrinol 2014;2014:289834.
33. Giannini R, Ugolini C, Poma AM, et al. Identification of two distinct molecular subtypes of non-invasive follicular neoplasm with papillary-like nuclear features by digital RNA counting. Thyroid 2017;27(10):1267–76.
34. Armstrong MJ, Yang H, Yip L, et al. PAX8/PPARgamma rearrangement in thyroid nodules predicts follicular-pattern carcinomas, in particular the encapsulated follicular variant of papillary carcinoma. Thyroid 2014;24(9):1369–74.
35. Wylie D, Beaudenon-Huibregtse S, Haynes BC, et al. Molecular classification of thyroid lesions by combined testing for miRNA gene expression and somatic gene alterations. J Pathol Clin Res 2016;2(2):93–103.
36. Nikiforov YE, Steward DL, Robinson-Smith TM, et al. Molecular testing for mutations in improving the fine-needle aspiration diagnosis of thyroid nodules. J Clin Endocrinol Metab 2009;94(6):2092–8.
37. American Thyroid Association (ATA) Guidelines Taskforce on Thyroid Nodules and Differentiated Thyroid Cancer, Cooper DS, Doherty GM, Haugen BR, et al. Revised American Thyroid Association management guidelines for patients with thyroid nodules and differentiated thyroid cancer. Thyroid 2009;19(11): 1167–214.
38. Yip L, Farris C, Kabaker AS, et al. Cost impact of molecular testing for indeterminate thyroid nodule fine-needle aspiration biopsies. J Clin Endocrinol Metab 2012;97(6):1905–12.
39. Yip L, Wharry LI, Armstrong MJ, et al. A clinical algorithm for fine-needle aspiration molecular testing effectively guides the appropriate extent of initial thyroidectomy. Ann Surg 2014;260(1):163–8.
40. Walsh PS, Wilde JI, Tom EY, et al. Analytical performance verification of a molecular diagnostic for cytology-indeterminate thyroid nodules. J Clin Endocrinol Metab 2012;97(12):E2297–306.
41. Alexander EK, Kennedy GC, Baloch ZW, et al. Preoperative diagnosis of benign thyroid nodules with indeterminate cytology. N Engl J Med 2012;367(8):705–15.
42. Nikiforova MN, Wald AI, Roy S, et al. Targeted next-generation sequencing panel (ThyroSeq) for detection of mutations in thyroid cancer. J Clin Endocrinol Metab 2013;98(11):E1852–60.
43. Nikiforov YE, Carty SE, Chiosea SI, et al. Highly accurate diagnosis of cancer in thyroid nodules with follicular neoplasm/suspicious for a follicular neoplasm cytology by ThyroSeq v2 next-generation sequencing assay. Cancer 2014; 120(23):3627–34.

44. Nikiforov YE, Carty SE, Chiosea SI, et al. Impact of the multi-gene ThyroSeq next-generation sequencing assay on cancer diagnosis in thyroid nodules with atypia of undetermined significance/follicular lesion of undetermined significance cytology. Thyroid 2015;25(11):1217–23.
45. Labourier E, Shifrin A, Busseniers AE, et al. Molecular testing for miRNA, mRNA, and DNA on fine-needle aspiration improves the preoperative diagnosis of thyroid nodules with indeterminate cytology. J Clin Endocrinol Metab 2015;100(7): 2743–50.
46. Lithwick-Yanai G, Dromi N, Shtabsky A, et al. Multicentre validation of a microRNA-based assay for diagnosing indeterminate thyroid nodules utilising fine needle aspirate smears. J Clin Pathol 2017;70(6):500–7.
47. National Comprehensive Cancer Network. Thyroid Carcinoma (Version 2.2018). Available at: http://www.nccn.org/professionals/physician_gls/pdf/thyroid.pdf. Accessed January 31, 2019.
48. Patel KN, Angell TE, Babiarz J, et al. Performance of a genomic sequencing classifier for the preoperative diagnosis of cytologically indeterminate thyroid nodules. JAMA Surg 2018;153(9):817–24.
49. Duh QY, Busaidy NL, Rahilly-Tierney C, et al. A systematic review of the methods of diagnostic accuracy studies of the afirma gene expression classifier. Thyroid 2017;27(10):1215–22.
50. Marti JL, Avadhani V, Donatelli LA, et al. Wide inter-institutional variation in performance of a molecular classifier for indeterminate thyroid nodules. Ann Surg Oncol 2015;22(12):3996–4001.
51. Brauner E, Holmes BJ, Krane JF, et al. Performance of the Afirma gene expression classifier in hurthle cell thyroid nodules differs from other indeterminate thyroid nodules. Thyroid 2015;25(7):789–96.
52. Ganly I, Ricarte Filho J, Eng S, et al. Genomic dissection of Hurthle cell carcinoma reveals a unique class of thyroid malignancy. J Clin Endocrinol Metab 2013;98(5):E962–72.
53. Steward DL, Carty SE, Sippel RS, et al. Performance of a multigene genomic classifier in thyroid nodules with indeterminate cytology: a prospective blinded multicenter study. JAMA Oncol 2018. [Epub ahead of print].
54. Zhang M, Lin O. Molecular testing of thyroid nodules: a review of current available tests for fine-needle aspiration specimens. Arch Pathol Lab Med 2016;140(12): 1338–44.
55. Vargas-Salas S, Martinez JR, Urra S, et al. Genetic testing for indeterminate thyroid cytology: review and meta-analysis. Endocr Relat Cancer 2018;25(3): R163–77.
56. Duick DS, Klopper JP, Diggans JC, et al. The impact of benign gene expression classifier test results on the endocrinologist-patient decision to operate on patients with thyroid nodules with indeterminate fine-needle aspiration cytopathology. Thyroid 2012;22(10):996–1001.
57. McCoy KL, Carty SE, Armstrong MJ, et al. Intraoperative pathologic examination in the era of molecular testing for differentiated thyroid cancer. J Am Coll Surg 2012;215(4):546–54.
58. Dedhia PH, Rubio GA, Cohen MS, et al. Potential effects of molecular testing of indeterminate thyroid nodule fine needle aspiration biopsy on thyroidectomy volume. World J Surg 2014;38(3):634–8.
59. Noureldine SI, Najafian A, Aragon Han P, et al. Evaluation of the effect of diagnostic molecular testing on the surgical decision-making process for patients with thyroid nodules. JAMA Otolaryngol Head Neck Surg 2016;142(7):676–82.

60. Livhits MJ, Kuo EJ, Leung AM, et al. Gene expression classifier versus targeted next-generation sequencing in the management of indeterminate thyroid nodules. J Clin Endocrinol Metab 2018;103(6):2261–8.
61. Raue F, Frank-Raue K. Thyroid cancer: risk-stratified management and individualized therapy. Clin Cancer Res 2016;22(20):5012–21.
62. Noureldine SI, Olson MT, Agrawal N, et al. Effect of gene expression classifier molecular testing on the surgical decision-making process for patients with thyroid nodules. JAMA Otolaryngol Head Neck Surg 2015;141(12):1082–8.
63. Elsheikh TM, Asa SL, Chan JK, et al. Interobserver and intraobserver variation among experts in the diagnosis of thyroid follicular lesions with borderline nuclear features of papillary carcinoma. Am J Clin Pathol 2008;130(5):736–44.
64. Nikiforov YE, Seethala RR, Tallini G, et al. Nomenclature revision for encapsulated follicular variant of papillary thyroid carcinoma: a paradigm shift to reduce overtreatment of indolent tumors. JAMA Oncol 2016;2(8):1023–9.
65. Faquin WC, Wong LQ, Afrogheh AH, et al. Impact of reclassifying noninvasive follicular variant of papillary thyroid carcinoma on the risk of malignancy in The Bethesda System for Reporting Thyroid Cytopathology. Cancer Cytopathol 2016;124(3):181–7.
66. Strickland KC, Howitt BE, Marqusee E, et al. The impact of noninvasive follicular variant of papillary thyroid carcinoma on rates of malignancy for fine-needle aspiration diagnostic categories. Thyroid 2015;25(9):987–92.
67. Alves VAF, Kakudo K, LiVolsi V, et al. Noninvasive follicular thyroid neoplasm with papillary-like nuclear features (NIFTP): achieving better agreement by refining diagnostic criteria. Clinics (Sao Paulo) 2018;73:e576.
68. Lee L, How J, Tabah RJ, et al. Cost-effectiveness of molecular testing for thyroid nodules with atypia of undetermined significance cytology. J Clin Endocrinol Metab 2014;99(8):2674–82.
69. Shapiro S, Pharaon M, Kellermeyer B. Cost-effectiveness of gene expression classifier testing of indeterminate thyroid nodules utilizing a real cohort comparator. Otolaryngol Head Neck Surg 2017;157(4):596–601.
70. Wu JX, Lam R, Levin M, et al. Effect of malignancy rates on cost-effectiveness of routine gene expression classifier testing for indeterminate thyroid nodules. Surgery 2016;159(1):118–26.
71. Balentine CJ, Vanness DJ, Schneider DF. Cost-effectiveness of lobectomy versus genetic testing (Afirma(R)) for indeterminate thyroid nodules: considering the costs of surveillance. Surgery 2018;163(1):88–96.
72. Nishino M, Nikiforova M. Update on molecular testing for cytologically indeterminate thyroid nodules. Arch Pathol Lab Med 2018;142(4):446–57.

Extent of Surgery for Low-Risk Differentiated Thyroid Cancer

Alexandria D. McDow, MD[a], Susan C. Pitt, MD, MPHS[b,*]

KEYWORDS

- Thyroid cancer • Thyroidectomy • Thyroid lobectomy • Surgery
- Extent of resection • Low-risk thyroid cancer • Differentiated thyroid cancer
- Active surveillance

KEY POINTS

- The incidence of thyroid cancer is rising, yet mortality remains stable.
- Surgical management of very low-risk and low-risk differentiated thyroid cancer remains controversial.
- In appropriate patients, papillary thyroid microcarcinoma may be managed with either thyroid lobectomy or active surveillance with no difference in overall survival.
- Both thyroid lobectomy and total thyroidectomy are appropriate surgeries for low-risk differentiated thyroid cancer measuring 1 cm to 4 cm. Multiple factors must be considered when deciding between the 2 approaches.

INTRODUCTION

Thyroid cancer is the fifth most common cancer in women and represents 3.1% of all new cancer cases in the United States.[1,2] Currently, an estimated 53,990 new cases of thyroid cancer are diagnosed each year and 2060 die from the disease. In 1975, the incidence of thyroid cancer was 4.9 per 100,000 people and remained relatively stable until the early 1990s, at which time the incidence increased significantly.[3] By 2009, the incidence rose to 14.3 per 100,000 people.[3] Despite this rise, thyroid cancer mortality has remained stable at approximately 0.5 deaths per 100,000 people.[2,3] Similar increases in incidence have been observed in many other countries throughout the world, particularly when screening is used.[4,5]

The increasing incidence of thyroid cancer over the past 40 years is largely attributed to overdiagnosis of small differentiated tumors.[3–9] There has also been a true

Disclosure Statement: The authors have nothing to disclose.

[a] Section of Endocrine Surgery, Department of Surgery, Indiana University, 545 Barnhill Drive EH 537, Indianapolis, IN 46202, USA; [b] Division of Endocrine Surgery, Department of Surgery, University of Wisconsin-Madison, 600 Highland Avenue, CSC K4/738, Madison, WI 53792-7375, USA
* Corresponding author.
E-mail address: pitt@surgery.wisc.edu

Surg Clin N Am 99 (2019) 599–610
https://doi.org/10.1016/j.suc.2019.04.003 surgical.theclinics.com
0039-6109/19/

increase, however, in the incidence secondary to radiation and unrecognized environmental exposure.[10] Overdiagnosis in the setting of thyroid cancer refers to the detection of indolent or very slow-growing cancers that are unlikely to cause symptoms or death.[3,9] Overdiagnosis is believed to result from several factors, including increased use of cervical ultrasonography and other cross-sectional imaging, the development of fine-needle aspiration, and increased scrutiny of thyroid specimens after surgical resection. For patients with thyroid cancer, overdiagnosis is detrimental when it leads to overtreatment where the risks of harm or complications from surgery outweigh the survival benefit. To prevent overtreatment, the extent of surgery recommended for patients with low-risk differentiated thyroid cancer (DTC) currently takes a less-is-more approach.

Risk of Recurrence

Historically, a vast majority of patients with low-risk DTC were treated with total thyroidectomy, radioactive iodine (RAI), and thyroid hormone suppression therapy.[11] Now, treatment is more individualized and based on multiple factors, including risk of recurrence and survival. The American Thyroid Association (ATA) guidelines reviewed in this article propose a 3-tiered risk stratification system for DTC (**Fig. 1**).[12] Patients are categorized as having low risk, intermediate risk, or high risk of recurrence.[12] Low risk includes intrathyroidal DTC without evidence of extrathyroidal extension (ETE), vascular invasion, or metastasis.[12] Intermediate risk is defined as 1 or more of the following: microscopic ETE, cervical lymph node metastases,

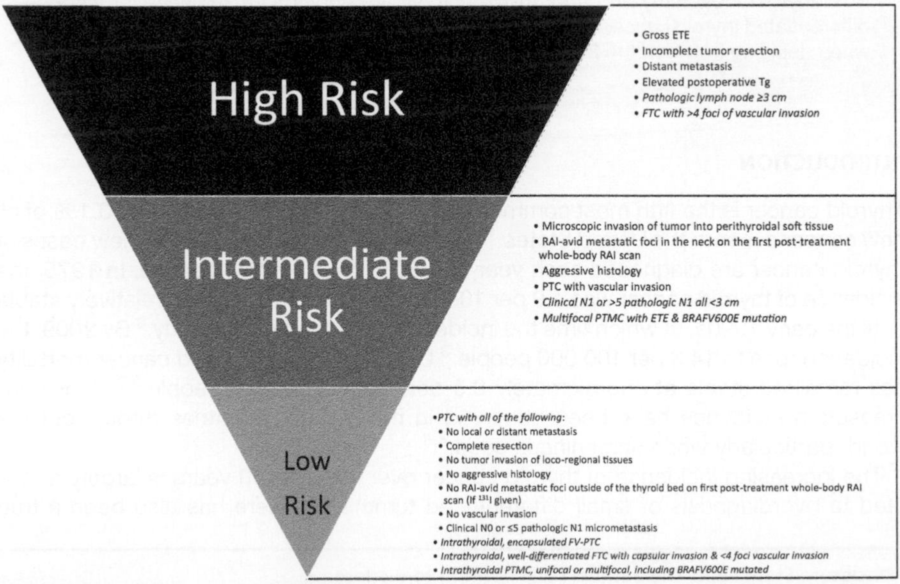

Fig. 1. ATA 2009 risk stratification system for structural disease recurrence DTC with proposed modifications (italics). FTC, follicular thyroid cancer; FV-PTC, follicular-variant papillary thyroid cancer; N0, no evidence of regional lymph node metastasis; N1, metastasis to regional lymph node; PTC, papillary thyroid cancer; PTMC, papillary thyroid microcarcinoma; Tg, thyroglobulin. (*Adapted from* Haugen BR, Alexander EK, Bible KC, et al. 2015 American Thyroid Association Management Guidelines for adult patients with thyroid nodules and differentiated thyroid cancer: The American Thyroid Association Guidelines Task Force on Thyroid Nodules and Differentiated Thyroid Cancer. Thyroid 2016;26(1):1–133, with permission.)

extrathyroidal disease in the neck avid to RAI, vascular invasion, and aggressive tumor histology.[12] Cancers that are at high risk of recurrence are characterized by gross ETE, incomplete tumor resection, distant metastatic disease, or inappropriate postoperative serum thyroglobulin level.[12] The most recent ATA guidelines describe an additional category of disease considered to be at very low risk of recurrence.[12] These tumors are defined as papillary thyroid cancers measuring 1 cm or smaller without clinically evident metastases or local invasion and without cytologic or molecular evidence of aggressive histology.

Goals of Treatment

When recommending treatment of patients with DTC, the 2015 ATA guidelines identify 5 goals of initial therapy:

1. Improve overall and disease-specific survival.
2. Reduce the risk of persistent/recurrent disease.
3. Permit accurate staging.
4. Minimize treatment-related morbidity.
5. Minimize unnecessary therapy.[12]

This article explores the recommended extent of surgery for very low-risk and low-risk DTC. This topic has been debated by experts for decades and continues to be widely debated today. This article critically examines the literature and discusses the controversy over the appropriate extent of resection according to risk of recurrence and size of the cancer.

VERY LOW-RISK DIFFERENTIATED THYROID CANCER

Patients with very low-risk DTC have 2 main management options: active surveillance and thyroid lobectomy.[12] If surgical resection is chosen for a thyroid cancer 1 cm or smaller with no high-risk features, thyroid lobectomy is the preferred treatment unless there are clear indications for resection of the contralateral lobe.[12] Total thyroidectomy should be reserved for patients at risk of more aggressive disease, such as those with a history of head and neck radiation, positive family history of thyroid cancer, or clinically detectable cervical lymph node metastasis.[12] These recommendations are based on evidence indicating that most very low-risk papillary cancers, or papillary microcarcinomas, are nonprogressive and do not lead to harm or decrease survival.[13–16]

Active surveillance is a nonsurgical management option for patients with very low-risk DTC that was newly endorsed by the 2015 ATA guidelines. Evidence supporting active surveillance originated in Japan with Miyauchi,[14] who performed an observational trial at Kuma Hospital of more than 2000 patients with very low-risk papillary thyroid cancer who underwent either active surveillance or immediate surgery. Eligible patients included those with papillary microcarcinoma without any of the following features: lymph node or distant metastasis, ETE, high-grade cytology, growth during a previous observation, location near the recurrent laryngeal nerve, and attachment to the trachea.[14] Of the 1235 patients who were surveilled with serial ultrasound examinations, 8% had tumors increase in size by 3 mm or more over 10 years, and 3.8% developed novel lymph node metastasis. Ultimately, 15% of patients enrolled in the study underwent surgery for either progression of disease or change in patient preference. All patients who experienced progression of disease were treated successfully with surgery, and none of the patients in the study had recurrence or died from their thyroid cancer. Alternatively, patients who underwent immediate surgery had a significantly increased rate of temporary vocal cord paralysis (4.1% vs 0.6%, $P<.0001$) as well as temporary and permanent hypoparathyroidism (16.7% vs 2.8%, $P<.0001$, and 1.6% vs 0.08%, $P<.0001$, respectively), compared with patients who underwent active surveillance. After this landmark observational study, Tuttle and colleagues[15] demonstrated similar results with patients in the United States who had thyroid nodules less than or equal to 1.5 cm with a cytologic diagnosis of papillary or suspicious for papillary thyroid cancer. These and other studies demonstrate that active surveillance is a viable management option with excellent oncologic outcomes for select patients and allows patients to avoid potentially unnecessary surgical risk.[12,17,18] Although protocols vary between institutions, active surveillance entails closely monitoring the known thyroid cancer with serial ultrasounds performed every 6 months for 1 year to 2 years followed by annual ultrasound examinations to monitor for growth or spread.[14,15]

LOW-RISK DIFFERENTIATED THYROID CANCER: 1 CM TO 4 CM

The recommended extent of surgery for patients with DTC measuring 1 cm to 4 cm is more controversial than that of very low-risk tumors. The surgical options for treatment of patients with 1 cm to 4 cm low-risk DTC include both the more traditional approach of total thyroidectomy and the newly endorsed thyroid lobectomy.[12] Arguments are explored for total thyroidectomy versus thyroid lobectomy for patients with DTC measuring 1 cm to 4 cm without high-risk features: gross ETE, incomplete tumor resection, distant metastasis, lymph node greater than 3 cm, and follicular thyroid cancer with extensive vascular invasion.[12] Additional factors to consider in the decision-making process also are discussed.

Arguments for Total Thyroidectomy

Multifocality and contralateral disease

One clear benefit of total thyroidectomy is the ability to eradicate possible contralateral disease if the cancer is multifocal. Previous reports reveal multifocality, the presence of 2 or more anatomically separate foci of cancer within the thyroid gland, can be present in 18% to 87% of cases.[19] Pyo and colleagues[20] investigated the impact of multifocal papillary thyroid cancer on lymph node metastasis and found that the greater total combined surface area of each tumor predicts lymph node metastasis and tumor behavior even in papillary microcarcinomas. Mazeh and colleagues[21] reported 57% of patients with papillary thyroid cancer measuring 0.3 cm to 7.0 cm have multifocal disease. This group further demonstrated that pathologic examination of the entire gland as opposed to representative sections significantly increases the incidence of contralateral disease, which was present in 71% of patients.[21] The presence of multifocality in 1 lobe has also been shown to be a risk factor for papillary thyroid cancer in the contralateral lobe and is unrelated to tumor size.[21,22] The European Society of Endocrine Surgeons consensus statement recommends total thyroidectomy in the setting of multifocality to reduce the risk of local recurrence.[19]

Potential for second surgery

Another benefit of total thyroidectomy is avoiding the need for a second surgery or a completion thyroidectomy. The decision to perform a total thyroidectomy or lobectomy for patients with low-risk DTC is complex and can result in either an oncologically excessive or oncologically inadequate resection.[23,24] Those who initially undergo a thyroid lobectomy are at risk of needing a completion thyroidectomy and second general anesthetic if any of the following is found on final pathology: gross ETE, metastasis to regional lymph nodes, vascular invasion, or aggressive histologic variants.[25] Dhir and colleagues[25] found that after thyroid lobectomy, 53% of patients have intermediate-risk disease on final histopathology and, thus, require completion thyroidectomy. Other investigators have reported that the proportion of patients requiring completion thyroidectomy is as low as 9.3%.[23,26,27] Total thyroidectomy allows for a single surgery and facilitates treatment with RAI for patients found at intermediate risk or high risk of recurrence.

Adequacy of resection

An additional benefit of a single-stage total thyroidectomy is that a single surgery may provide a more oncologically adequate resection. Oltmann and colleagues[28] examined postoperative RAI uptake scans and demonstrated significantly higher thyroid remnant uptake after completion thyroidectomy compared with total thyroidectomy. This finding suggests single-stage total thyroidectomy may be more oncologically adequate than lobectomy followed by completion thyroidectomy.[28] Unpublished data from the authors' group (Dedhia et al, 2018) indicate, however, that the 6-week unstimulated thyroglobulin levels do not differ between patients undergoing initial total thyroidectomy compared with those undergoing lobectomy followed by completion thyroidectomy. Therefore, the degree to which total thyroidectomy provides a better oncologic surgery is unclear.

Detection of residual or recurrent thyroid cancer

Total thyroidectomy also has the benefit of facilitating detection of persistent or recurrent thyroid cancer. The ATA guidelines recommend routine use of serum thyroglobulin and either a neck ultrasound or whole-body scan to assess postoperative disease status after total thyroidectomy (**Fig. 2**A).[12] Thyroglobulin levels facilitate the ability to assess the adequacy and completeness of surgical resection. If detectable immediately after a total thyroidectomy, the patient may have persistent or residual thyroid cancer.

On the other hand, when thyroid lobectomy is performed, serum thyroglobulin is less useful and uptake scans no longer are recommended. The detection of persistent or recurrent disease in postlobectomy patients is based primarily on ultrasonography (**Fig. 2**B). Because serum thyroglobulin levels increase gradually after lobectomy in patients with and those without recurrent disease, interpreting thyroglobulin levels after lobectomy can be challenging and, at times, of limited value for predicting recurrence.[29] In addition, RAI uptake scans cannot be performed because of the residual thyroid lobe. Therefore, ultrasonography is the mainstay of detection of recurrence after thyroid lobectomy, which also has its challenges. Previous studies suggest that a majority of nonspecialist-performed ultrasounds do not appropriately evaluate lymph nodes.[30] Ultrasound performance by high-volume endocrine surgeons is more accurate than those performed by nonspecialists.[30] Keeping the limitations of surveillance of ultrasound in mind, many investigators argue that total thyroidectomy allows for easier detection of recurrent disease.

Arguments for Thyroid Lobectomy

Avoidance of thyroid hormone replacement

Although total thyroidectomy offers several benefits for treating patients with low-risk DTC measuring 1 cm to 4 cm, thyroid lobectomy also has several advantages. One major advantage of thyroid lobectomy is that patients may remain euthyroid and not require thyroid hormone supplementation.[31] The proportion of patients who require thyroid hormone supplementation, however, is controversial. Cox and colleagues[32] recently showed that up to 73% of patients who have a lobectomy may require thyroid hormone supplementation because they have a

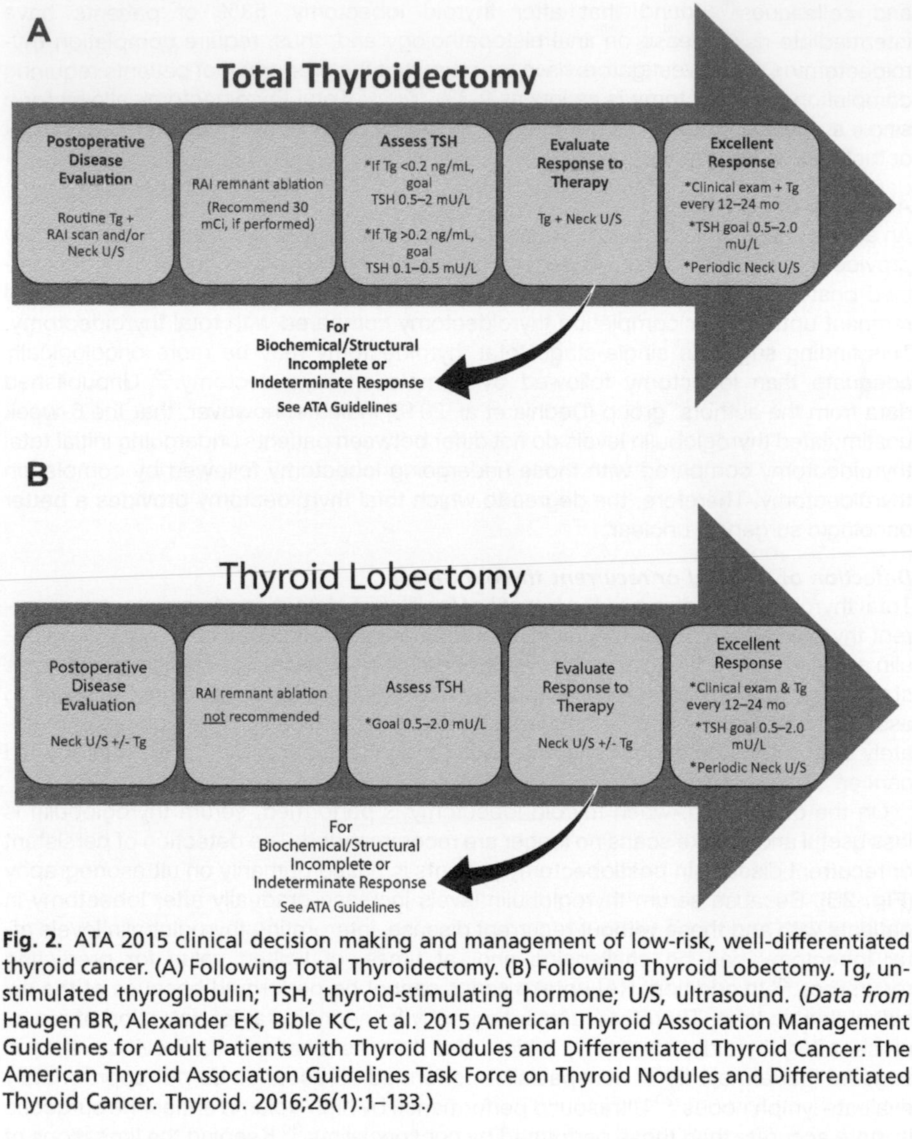

Fig. 2. ATA 2015 clinical decision making and management of low-risk, well-differentiated thyroid cancer. (A) Following Total Thyroidectomy. (B) Following Thyroid Lobectomy. Tg, unstimulated thyroglobulin; TSH, thyroid-stimulating hormone; U/S, ultrasound. (*Data from* Haugen BR, Alexander EK, Bible KC, et al. 2015 American Thyroid Association Management Guidelines for Adult Patients with Thyroid Nodules and Differentiated Thyroid Cancer: The American Thyroid Association Guidelines Task Force on Thyroid Nodules and Differentiated Thyroid Cancer. Thyroid. 2016;26(1):1–133.)

thyroid-stimulating hormone level greater than 2 mIU/L at some point during the first postoperative year. The 2015 ATA guidelines recommend maintaining the thyroid-stimulating hormone level less than 2 mIU/L postoperatively in patients with low-risk DTC.[33] Whether or not these patients require hormone supplementation long term is unclear.

Little impact on quality of life

Another potential benefit of lobectomy is the lack of impact on quality of life, which may or may not be related to thyroid hormone changes. Although some patients notice little difference in quality of life after complete removal of the thyroid, others report weight gain, fatigue, dry or coarse skin, extremity edema, and asthenia despite having a euthyroid state.[34] Multiple studies demonstrate these symptoms can lead to a reduction in overall quality of life.[34,35] Rosato and colleagues[35] explored the prevalence of asthenia, the reduced ability to perform mental and physical work, after thyroid lobectomy and total thyroidectomy. In their study, no patients experienced asthenia after thyroid lobectomy, whereas the incidence of asthenia after total thyroidectomy was significantly higher at 25%.[35] Unpublished data from the authors' group (Dedhia et al, 2018) suggest that patients experience few changes in quality of life after lobectomy when assessed by semistructured interviews and health-related quality-of-life tests. More data are needed, however, to determine if there are real differences in quality of life in lobectomy patients compared with those undergoing total thyroidectomy.

Decreased risks of complications

An additional and less debatable benefit of thyroid lobectomy is that patients have a decreased risk of postoperative complications compared with total thyroidectomy. As expected, the risk of hypocalcemia is significantly higher after total thyroidectomy compared with thyroid lobectomy because there is no risk to the contralateral parathyroid glands after lobectomy.[36] The risks of hematoma, seroma, fever, nausea, vomiting, dehydration, urinary retention, and urinary tract infection also are significantly lower after lobectomy.[36] It is well known that patients can develop voice and throat dysfunction after thyroid surgery. Ryu and colleagues[37] demonstrated 14% to 83% of patients developed some element of voice changes or throat dysfunction postoperatively, despite no evidence of laryngeal nerve injury. In this study, patients experience less vocal and throat dysfunction after thyroid lobectomy compared with total thyroidectomy.[37] Patients were less likely to experience voice roughness, jitter, and strain.

Equivalent recurrence and survival

Although minimizing treatment-related morbidity is incredibly important and an advantage of thyroid lobectomy, the primary goal of all cancer treatment is to improve overall and disease-specific survival while reducing recurrence. For patients with low-risk DTC measuring 1 cm to 4 cm, thyroid lobectomy and total thyroidectomy have been shown in multiple studies to have equivalent survival and recurrence, although this area is controversial.[38–42] Although several studies demonstrate equivalent outcomes between the 2 surgical approaches, Bilimoria and colleagues[43] reported in 2007 that patients with papillary thyroid cancer greater than or equal to 1 cm who underwent a lobectomy had an increased risk of recurrence and decrease in survival at 10 years compared with those who underwent total thyroidectomy. The study did not account for multiple confounding factors, however, such as ETE, presence of aggressive histologic variants of papillary thyroid cancer, multifocality, patient comorbidities, or adequacy of resection. Subsequently, Adam and colleagues[38,40] and Mendelsohn and colleagues[39] attempted to account for these confounders and revealed no difference in survival between lobectomy and total thyroidectomy in patients with papillary thyroid cancer using multivariable and Cox proportional hazards models. Nixon and colleagues[41] also explored this controversy and found no difference in overall survival and disease-specific survival as well as no difference in recurrence-free survival. A recent systematic review of the literature on this topic similarly concluded that a majority of data support comparable oncologic outcomes between lobectomy and total thyroidectomy in patients with papillary thyroid cancer measuring 1 cm to 4 cm.[42]

Additional Considerations

As described previously, the decision to perform a total thyroidectomy or thyroid lobectomy for low-risk DTC measuring 1 cm to 4 cm is complex. There are several advantages and disadvantages of each approach. Additional factors that may influence decision making about the appropriate extent of surgery for patients with these tumors are explored.

Surgeon-performed ultrasonography

Cervical ultrasonography is paramount to preoperative surgical planning and should be considered when determining the appropriate extent of surgery. Cervical ultrasonography should examine thyroid nodule features, including location and evidence of local invasion or intrathoracic extension, as well as investigate contralateral nodules and survey cervical lymph nodes in the central and lateral compartments.[30] Carneiro-Pla and Amin[30] revealed that surgeon-performed ultrasonography altered the preoperative management of 45% of patients due to identification of central or lateral lymph node metastasis or other high-risk features that were not mentioned on preconsultation ultrasound. Other studies have also demonstrated the importance of obtaining a high-quality ultrasound to reduce the risk of an oncologically inadequate resection.

Molecular testing

Molecular testing is another facet of the preoperative evaluation of patients with DTC that should be considered when deciding on the appropriate extent of surgery. Although not all patients will or need to undergo molecular testing of thyroid nodules, the use of molecular testing for indeterminate nodules is increasing. Several studies have assessed the use of molecular testing to aid in decision-making regarding extent of surgery for indeterminate thyroid nodules and are discussed in more depth in Janeil Mitchell's and Linwah Yip's article, "Decision-Making in Indeterminate Thyroid Nodules and the Role of Molecular Testing," in this issue. Studies examining the value of molecular markers, however, in therapeutic decision making for patients with known thyroid cancer are lacking.[44] Because the molecular status of an individual cancer can help predict tumor biology, the results of any testing should play a role in the decision to perform a total thyroidectomy or lobectomy. For instance, a patient with a known BRAF mutation, which has a strong association with ETE, lymph node metastasis, advanced stage, recurrent or persistent disease, and loss of RAI avidity, likely should undergo a total thyroidectomy.[44] Similarly, TERT promoter mutations have been associated with advanced or aggressive thyroid cancer, whereas patients with RET/PTC rearrangement may have a better prognosis.[44] Because molecular testing offers important prognostic information, it may play a bigger role in decision making about the extent of surgery for thyroid cancer in the future.

Cost effectiveness

Another factor that may contribute to the decision to perform a total thyroidectomy or thyroid lobectomy is cost effectiveness, particularly in lieu of the current health care system. Several studies have examined the cost effectiveness of total thyroidectomy versus lobectomy with varying results. Corso and colleagues[45] performed a cost-utility analysis in patients with indeterminate thyroid nodules and found total thyroidectomy to be more cost saving when considering the risks of reoperation, recurrence, or complications, such as recurrent laryngeal nerve injury or hypoparathyroidism. When examining the surgical approach for patients with "suspicious for papillary thyroid cancer" on fine-needle aspiration, Leiker and colleagues[46] similarly found total thyroidectomy the most cost effective. Conversely, Lang and Wong[47] performed a

Markov module of patients with low-risk, 1 cm to 4 cm papillary thyroid cancer without clinically apparent high-risk features after the emergence of the most recent ATA guidelines. This study identified initial lobectomy as the most cost-effective long-term strategy despite incorporating the risk of locoregional recurrence and potential for completion thyroidectomy.[47] Although total costs in this study included costs of procedures, complications, and hospitalization, they did not include indirect costs, such as loss of productivity or wages.[47] Currently, data looking at such direct costs to patients are lacking but are needed. Patients with thyroid cancer are known to have an increased risk of bankruptcy compared with the population and are at greater risk than patients with other cancers, except lung cancer.[48]

Patient preference

The decision about the appropriate extent of surgery for patients with low-risk DTC 1 cm to 4 cm also should consider individual patient preference. Surgeons should use a shared decision-making process to understanding each patient's values and preferences and align them with the best overall treatment strategy. To reach a shared decision, providers must have a firm grasp of the literature to articulate the pros and cons of each approach in a manner that takes a patient's unique presentation and preferences into account. There is a fine balance between avoiding undertreatment of a clinically significant cancer and overtreatment of indolent lesions.

LOW-RISK DIFFERENTIATED THYROID CANCER: GREATER THAN 4 CM

Unlike small low-risk nodules, the most recent ATA guidelines continue to recommend total thyroidectomy for DTC greater than 4 cm.[12] Although not explored in this article, total thyroidectomy also is recommended for cancers with any high-risk features, including gross ETE or clinically apparent metastatic disease to lymph nodes or distant sites.[12] One of the driving factors for this recommendation is the ability to perform RAI remnant ablation postoperatively. Cancers greater than 4 cm were previously considered intermediate risk. Ruel and colleagues[49] performed the first national study examining the impact of RAI on overall survival in patients with intermediate-risk disease. This study included patients with tumor size greater than 4 cm with no other concerning features as well as tumors with or without minimal ETE and with or without lymph node metastasis.[48] Their results concluded that there is a reduced risk of death when RAI is administered in intermediate-risk cancers.[49] Both patients who received RAI and those who did not, however, had a very high overall survival.[49] Therefore, the question remains whether this bears clinical significance. With the new American Joint Committee on Cancer staging system, cancers greater than 4 cm without gross ETE are now considered stage II, or low-risk of death.[49] These new staging guidelines are clear, however, that this does not necessarily denote risk of recurrence.[50] More recently, tumors greater than 4 cm confined to the thyroid (T3a) also are considered low risk for recurrence in the ATA guidelines.[12] Further studies are needed to assess whether RAI decreases recurrence or survival based on size alone. These results may have an impact on whether total thyroidectomy is recommended for all cancers greater than 4 cm in the future.

SUMMARY

In conclusion, the appropriate extent of surgery for patients with low-risk DTC is complex and constantly under debate, which makes caring for these patients exciting and dynamic. Several factors should be considered in the decision-making process, including multifocality, contralateral disease, the potential for a seconding surgery, postoperative surveillance, the need for thyroid hormone replacement, quality of life, risk of complications, ultrasound findings, molecular test results, and costs. Ultimately, understanding what is most important to each patient is critical to aligning the treatment decision with patient preferences and values. Therefore, providers should have an in-depth understanding of the pros and cons of each treatment option—active surveillance, lobectomy, and total thyroidectomy—and seek to elicit patients' treatment goals to reach shared decisions.

REFERENCES

1. Siegel RL, Miller KD, Jemal A. Cancer statistics, 2018. CA Cancer J Clin 2018; 68(1):7–30.
2. National Cancer Institute Surveillance. Epidemiology, and end results program. cancer stat facts: thyroid cancer 2018. Available at: https://seer.cancer.gov/statfacts/html/thyro.html. Accessed November 1, 2018.
3. Davies L, Welch G. Current thyroid cancer trends in the Unites States. JAMA Otolaryngol Head Neck Surg 2014;140(4):317–22.
4. Vaccarella S, Franceschi S, Bray F, et al. Worldwide thyroid-cancer epidemic? The increasing impact of overdiagnosis. N Engl J Med 2016;375(7):614–7.
5. Pellegriti G, Frasca F, Regalbuto C, et al. Worldwide increasing incidence of thyroid cancer: update of epidemiology and risk factors. J Cancer Epidemiol 2013; 2013:965212.
6. Brito JP, Morris JC, Montori VM. Thyroid cancer: zealous imaging has increased detection and treatment of low risk tumors. BMJ 2013;347:f4706.
7. Enewold L, Zhu K, Ron E, et al. Rising thyroid cancer incidence in the United States by demographic and tumor characteristics, 1980-2005. Cancer Epidemiol Biomarkers Prev 2009;18(3):784–91.
8. Hall SF, Irish J, Groome P, et al. Access, excess, and overdiagnosis: the case for thyroid cancer. Cancer Med 2014;3(1):154–61.
9. Davies L. Overdiagnosis of thyroid cancer. BMJ 2016;355:i6312.
10. Hoffman K, Lorenzo A, Butt CM, et al. Exposure to flame retardant chemicals and occurrence and severity of papillary thyroid cancer: a case-control study. Environ Int 2017;107:235–42.
11. Iñiguez-Ariza NM, Brito JP. Management of low-risk papillary thyroid cancer. Endocrinol Metab (Seoul) 2018;33(2):185–94.
12. Haugen BR, Alexander EK, Bible KC, et al. 2015 American Thyroid Association Management guidelines for adult patients with thyroid nodules and differentiated thyroid cancer: the American Thyroid Association Guidelines task force on thyroid nodules and differentiated thyroid cancer. Thyroid 2016;26(1):1–133.
13. Oda H, Miyauchi A, Ito Y, et al. Incidences of unfavorable events in the management of low-risk papillary thyroid microcarcinoma of the thyroid by active surveillance versus immediate surgery. Thyroid 2016;26(1):150–5.
14. Miyauchi A. Clinical trials of active surveillance of papillary microcarcinoma of the thyroid. World J Surg 2016;40(3):516–22.
15. Tuttle RM, Fagin JA, Minkowitz G, et al. Natural history of tumor volume kinetics of papillary thyroid cancers during active surveillance. JAMA Otolaryngol Head Neck Surg 2017;143(10):1015–20.
16. Roman BR, Morris LG, Davies L. The thyroid cancer epidemic, 2017 perspective. Curr Opin Endocrinol Diabetes Obes 2017;24(5):332–6.
17. Ito Y, Miyauchi A, Kihara M, et al. Patient age is significantly related to the progression of papillary microcarcinoma of the thyroid under observation. Thyroid 2014;24(1):27–34.

18. Sugitani I, Toda K, Yamada K, et al. Three distinctly different kinds of papillary thyroid microcarcinoma should be recognized: our treatment strategies and outcomes. World J Surg 2010;34(6):1222–31.
19. Iacobone M, Jansson S, Barczynski M, et al. Multifocal papillary thyroid carcinoma – a consensus report of the European Society of Endocrine Surgeons (ESES). Langenbecks Arch Surg 2014;399(2):141–54.
20. Pyo JS, Sohn JH, Kang G, et al. Total surface area is useful for differentiating between aggressive and favorable multifocal papillary thyroid carcinomas. Yonsei Med J 2015;56(2):355–61.
21. Mazeh H, Samet Y, Hochstein D, et al. Multifocality in well-differentiated thyroid carcinomas calls for total thyroidectomy. Am J Surg 2011;201(6):770–5.
22. Pitt SC, Sippel RS, Chen H. Contralateral papillary thyroid cancer: does size matter? Am J Surg 2009;197(3):342–7.
23. Schneider DF, Cherney Stafford LM, Brys N, et al. Gauging the extent of thyroidectomy for indeterminate thyroid nodules: an oncologic perspective. Endocr Pract 2017;23(4):442–50.
24. Pitt SC, Lubitz CC. Complex decision making in thyroid cancer: costs and consequences—Is less more? Surgery 2017;161(1):134–6.
25. Dhir M, McCoy KL, Ohori NP, et al. Correct extent of thyroidectomy is poorly predicted preoperatively by the guidelines of the American Thyroid Association for low and intermediate risk thyroid cancers. Surgery 2018;163(1):81–7.
26. Kluijfhout WP, Pasternak JD, Drake FT, et al. Application of the new American Thyroid Association guidelines leads to a substantial rate of completion total thyroidectomy to enable adjuvant radioactive iodine. Surgery 2017;161(1):127–33.
27. Hirshoren N, Kaganov K, Weinberger JM, et al. Thyroidectomy practice after implementation of the 2015 American Thyroid Association Guidelines on surgical options for patients with well-differentiated thyroid carcinoma. JAMA Otolaryngol Head Neck Surg 2018;144(5):427–32.
28. Oltmann SC, Schneider DF, Leverson G, et al. Radioactive iodine remnant uptake after completion thyroidectomy: not such a complete cancer operation. Ann Surg Oncol 2014;21(4):1379–83.
29. Park S, Jeon MJ, Oh HS, et al. Changes in serum thyroglobulin levels after lobectomy in patients with low-risk papillary thyroid cancer. Thyroid 2018;28(8):997–1003.
30. Carneiro-Pla D, Amin S. Comparison between pre-consultation ultrasonography and office surgeon-performed ultrasound in patients with thyroid cancer. World J Surg 2014;38(3):622–7.
31. Stoll SJ, Pitt SC, Liu J, et al. Thyroid hormone replacement after thyroid lobectomy. Surgery 2009;146(4):554–8.
32. Cox C, Bosley M, Southerland LB, et al. Lobectomy for treatment of differentiated thyroid cancer: can patients avoid postoperative thyroid hormone supplementation and be compliant with the American Thyroid Association guidelines? Surgery 2018;163(1):75–80.
33. Lim H, Devessa SS, Sosa JA, et al. Trends in thyroid cancer incidence and mortality in the United States, 1974-2013. JAMA 2017;317(13):1338–48.
34. Tan NC, Chew RQ, Subramanian RC, et al. Patients on levothyroxine replacement in the community: association between hypothyroidism symptoms, co-morbidities and their quality of life. Fam Pract 2018. https://doi.org/10.1093/fampra/cmy064.
35. Rosato L, Pacini F, Panier Suffat L, et al. Post-thyroidectomy chronic asthenia: self-deception or disease? Endocrine 2015;48(2):615–20.

36. Orosco RK, Lin HW, Bhattacharyya N. Ambulatory thyroidectomy: a multistate study of revisits and complications. Otolaryngol Head Neck Surg 2015;152(6): 1017–23.
37. Ryu J, Ryu YM, Jung YS, et al. Extent of thyroidectomy affects vocal and throat functions: a prospective observational study of lobectomy versus total thyroidectomy. Surgery 2013;154(3):611–20.
38. Adam MA, Pura J, Gu L, et al. Extent of surgery for papillary thyroid cancer is not associated with survival: an analysis of 61,775 patients. Ann Surg 2014;260(4): 601–5.
39. Mendelsohn AH, Elashoff DA, Abemayor E, et al. Surgery for papillary thyroid carcinoma: is lobectomy enough? Arch Otolaryngol Head Neck Surg 2010;136(11): 1055–61.
40. Adam MA, Pura J, Goffredo P, et al. Impact of extent of surgery on survival for papillary thyroid cancer patients younger than 45 years. J Clin Endocrinol Metab 2015;100(1):115–21.
41. Nixon IJ, Ganly I, Patel SG, et al. Thyroid lobectomy for treatment of well differentiated intrathyroid malignancy. Surgery 2012;151(4):571–9.
42. Gartland RM, Lubitz CC. Impact of extent of surgery on tumor recurrence and survival for papillary thyroid cancer patients. Ann Surg Oncol 2018;25(9):2520–5.
43. Bilimoria KY, Bentrem DJ, Ko CY, et al. Extent of surgery affects survival for papillary thyroid cancer. Ann Surg 2007;246(3):375–81.
44. Ozgursoy OB, Eisele DW, Tufano RP. The prognostic implications from molecular testing of thyroid cancer. Otolaryngol Clin North Am 2014;47(4):595–607.
45. Corso C, Gomez X, Sanabria A, et al. Total thyroidectomy versus hemithyroidectomy for patients with follicular neoplasm. A cost-utility analysis. Int J Surg 2014; 12(8):837–42.
46. Leiker AJ, Yen TW, Cheung K, et al. Cost analysis of thyroid lobectomy and intraoperative frozen section versus total thyroidectomy in patients with a cytologic diagnosis of “suspicious for papillary thyroid cancer”. Surgery 2013;154(6): 1307–13.
47. Lang BH, Wong CKH. Lobectomy is a more cost-effective option than total thyroidectomy for 1 to 4 cm papillary thyroid carcinoma that do not possess clinically recognizable high-risk features. Ann Surg Oncol 2016;23(11):3641–52.
48. Ramsey S, Blough D, Kirchhoff A, et al. Washington State cancer patients found to be at greater risk for bankruptcy than people without a cancer diagnosis. Health Aff 2013;32(6):1143–52.
49. Ruel E, Thomas S, Dinan M, et al. Adjuvant radioactive iodine therapy is associated with improved survival for patients with intermediate-risk papillary thyroid cancer. J Clin Endocrinol Metab 2015;100(4):1529–36.
50. Tuttle RM, Haugen B, Perrier ND. Updated American Joint Committee on cancer/tumor-node-metastasis staging system for differentiated and anaplastic thyroid cancer (eighth edition): what changed and why? Thyroid 2017;27(6):751–6.

Management of Nodal Disease in Thyroid Cancer

Mamoona Khokhar, MD, Mira Milas, MD*

KEYWORDS

- Thyroid cancer • Lymph nodes • Lymphadenopathy • Metastatic disease
- Ultrasound • Neck dissection • Percutaneous ethanol ablation

KEY POINTS

- A preoperative ultrasound evaluating central and lateral neck lymph nodes is recommended for all patients undergoing thyroidectomy when cytology is suspicious for malignancy or malignant.
- Sonographically abnormal lymph nodes ≥8 to 10 mm in smallest diameter should undergo an ultrasound-guided fine-needle aspiration, with or without thyroglobulin (Tg) washout.
- A therapeutic central neck dissection should accompany total thyroidectomy in patients with clinically involved central neck lymph nodes, and a therapeutic lateral neck dissection should be performed for patients with biopsy-proven lateral lymph node disease.
- Following initial operative intervention, an ultrasound evaluating central and lateral neck lymph nodes should be performed at 6 to 12 months and then periodically, depending on the patient's Tg status and recurrence risk.
- A therapeutic central and/or lateral neck dissection in a previously operated compartment is more complex and thus should be performed only after consideration of multiple clinical factors that include, among others, biopsy-proven persistent or recurrent disease for central neck nodes ≥8 mm and lateral neck nodes ≥10 mm in smallest dimension that can be localized on anatomic imaging.

INTRODUCTION

Cervical lymph node metastases are present in 20% to 50% of patients with differentiated thyroid cancer (DTC) and 11% to 93% of patients with medullary thyroid cancer (MTC).[1–7] Nodal metastases may be present even when the primary tumor is small and intrathyroidal.[8] Micrometastases (<2 mm) may be present in up to 90% of patients, although the clinical implication of micrometastases is likely less significant than that of macrometastases.[9,10]

The authors have nothing to disclose.
Division of Endocrine Surgery, University of Arizona College of Medicine–Phoenix, Banner University Medical Center Phoenix, 1441 North 12th Street, 2nd Floor, Phoenix, AZ 85006, USA
* Corresponding author.
E-mail address: Mira.Milas@bannerhealth.com

Surg Clin N Am 99 (2019) 611–632
https://doi.org/10.1016/j.suc.2019.04.004
surgical.theclinics.com

The goals of initial therapy for patients with thyroid cancer are to (1) improve disease-specific and overall survival, (2) reduce the risk of persistent and recurrent disease, and (3) allow accurate disease staging, all while minimizing treatment-related morbidity. The completeness of surgical resection, including clinically significant lymph node metastases, is an important determinant of outcome because it affects all three of the above objectives. Metastatic lymph nodes represent the most common site of persistent and recurrent disease.[11–13] This review delineates the management of nodal disease in thyroid cancer, primarily as it applies to DTC because this is the vastly more common thyroid malignancy, and for MTC, because it is relevant and unique.

PREOPERATIVE NODAL EVALUATION

Preoperative ultrasound (US) is reported to identify suspicious cervical lymph nodes in 20% to 31% of patients and alters surgical approach in up to 20% of patients.[4,14,15] Per the 2015 American Thyroid Association (ATA) Thyroid Nodule and DTC Guidelines[16]:

- A preoperative US evaluating central and lateral neck lymph nodes is recommended for all patients undergoing thyroidectomy when cytology indicates cells suspicious for malignancy or frankly malignant.
- Sonographically abnormal lymph nodes ≥8 to 10 mm in smallest diameter should undergo US-guided fine-needle aspiration (FNA).
- The addition of FNA-thyroglobulin (Tg) washout in the evaluation of suspicious cervical lymph nodes may be appropriate.
- Preoperative cross-sectional imaging (computed tomography [CT], MRI) with intravenous (IV) contrast is recommended as an adjunct to US for patients with clinical suspicion for advanced disease, including clinically apparent disperse or bulky lymph node disease.

Preoperative Nodal Evaluation with Ultrasound

Sonographic features of lymph nodes that are suggestive of malignant involvement include enlargement, loss of fatty hilum, round shape, hyperechogenicity (reflecting infiltrative growth within lymph nodes, which are typically hypoechoic), cystic change, peripheral vascularity, and microcalcifications (**Fig. 1**).[16] No single US feature is adequately sensitive to prove by itself that a lymph node harbors metastatic thyroid cancer.[16] Although the absence of a fatty hilum has a reported sensitivity of 100%, it has a low specificity of 29%.[17,18] Microcalcifications have the highest specificity (93%–100%), and any lymph node with microcalcifications should be considered abnormal. Cystic change similarly has a high specificity of 91% to 100%, and lymph nodes with predominantly cystic or cystic/solid architecture should also be considered abnormal.[16] One study correlating sonographic features and histologic outcomes found that the most specific features for nodal metastases were short axis greater than 5 mm (96%; this feature has not been confirmed by other studies), cystic changes (100%), punctate hyperechoic areas (100%), and peripheral vascularity (82%). Peripheral vascularity was reported to have a sensitivity of 82%, whereas the remaining features had sensitivities of less than 60%.[19]

Lymph node location is also a consideration in the evaluation and treatment of thyroid cancer. Lymph node metastases are more likely to occur in level III, level IV, and level VI than level II (**Fig. 2**A, B).[18–20] Upper pole papillary thyroid cancers, however, are more likely to demonstrate "skip metastases" to level II and level III.[21]

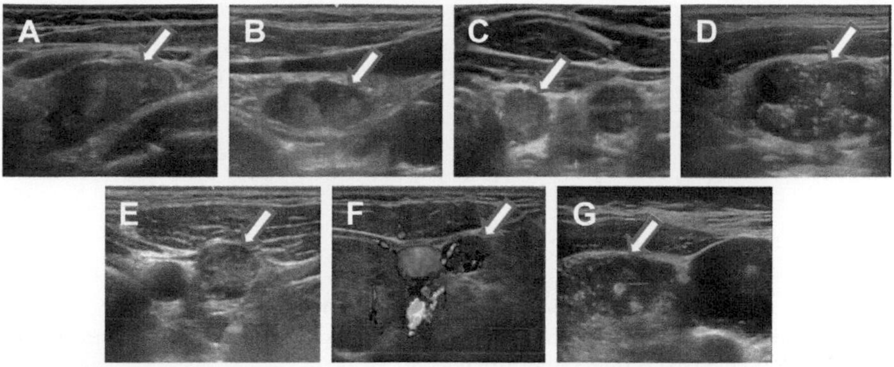

Fig. 1. Sonographic features of lymph nodes suggestive of malignant involvement. Arrows are directed at lymph nodes of interest. (*A*) Enlargement, (*B*) loss of fatty hilum, (*C*) round shape, (*D*) hyperechogenicity, (*E*) cystic change, (*F*) peripheral vascularity, (*G*) microcalcifications. (*Adapted from* Haugen B, Alexander E, Bible K, et al. 2015 American Thyroid Association management guidelines for adult patient with thyroid nodules and differentiated thyroid cancer. Thyroid. 2016; 26(1):1-133, with permission.)

Preoperative Nodal Evaluation with Fine-Needle Aspiration

As a general principle, sonographically abnormal lymph nodes should undergo a US-guided FNA to confirm malignancy (**Fig. 3**).[16] Before initial thyroidectomy for DTC and MTC, FNA of abnormal lateral neck lymph nodes is essential. In contrast, abnormal central neck lymph nodes detected before initial thyroidectomy usually do not require FNA. It is helpful that the surgeon is alerted to the possibility of central neck nodal disease, and these nodes are then assessed carefully intraoperatively by palpation, inspection, and frozen section. In MTC, initial operative intervention requires prophylactic removal of central neck lymph nodes, and preoperative FNA of these nodes is therefore irrelevant. In contrast, reoperative surgery for persistent or recurrent nodal disease, in either the central or the lateral neck, requires preoperative FNA confirmation of malignancy.

FNA-Tg washout may also be used in the evaluation of suspicious cervical lymph nodes. A Tg of less than 1 ng/mL is reassuring, whereas the probability of nodal disease increases with higher Tg levels.[22] Tg washout may be particularly useful

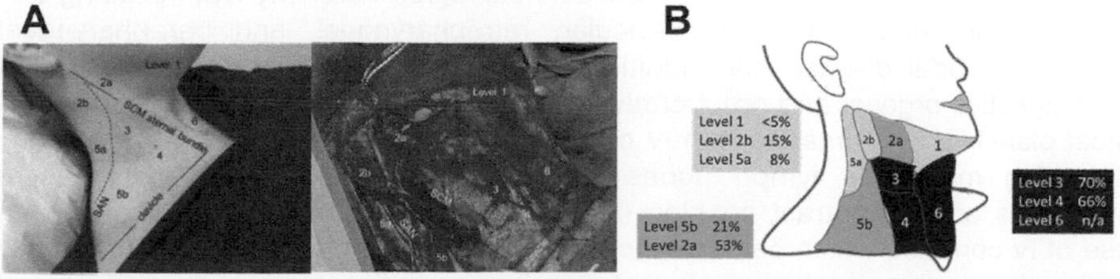

Fig. 2. (*A*) Cervical lymph node compartments. (*B*) Cervical lymph node compartments with approximate rate of involvement with DTC metastasis. ([A] *Courtesy of* Zvonimir L. Milas (Carolinas Medical Center, Levine Cancer Center and University of North Carolina, Charlotte, NC); [B] *Redrawn from* Eskander A, Merdad M, Freeman J, et al. Pattern of spread to the lateral neck in metastatic well-differentiated thyroid cancer: a systematic review and meta-analysis. Thyroid. 2013; 23:583–592.)

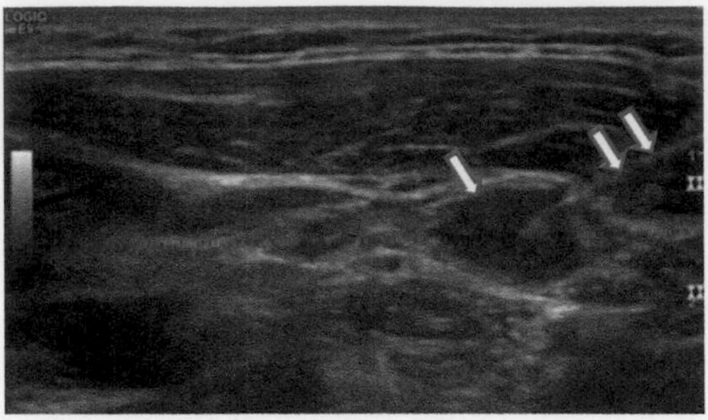

Fig. 3. US-guided FNA of lymph node. The single arrow is directed at the lymph node of interest. The double arrow is directed at the needle.

in cases where lymph nodes are cystic, where cytology is inadequate, or where there are divergent sonographic and cytologic findings.[23] False positive Tg washout may occur, particularly in the central compartment when the thyroid gland is still present.[24,25] One systematic review concluded that Tg washout greater than 32 ng/mL has the best sensitivity and specificity in patients with an intact thyroid gland.[25] Other studies suggest that Tg washout levels must be interpreted based on serum thyroid stimulating hormone (TSH) and Tg. Different Tg washout levels apply to postoperative patients without a thyroid gland. There is currently no standardization of Tg washout procedures or assays, making this diagnostic tool difficult to interpret at times.[26]

The performance of a Tg washout, however, is straightforward. Sterile saline is drawn through the same needle and syringe that sampled the abnormal lymph node, capturing any residual material in the needle hub. This fluid is then deposited in a test tube. The test tube should always be accompanied with explicit directions about the assay requested (Tg) and description of source (tissue, not blood), because many hospital laboratories lack familiarity with the process and handle such a specimen as an esoteric send-out laboratory test. In the authors' experience, despite such logistical challenges, it is always advisable to collect a sample for Tg measurement and warranted especially for cystic lymph nodes.

Preoperative Nodal Evaluation with Cross-Sectional Imaging

Patients presenting with disperse or bulky lymph node disease on US may have nodal involvement in areas beyond the cervical region visible by US, including disease in the mediastinal, infraclavicular, retropharyngeal, and parapharyngeal spaces.[16] Nodal disease may additionally extend into muscle, vasculature, and aerodigestive organs, and preoperative knowledge of these factors influences surgical planning.[27] CT images with IV contrast provide clear delineation of anatomy, detecting metastatic lymph nodes that may otherwise blend with adjacent structures on noncontrast imaging (**Fig. 4**). Clinicians do not need to avoid the use of IV contrast, which contains iodine, out of concern of affecting postoperative radioactive iodine ablation (RAI) therapy. Some studies suggest that combined mapping with US and CT may be superior to US alone, particularly in the central neck.[28] The sensitivities of MRI and PET for detection of nodal metastases are, in comparison, demonstrably low (30%–40%).[29] Although all patients should have a preoperative neck US, addition of routine cross-sectional imaging remains surgeon preference.

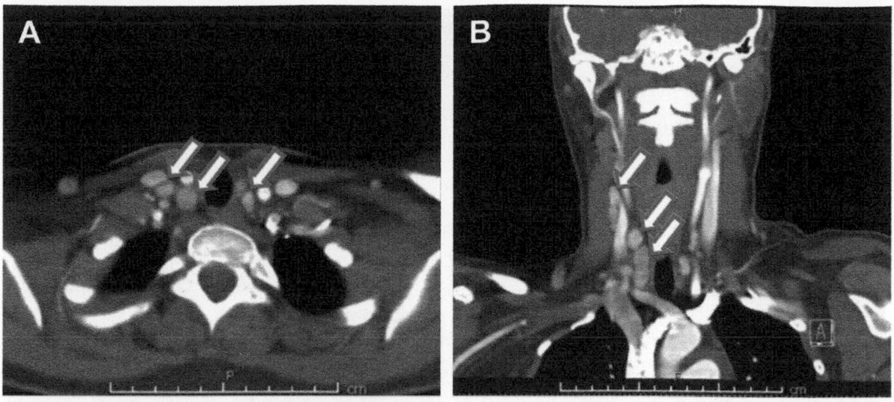

Fig. 4. Nodal disease on CT scan with IV contrast. Arrows are directed at lymph nodes. (*A*) Axial view, (*B*) coronal view.

OPERATIVE MANAGEMENT OF NODAL DISEASE

The most common site for nodal metastases is cervical level VI in the central neck (see **Fig. 2**A, B).[30] Per the 2015 ATA Guidelines for DTC (**Fig. 5**)[16]:

- A therapeutic central neck dissection (CND) should accompany total thyroidectomy in patients with clinically involved central neck lymph nodes (cN1) (**Fig. 6**A, B, D).
- A thyroidectomy without prophylactic CND is suitable for small (T1 or T2), noninvasive, clinically node negative (cN0) papillary thyroid cancers, and for most follicular cancers.

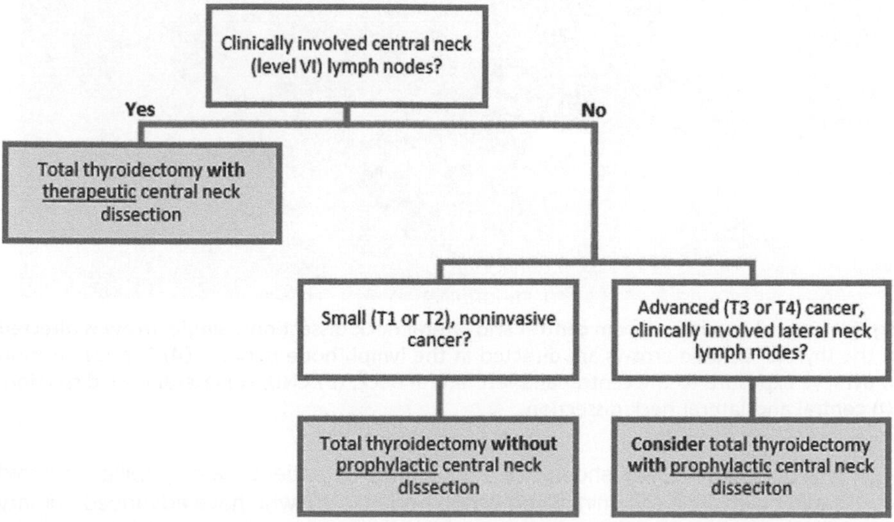

Fig. 5. Operative management of central neck nodal disease in DTC. (*Adapted from* Haugen B, Alexander E, Bible K, et al. 2015 American Thyroid Association management guidelines for adult patient with thyroid nodules and differentiated thyroid cancer. Thyroid. 2016; 26(1):1-133, with permission.)

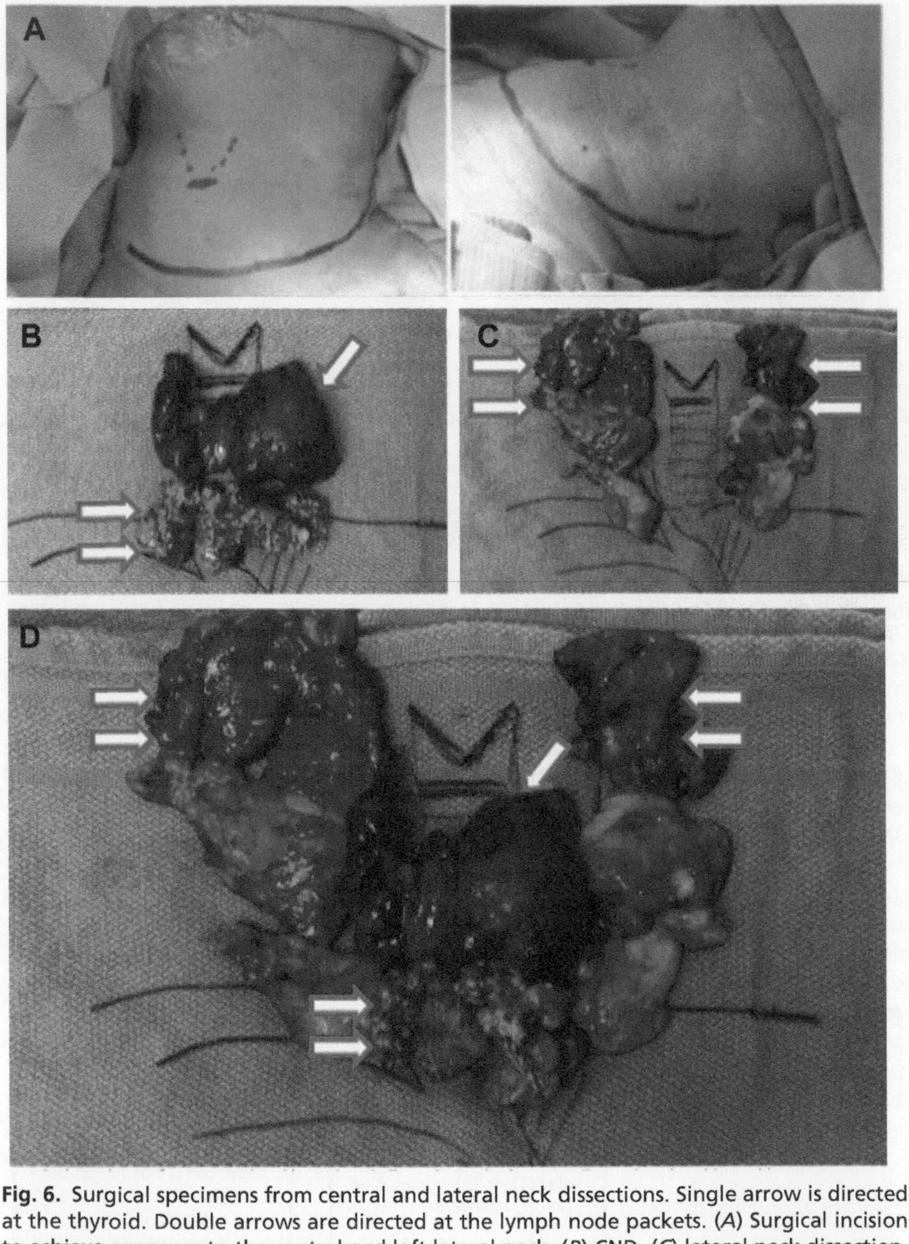

Fig. 6. Surgical specimens from central and lateral neck dissections. Single arrow is directed at the thyroid. Double arrows are directed at the lymph node packets. (*A*) Surgical incision to achieve exposure to the central and left lateral neck, (*B*) CND, (*C*) lateral neck dissection, (*D*) central and lateral neck dissection.

- A prophylactic CND should be considered in patients with papillary thyroid cancer with clinically uninvolved lymph nodes (cN0) who have advanced primary tumors (T3 or T4), who have clinically involved lateral neck nodes (cN1b), or if the information would be used to plan further therapy.
- Therapeutic lateral neck dissection should be performed for patients with biopsy-proven lateral lymph node disease (**Fig. 6**A, C, D).

The operative management of central and lateral nodal disease for MTC is slightly different (**Table 1**).[31] A prophylactic CND should accompany total thyroidectomy in patients with MTC. A prophylactic lateral neck dissection should be considered if there is no evidence of nodal metastases on imaging but there are aggressive disease features (eg, very elevated serum calcitonin).[31]

Operative Management of Central Neck Nodal Disease

Many patients have clinically negative (cN0) disease, where central compartment lymph nodes are not abnormal on preoperative imaging[5,14,32–34] or intraoperative inspection.[6] Although the role of therapeutic CND for cN1 disease is well defined,[35–38] the value of routine prophylactic CND for cN0 disease for DTC remains unclear. Although a CND can be performed with low morbidity by an experienced thyroid surgeon,[39–41] the benefit for an individual patient depends on the utility of the information gained.[41,42]

Some studies have reported that prophylactic CND for DTC may improve postintervention Tg,[34,43] local recurrence,[34,44] and disease-specific survival.[45] Other research suggests that prophylactic CND may guide the use of adjuvant RAI[33,37,40,46] and the estimation of recurrence risk.[46–48] Such studies, however, are based on largely limited data. In addition, several other papers have demonstrated that prophylactic CND confers no improvement in long-term outcome, while increasing the risk of temporary morbidity like hypocalcemia.[5,36,37,39,49–54] Although the removal of clinically negative central neck nodes (cN0) diagnoses a substantial number of patients with pathologically positive central neck disease (pN1a), the impact this has on long-term outcome is small.[55,56] It is, therefore, important to consider whether this information will affect the medical team's subsequent decisions regarding adjuvant therapy.

The presence of the BRAF V600E mutation may be associated with the risk of nodal disease.[57–59] The mutation, however, has a limited positive predictive value for recurrence, so mutation status should not impact the decision to perform a prophylactic CND.[60]

Surgeons may choose to perform prophylactic CND on patients with features that confer an increased risk for metastases or recurrence: very young or older age, larger tumor size, multifocal disease, extrathyroidal extension, or known lateral neck disease.[34,41,43] Some may use prophylactic CND in patients with better prognostic features because the nodal staging information gained would be used to guide decisions regarding adjuvant therapy.[33,40,46] Still other investigators report the use a selective approach, performing CND only for patients with clinically evident disease on preoperative examination, preoperative imaging, or intraoperative findings.[6,49,61]

The pathologic information gained from a prophylactic CND must be used cautiously for staging. Microscopic nodal metastases occur frequently, so

Table 1
Operative management of central and lateral neck nodal disease in differentiated thyroid cancer and medullary thyroid cancer

	DTC	MTC
Total thyroidectomy	Most often	Always
Therapeutic CND	Always	Always
Therapeutic lateral neck dissection	Always	Always
Prophylactic CND	Sometimes	Always
Prophylactic lateral neck dissection	Never	Sometimes

prophylactic CND often converts patients from clinically negative (cN0) to pathologically positive (pN1a) disease.[5,33,34,36,37] Microscopic nodal metastases, however, do not carry the same recurrence risk as macroscopic disease.[6] This "upstaging" may, therefore, lead to excess RAI use and increased patient follow-up. The demonstration of negative central neck nodes by prophylactic CND, on the other hand, may decrease RAI use by some groups.[33,40,46]

For MTC, prophylactic CND is advised at the time of initial total thyroidectomy, and therapeutic CND is absolutely mandated when lymph nodes are clearly diseased. MTC has different biology and tumor markers (calcitonin and carcinoembryonic antigen) than DTC, and RAI is not applicable. Initial nodal clearance, even if apparently prophylactic, therefore provides a unique and significant benefit.[31]

Operative Management of Lateral Neck Nodal Disease

Thyroid cancer may also involve lymph nodes in the lateral neck (levels II-V) (see **Fig. 2**) as well as the anterior mediastinum (level VII) and submental area (level I).[2,6,62,63] Patients with clinically involved lateral neck disease, proven on preoperative US and nodal FNA (with/without Tg washout), should undergo a comprehensive lateral neck dissection. Such compartmental nodal dissection, as opposed to targeted "berry-picking" of individual diseased lymph nodes, may reduce risk of recurrence and possibly mortality.[64–66]

It should be noted that prophylactic lateral neck dissection does have consideration in MTC (see **Table 1**). Once performed quite routinely, it is currently recommended in the more limited setting of large upper thyroid pole tumors, baseline preoperative calcitonin levels greater than 200 pg/mL, and bulky central neck nodal disease.[33] In the United States, prophylactic lateral neck dissection for DTC, in comparison, is not routine and not advised.

Operative Techniques of Cervical Node Dissection

Contemporary peer-reviewed literature provides access to operative demonstrations of both central and lateral neck dissections.[67] These real-time video demonstrations can enhance understanding of the evaluation and management of lymph nodes with visual details. The following sources contain multiple helpful examples of cervical lymph node dissections that can be directly queried on their peer-reviewed websites: ATA-associated VideoEndocrinology (www.thyroid.org/videoendocrinology-featured-articles/ and directly from the publisher at https://home.liebertpub.com/videoendocrinology) and American College of Surgeons Video Library (www.facs.org/education/division-of-education/publications/videolibrary). A comprehensive lateral neck dissection cine-video[67] clearly illustrates the cervical levels and anatomic structures encountered during surgery.

NODAL DISEASE IN POSTOPERATIVE STAGING AND RISK STRATIFICATION

Accurate staging is critical for tailoring treatment, establishing surveillance, and determining prognosis. Nodal metastases are used in the staging of thyroid cancer, as defined by the American Joint Committee on Cancer (AJCC) 8th Edition TNM Classification (**Fig. 7**).[68] For both DTC and MTC, TNM staging is fundamentally designed for prognosis of survival. In the modified 2009 ATA Initial Risk Stratification system for DTC, patients with cervical lymph node metastases are classified as low, intermediate, or high risk (**Fig. 8**).[16] This classification in turn helps define the prognosis and risk of structural recurrence (**Fig. 9**).[16] Characteristics of nodal metastases, such as the presence of clinically evident, multiple, large metastases, or extranodal extension, aid in

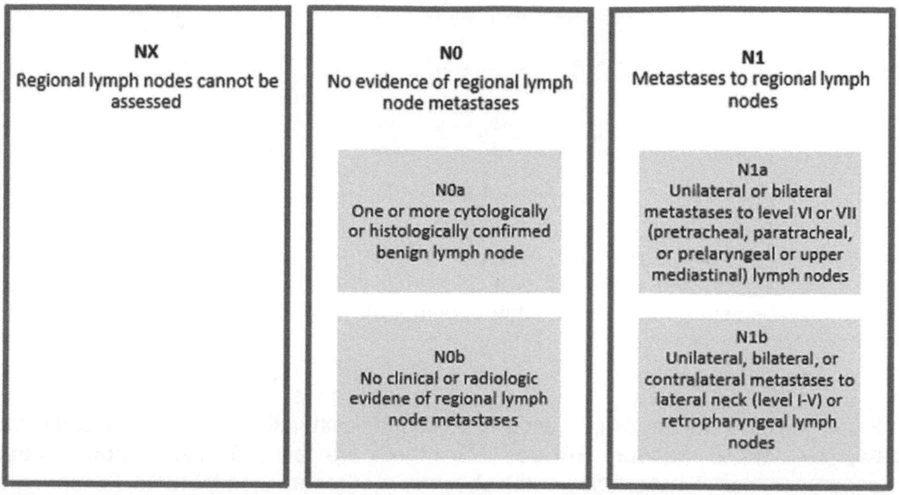

Fig. 7. 2018 AJCC/TNM Thyroid Cancer Staging System definitions of lymph node status. (*Data from* Tuttle R, Haugen B, Perrier N. Updated American Joint Committee on Cancer/Tumor-Node-Metastases Staging System for Differentiated and Anaplastic Thyroid Cancer (Eighth Edition): What Changed and Why. Thyroid. 2017; 26(6):751-756.)

the delineation of recurrence risk.[63,69] A comparable separate risk stratification system does not exist for MTC.

A Surveillance, Epidemiology, and End Results (SEER) database study reported an all-cause survival at 14 years of 82% for papillary thyroid cancer without nodal metastases versus 79% with nodal metastases ($P<.05$).[35] A National Cancer Database and SEER analysis showed an increased risk of death in patients younger than 45 years with lymph node metastases compared with those without nodal involvement. The study further found that, in this age group, having incrementally more involved lymph nodes up to 6 confers additional mortality risk.[70]

Risk stratification can be used to guide individualized treatment, including the following: (1) The need for and degree of RAI, TSH suppression, external beam radiation, and systemic therapy, and (2) The intensity and type of follow-up studies required for evaluating response to therapy.[16]

For DTCs that are ATA low- to intermediate-risk, T1-3 cancers, the presence of lymph node metastases may impact decision making regarding postoperative RAI (**Fig. 10**).[16] Postoperative RAI may be considered in cancers with central compartment lymph node metastases. It is generally favored when features confer a higher risk of persistent or recurrent disease: increasing number of clinically evident or large

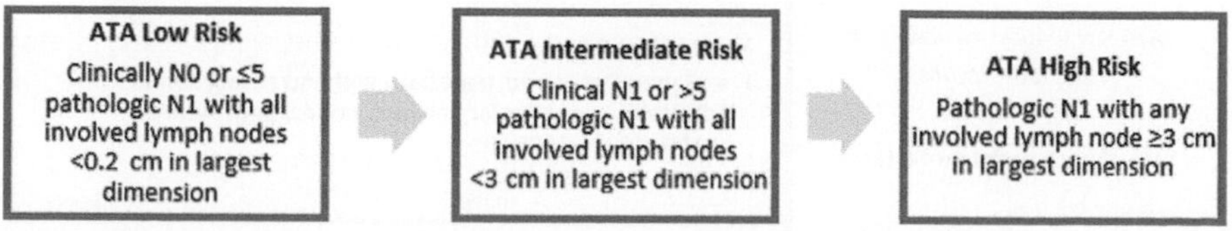

Fig. 8. 2009 ATA Initial Risk Stratification System definitions of lymph node status. (*Data from* Haugen B, Alexander E, Bible K, et al. 2015 American Thyroid Association management guidelines for adult patient with thyroid nodules and differentiated thyroid cancer. Thyroid. 2016; 26(1):1–133.)

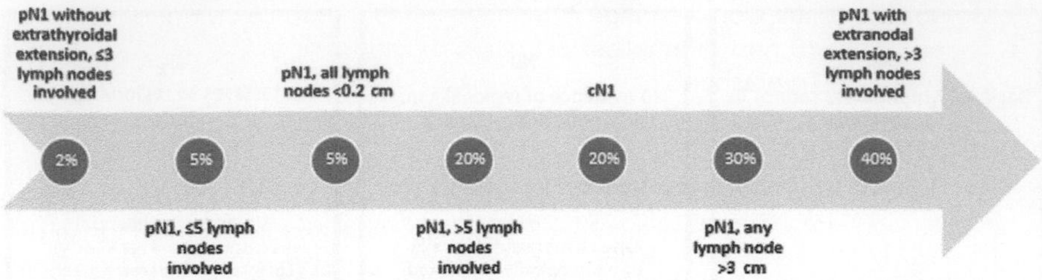

Fig. 9. 2015 ATA Thyroid Nodule Guidelines risk of structural recurrence based on lymph node status. (*Data from* Haugen B, Alexander E, Bible K, et al. 2015 American Thyroid Association management guidelines for adult patient with thyroid nodules and differentiated thyroid cancer. Thyroid. 2016; 26(1):1–133.)

(>2-3 cm) lymph nodes, or presence of extranodal extension. There are insufficient data, however, to mandate RAI use when there are few (<5) microscopic central compartment nodal metastases, in the absence of other adverse features. For cancers with lateral compartment lymph node metastases, postoperative RAI is generally favored when there are an increasing number of clinically evident or large lymph nodes, or if there is extranodal extension. Advancing age may also favor RAI use in patients with central or lateral nodal metastases.[16]

POSTOPERATIVE NODAL EVALUATION

Accurate surveillance for recurrence is a major goal of long-term follow-up, and this includes evaluation for nodal disease. Per the 2015 ATA Guidelines for DTC[16]:

- Following initial operative intervention, US evaluating central and lateral neck lymph nodes should be performed at 6 to 12 months and then periodically, depending on the patient's Tg status and recurrence risk.

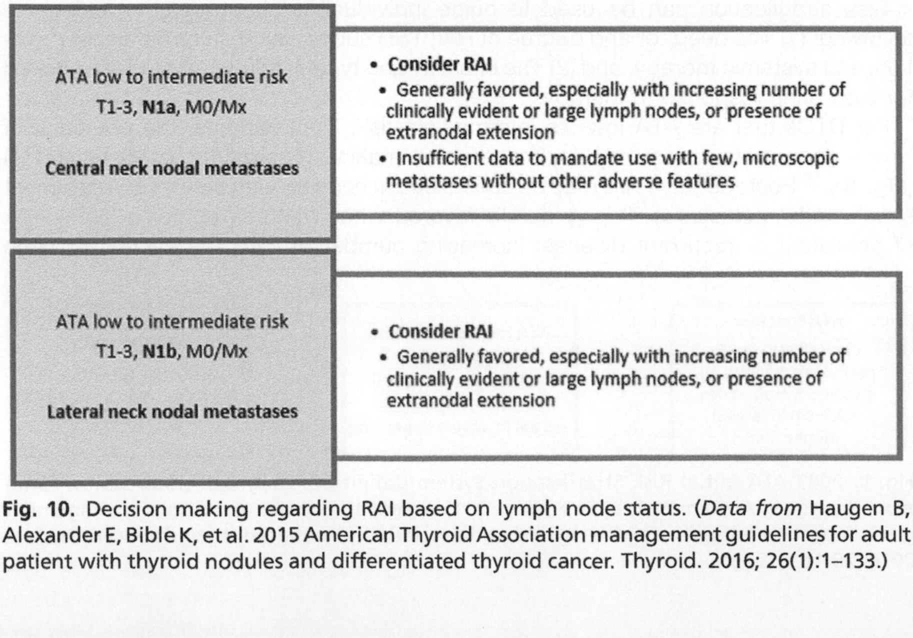

Fig. 10. Decision making regarding RAI based on lymph node status. (*Data from* Haugen B, Alexander E, Bible K, et al. 2015 American Thyroid Association management guidelines for adult patient with thyroid nodules and differentiated thyroid cancer. Thyroid. 2016; 26(1):1–133.)

- If a positive result would change management, sonographically abnormal lymph nodes ≥8 to 10 mm in smallest diameter should undergo US-guided FNA for cytology and Tg washout.
- Sonographically abnormal lymph nodes less than 8 to 10 mm in smallest diameter may be followed without biopsy, with consideration for FNA or intervention if there is growth or threat to vital structures.
- Cross-sectional imaging (CT, MRI) with IV contrast should be considered an adjunct to neck US for patients with disperse or bulky recurrent nodal disease. It may also be used when US may not be adequately visualizing nodal disease (ie, high Tg with negative neck US).

Postoperative Nodal Evaluation with Ultrasound

US is highly sensitive in the detection of nodal recurrences in patients with DTC.[4,71,72] A study correlating sonographic findings and pathology results found that lymph nodes with a hyperechoic hilum are reassuring. Lymph nodes greater than 7 mm in smallest diameter with hyperechoic foci or cystic components, on the other hand, should be considered malignant. The type of nodal vascularization was also found to be highly sensitive and specific, with central vascularity being reassuring and peripheral vascularity being concerning. Because no single US feature is adequately sensitive to confirm metastases within lymph nodes, the study suggests that round shape, hypoechoic appearance, or loss of fatty hilum in isolation does not justify FNA.[19]

Surveillance US should be interpreted in the context of previous clinical and pathologic data for the individual patient. Recurrence risk is closely related to initial lymph node status. Most nodal recurrences occur in already involved compartments. The risk of recurrence increases if there was a greater number of involved lymph nodes or a higher number of nodes with extranodal extension.[63] ATA low- to intermediate-risk DTC patients with undetectable Tg have a low risk of lymph node recurrence (<2%). The risk is much higher in patients with a detectable or high Tg. Although surveillance US can detect nodal disease as small as 2 to 3 mm, where Tg may be undetectable or low, the benefit of this early detection is not demonstrated.[73,74]

Postoperative Nodal Evaluation with Fine-Needle Aspiration

FNA with Tg washout should be performed for suspicious lymph nodes ≥8 to 10 mm in smallest diameter.[16] US guidance may assist in the success of FNA, particularly for small and/or deep lymph nodes. Cytology, however, misses up to 20% of nodal metastases. The addition of Tg washout to cytology increases sensitivity.[75–77] Tg washout levels greater than 10 ng/mL are highly suspicious. Concentrations between 1 and 10 ng/mL are moderately suspicious. In these patients, comparison between serum and washout Tg should be considered.[22,24,78]

Up to half of FNAs performed on sonographically suspicious lymph nodes are benign. The selection of patients for nodal biopsy may, therefore, need to be improved.[22,78,79] Sonographically nonsuspicious nodes, and small nodes less than 8 to 10 mm in smallest diameter, can be monitored. In addition, cytologic evaluation should not be pursued if the results will not impact evaluation or treatment.[16]

Postoperative Nodal Evaluation with Cross-Sectional Imaging

A CT scan may complement surveillance US in the detection of recurrent disease.[28,80,81] Cross-sectional imaging should be used in patients with diffuse or bulky recurrent nodal disease, where US may not completely delineate pathologic condition. In addition, in patients with a high or rising Tg or Tg antibody level and no structural disease visualized on US or RAI, CT should be considered. Cross-sectional imaging aids in defining nodal disease and its relationship to vital structures, which is critical before revision surgery is contemplated.[16]

MANAGEMENT OF PERSISTENT AND RECURRENT NODAL DISEASE

Persistent or recurrent nodal disease may be a significant source of patient and physician anxiety.[82] Per the 2015 ATA Guidelines for DTC[16]:

- A therapeutic central and/or lateral neck dissection in a previously operated compartment should be performed for biopsy-proven persistent or recurrent disease for central neck nodes ≥8 mm and lateral neck nodes ≥10 mm in smallest dimension that can be localized on anatomic imaging.
- Smaller lesions may be managed with active surveillance, with consideration for FNA or intervention if there is disease progression.
- Other treatment modalities, such as percutaneous ethanol injection (PEI) and radiofrequency ablation (RFA), may be considered for the treatment of nodal metastases in patients who are poor surgical candidates.

Operative Management of Persistent or Recurrent Nodal Disease

Although observational studies suggest that low-volume recurrent nodal disease may be indolent and monitored,[83,84] bulky or invasive nodal recurrences should be surgically managed.[85–89] The decision to pursue an operative intervention for recurrent nodal disease must balance the risks of revision surgery with the fact surgical resection is generally the optimal treatment for macroscopic nodal disease (**Fig. 11**).[16] The availability and utilization of surgeons with expertise in performing revision nodal surgery are also critical. The decision for reoperative surgery should involve collaboration between surgery, endocrinology, and the patient.[90]

Given the risks of revision nodal surgery, it is mandatory to have a clearly defined radiographic target. Clinically apparent, macroscopic disease must be recognized on US and/or cross-sectional imaging. Operative risks are related to nodal location and whether a compartment has been previously dissected, so targets must be defined on high-resolution anatomic studies (US or CT with IV contrast) to facilitate mapping and localization.[27,28]

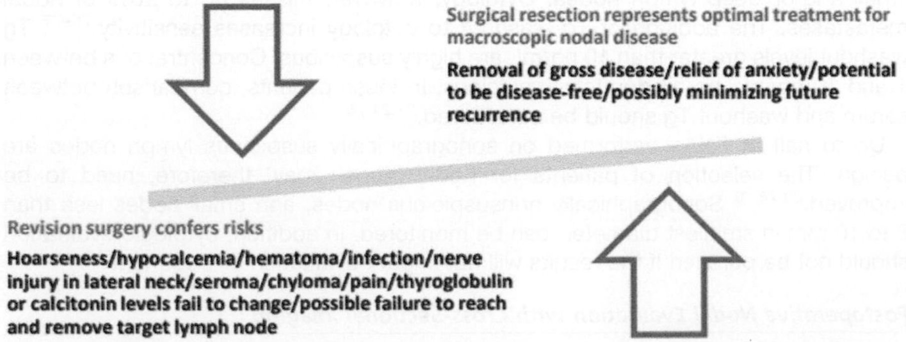
Surgical resection represents optimal treatment for macroscopic nodal disease
Removal of gross disease/relief of anxiety/potential to be disease-free/possibly minimizing future recurrence
Revision surgery confers risks
Hoarseness/hypocalcemia/hematoma/infection/nerve injury in lateral neck/seroma/chyloma/pain/thyroglobulin or calcitonin levels fail to change/possible failure to reach and remove target lymph node

Fig. 11. Decision making regarding operative management of persistent or recurrent nodal disease. (*Data from* Haugen B, Alexander E, Bible K, et al. 2015 American Thyroid Association management guidelines for adult patient with thyroid nodules and differentiated thyroid cancer. Thyroid. 2016; 26(1):1–133.)

Surgery should be considered for malignant central neck nodes ≥8 mm and lateral neck nodes ≥10 mm in smallest dimension that have undergone an FNA and can be localized on US and/or CT with IV contrast.[28,91–93] Smaller lesions may be managed with active surveillance, pursuing FNA and intervention in the event of disease progression.[16]

Factors in addition to nodal size, however, must be considered in the decision making for operative intervention. These factors include the proximity of nodal disease to vital structures as well as the function status of the vocal cords. Characteristics of the primary tumor, such as high-grade histology, presence of mutational markers associated with aggressive behavior, Tg doubling time, RAI avidity, and PET avidity, should also be considered. Patient comorbidities, compliance, and emotional concerns also impact decision making.[16] Although the decision to operate on nodal recurrences should be made with an appreciation of the presence and progression of distant disease, it may still be undertaken in the setting of known distant metastases for prevention or palliation of symptoms.[90]

In selected patients, nodal metastases greater than 8 to 10 mm can be actively surveyed with clinical and radiographic follow-up, using a systematic multidisciplinary approach. If these lesions remain stable, surveillance may be maintained. If there is progression, surgery may be considered.[16]

Focal "berry-picking" carries an increased risk of recurrence. Compartmental surgery is, therefore, recommended for nodal metastases.[94,95] The plan for compartmental dissection must be modified and limited, however, based on intraoperative findings that impact risk/benefit, such as significant scarring or distorted anatomy. Reoperative CND typically involves at least 1 paratracheal region with prelaryngeal and pretracheal subcompartments. Revision lateral neck dissection usually comprises levels II, III, and IV (see **Fig. 2**).[16] Because of the risk of bilateral recurrent laryngeal nerve injury and permanent hypoparathyroidism, revision bilateral neck dissection should only be offered when mandated by disease distribution.[16]

Series indicate that basal Tg decreases by 60% to 90% after compartment dissection for recurrent nodal disease. Only 30% to 50% of patients, however, have undetectable Tg after operative intervention. Although it is difficult to predict which patients will respond with Tg reduction,[20,92,96–112] studies suggest that revision surgery results in high clearance of structural disease in more than 80% of patients.[93,111]

Radioactive Iodine Ablation for Management of Persistent or Recurrent Nodal Disease

Regional nodal DTC metastases recognized on diagnostic whole body scan may be treated with RAI in patients with low-volume disease or in combination with surgery. Operative intervention, however, is preferred if the nodal disease is amenable to surgery or is bulky in nature. Adjuvant RAI is used after surgery for nodal disease if residual RAI-avid disease is suspected or present.[16] The benefit of empiric RAI for non-RAI-avid structural disease is unlikely significant. It is, therefore, not generally recommended.[113]

Percutaneous Ethanol Injection for Management of Persistent or Recurrent Nodal Disease

PEI as a nonsurgical treatment for metastatic nodal disease is gaining interest. Most research using PEI limited its use to patients who had previously undergone neck dissection or RAI, had biopsy-proven nodal disease, and had no known distant metastases.[16]

In a retrospective study that treated 63 patients with 109 metastatic nodes, 92 lymph nodes (84%) were successfully ablated, with a mean follow-up of 38 months.

Nodal metastases typically required 1 to 3 treatment sessions. Minor complications included pain at the injection site. No major complications were reported.[114] Another retrospective study examined 25 patients who had 37 lymph nodes ablated. All nodal metastases were successfully ablated, defined by lack of flow on US, in 1 to 5 sessions. Mean follow-up was 65 months. Serum Tg reduced in most patients and decreased to less than 2.4 ng/mL in 82% of patients. Most lymph nodes decreased in size, and 46% disappeared. No long-term complications were reported.[115] Such studies are limited by small patient numbers, short follow-up, as well as the fact that many patients had small lymph nodes measuring less than 5 to 8 mm.[16]

The ATA Guidelines conclude that PEI should be considered in patients who are poor surgical candidates, with the following considerations. Many patients will require more than 1 treatment. Large lymph nodes (>2 cm) may be difficult to treat with PEI. In deciding the optimal strategy for nodal metastases, previously used treatment modalities must also be taken into consideration. Compartmental dissection remains the first-line treatment for patients with thyroid cancer with clinically apparent and progressive nodal metastases.[16]

Radiofrequency or Laser Ablation for Management of Persistent or Recurrent Nodal Disease

RFA for recurrent DTC has been reported to achieve a volume reduction between 55% and 95%.[116,117] Forty percent to 60% of cases had disappearance of metastatic disease.[117–119] Multiple treatment sessions are often required. Reported complications include discomfort, burns, and voice changes.[120] Like PEI, RFA may be most useful in patients who are high-risk operative candidates, or in patients refusing additional operative intervention. It should not be considered a standard alternative to compartmental dissection.[119–121] US-guided laser ablation of nodal metastases has also been described.[122]

Other Therapies for Management of Persistent or Recurrent Nodal Disease

Although stereotactic radiotherapy can be used to treat isolated metastatic disease, it should not be favored with patients who have resectable nodal metastases.[16] External beam radiation therapy may be used for locoregional DTC recurrences that are not resectable, or for disease with extranodal extension or soft tissue involvement. Studies suggest efficacy, but this research is retrospective and limited in its numbers.[123,124] Systemic therapies (eg, cytotoxic chemotherapy or kinase inhibiters) are only considered once all surgical and radiation therapies for both DTC and MTC have been exhausted.[15]

SUMMARY

Cervical lymph node metastases are present in a considerable number of patients with thyroid cancer, and residual metastatic lymph nodes represent the most common site of persistent and recurrent disease. Preoperative evaluation of cervical lymph nodes by US is, therefore, of paramount importance. Therapeutic compartmental dissection should be pursued for clinically involved central neck disease and biopsy-proven lateral neck disease in both DTC and MTC. Pathologic nodal status assists in determining risk of recurrence, which in turn helps in tailoring treatment, establishing surveillance, and determining prognosis. After initial operative intervention, the sonographic surveillance of cervical lymph nodes is recommended. A therapeutic central and/or lateral neck dissection in a previously operated compartment is more complex; thus, it is applied only after consideration of multiple clinical factors that include, among others, biopsy-proven persistent or recurrent disease for central neck nodes ≥8 mm and lateral neck nodes ≥10 mm in smallest dimension that can be localized on anatomic imaging.

REFERENCES

1. Grebe S, Hay I. Thyroid cancer nodal metastases: biologic significance and therapeutic considerations. Surg Oncol Clin Am 1996;5:43–63.
2. Scheumann G, Gim O, Wegener G, et al. Prognostic significance and surgical management of locoregional lymph node metastases in papillary thyroid cancer. World J Surg 1994;18:559–67.
3. Ito Y, Uruno T, Nakano K, et al. An observation trial without surgical treatment in patients with papillary microcarcinoma of the thyroid. Thyroid 2003;13:381–7.
4. Kouvaraki M, Shapiro S, Fornage B, et al. Role of preoperative ultrasonography in the surgical management of patients with thyroid cancer. Surgery 2003;134:946–54.
5. Hughes D, White M, Miller B, et al. Influence of prophylactic central lymph node dissection on postoperative thyroglobulin levels and radioiodine treatment in papillary thyroid cancer. Surgery 2010;148:1100–6.
6. Randolph G, Duh Q, Heller K, et al. The prognostic significance of nodal metastases from papillary thyroid carcinoma can be stratified based on the size and number of metastatic lymph nodes, as well as the presence of extranodal extension. Thyroid 2012;22:1144–52.
7. Machens A, Hinze R, Thmusche O, et al. Pattern of nodal metastasis for primary and reoperative thyroid cancer. World J Surg 2002;26:22–8.
8. Hay I, Grant C, van Heerden J, et al. Papillary thyroid microcarcinoma: a study of 535 cases observed in a 50-year period. Surgery 1992;112:1139–46.
9. Qubain S, Nakano S, Baba M, et al. Distribution of lymph node micrometastasis in pN0 well-differentiated thyroid carcinoma. Surgery 2002;131:249–56.
10. Arturi F, Russo D, Giuffrida D, et al. Early diagnosis by genetic analysis of differentiated thyroid cancer metastases in small lymph nodes. J Clin Endocrinol Metab 1997;82:1638–41.
11. Hay I, Bergstralh E, Goellner J, et al. Predicting outcome in papillary thyroid carcinoma: development of a reliable prognostic scoring system in a cohort of 1779 patients surgically treated at one institution during 1940 through 1989. Surgery 1993;114:1050–7.
12. Shah M, Hall F, Eski S, et al. Clinical course of thyroid carcinoma after neck dissection. Laryngoscope 2003;113:2102–7.
13. Wang T, Dubner S, Sznyter L, et al. Incidence of metastatic well-differentiated thyroid cancer in cervical lymph nodes. Arch Otolaryngol Head Neck Surg 2004;130:110–3.
14. Stulak J, Grant C, Farley D, et al. Value of preoperative ultrasonography in the surgical management of initial and reoperative papillary thyroid cancer. Arch Surg 2006;141:489–94.
15. O'Connel K, Yen T, Quiroz F, et al. The utility of routine preoperative cervical ultrasonography in patients undergoing thyroidectomy for differentiated thyroid cancer. Surgery 2013;154:697–701.
16. Haugen B, Alexander E, Bible K, et al. 2015 American Thyroid Association management guidelines for adult patient with thyroid nodules and differentiated thyroid cancer. Thyroid 2016;26(1):1–133.

17. Frasoldati A, Valcavi R. Challenges in neck ultrasonography: lymphadenopathy and parathyroid glands. Endocr Pract 2004;10:261–8.
18. Kuna S, Bracic I, Tesic V, et al. Ultrasonographic differentiation of benign from malignant neck lymphadenopathy in thyroid cancer. J Ultrasound Med 2006; 25:1531–7.
19. Leboulleux S, Girard E, Rose M, et al. Ultrasound criteria of malignancy for cervical lymph nodes in patients followed up for differentiated thyroid cancer. J Clin Endocrinol Metab 2007;92:3590–4.
20. Eskander A, Merdad M, Freeman J, et al. Pattern of spread to the lateral neck in metastatic well-differentiated thyroid cancer: a systematic review and meta-analysis. Thyroid 2013;23:583–92.
21. Park J, Lee Y, Kim B, et al. Skip lateral neck node metastases in papillary thyroid carcinoma. World J Surg 2012;36:743–7.
22. Snozek C, Chambers E, Reading C, et al. Serum thyroglobulin, high-resolution ultrasound, and lymph node thyroglobulin in diagnosis of differentiated thyroid carcinoma nodal metastases. J Clin Endocrinol Metab 2007;92:4278–81.
23. Chung J, Kim E, Lim H, et al. Optimal indication of thyroglobulin measurement in fine-needle aspiration for detecting lateral metastatic lymph nodes in patients with papillary thyroid carcinoma. Head Neck 2014;36:795–801.
24. Grani G, Fumarola A. Thyroglobulin in lymph node fine-needle aspiration washout: a systematic review and meta-analysis of diagnostic accuracy. J Clin Endocrinol Metab 2014;99:1970–82.
25. Pak K, Suh S, Hong H, et al. Diagnostic values of thyroglobulin measurement in fine-needle aspiration of lymph nodes in patients with thyroid cancer. Endocrine 2015;49:70–7.
26. Giovanella L, Bongiovanni M, Trimboli P. Diagnostic value of thyroglobulin assay in cervical lymph node fine-needle aspirations for metastatic differentiated thyroid cancer. Curr Opin Oncol 2013;25:6–13.
27. Yeh M, Bauer A, Bernet V, et al. American Thyroid Association statement on preoperative imaging for thyroid cancer surgery. Thyroid 2015;25:3–14.
28. Lesnik D, Cunanne M, Zurakowski D, et al. Papillary thyroid carcinoma nodal surgery directed by a preoperative radiographic map utilizing CT scan and ultrasound in all primary and reoperative patients. Head Neck 2014;36:191–202.
29. Jeogn H, Baek C, Son Y, et al. Integrated 18F-FDG PET/CT for the initial evaluation of cervical node level of patients with papillary thyroid carcinoma: comparison with ultrasound and contrast-enhanced CT. Clin Endocrinol (Oxf) 2006;65: 402–7.
30. Robbins K, Shaha A, Medina J, et al. Consensus statement on the classification and terminology of neck dissection. Arch Otolaryngol Head Neck Surg 2008; 134:536–8.
31. Wells A, Sylvia L, Henning D, et al. Revised American Thyroid Association guidelines for the management of medullary thyroid carcinoma. Thyroid 2016; 256:567–610.
32. Mulla M, Schulte K. Central cervical lymph node metastases in papillary thyroid cancer: a systematic review of imaging-guided and prophylactic removal of the central compartment. Clin Endocrinol (Oxf) 2012;76:131–6.
33. Hartle D, Leboullex S, Al Ghuzlan A, et al. Optimization of staging of the neck with prophylactic central and lateral neck dissection for papillary thyroid carcinoma. Ann Surg 2012;255:777–83.

34. Popadich A, Levin O, Lee J, et al. A multicenter cohort study of total thyroidectomy and routine central lymph node dissection for cN0 papillary thyroid cancer. Surgery 2011;150:1048–57.
35. Podnos Y, Smith D, Wagman L, et al. The implication of lymph node metastasis on survival in patients with well-differentiated thyroid cancer. Am Surg 2005;71:731–4.
36. Lang B, Wong K, Wan K, et al. Impact of routine unilateral central neck dissection on preablative and postablative stimulated thyroglobulin levels after total thyroidectomy in papillary thyroid carcinoma. Ann Surg Oncol 2012;19:60–7.
37. Wang T, Evans D, Fareau G, et al. Effect of prophylactic central compartment neck dissection on serum thyroglobulin and recommendations for adjuvant radioactive iodine in patients with differentiated thyroid cancer. Ann Surg Oncol 2012;19:4217–22.
38. Carty S, Cooper D, Doherty G, et al. Consensus statement on the terminology and classification of central neck dissection for thyroid cancer. Thyroid 2009;19:1153–8.
39. Chisholm E, Kulinskaya E, Tolley N. Systematic review and meta-analysis of the adverse effects of thyroidectomy combined with central neck dissection as compared to thyroidectomy alone. Laryngoscope 2009;119:1135–9.
40. Bonnet S, Hartl D, Leboulleux S, et al. Prophylactic lymph node dissection for papillary thyroid cancer less than 2cm: implications for radioiodine treatment. J Clin Endocrinol Metab 2009;94:1162–7.
41. Sancho J, Lennard T, Paunovic I, et al. Prophylactic central neck dissection in papillary thyroid cancer: a consensus report of the European Society of Endocrine Surgeons (ESES). Langenbecks Arch Surg 2014;399:155–63.
42. Zetoune T, Keutgen X, Buitrago D, et al. Prophylactic central neck dissection and local recurrence in papillary thyroid cancer. Ann Surg Oncol 2010;17:3287–93.
43. Sywak M, Cornford L, Roach P, et al. Routine ipsilateral level VI lymphadenectomy reduces postoperative thyroglobulin levels in papillary thyroid cancer. Surgery 2006;150:1000–5.
44. Hartl D, Mamelle E, Borget I, et al. Influence of prophylactic neck dissection on rate of retreatment for papillary thyroid carcinoma. World J Surg 2013;37:1951–8.
45. Barczynski M, Konturek A, Stopa M, et al. Prophylactic central neck dissection for papillary thyroid cancer. Br J Surg 2013;100:410–8.
46. Laird A, Gauger P, Miller B, et al. Evaluation of postoperative radioactive iodine scans in patients who underwent prophylactic central lymph node dissection. World J Surg 2012;36:1268–73.
47. Costa S, Guigliano G, Santoro L, et al. Role of prophylactic central neck dissection in cN0 papillary thyroid cancer. Acta Otorhinolaryngol Ital 2009;29:61–9.
48. Ryu I, Song C, Choi S, et al. Lymph node ratio of the central compartment is a significant predictor for locoregional recurrence after prophylactic central neck dissection in patients with thyroid papillary carcinoma. Ann Surg Oncol 2014;21:277–83.
49. Moreno M, Edeiken-Monroe B, Siegel E, et al. In papillary thyroid cancer, preoperative central neck ultrasound detects only macroscopic surgical disease, but negative findings predict excellent long-term regional control and survival. Thyroid 2012;22:347–55.

50. Yoo D, Ajmal S, Gowda S, et al. Level VI lymph node dissection dose not decrease radioiodine uptake in patients undergoing radioiodine ablation for differentiated thyroid cancer. World J Surg 2012;36:1255–61.
51. Roh J, Park J, Par C. Total thyroidectomy plus neck dissection in differentiated papillary thyroid carcinoma patients: patter of nodal metastasis, morbidity, recurrence, and postoperative levels of serum parathyroid hormone. Ann Surg 2007;245:604–10.
52. Cavicchi O, Piccin O, Caliceti U, et al. Transient hypoparathyroidism following thyroidectomy: a prospective study and multivariate analysis of 604 consecutive patients. Otolaryngol Head Neck Surg 2007;137:654–8.
53. Raffaelli M, De Crea C, Sessa L, et al. Prospective evaluation of total thyroidectomy versus ipsilateral versus bilateral central neck dissection in patients with clinically node negative papillary thyroid carcinoma. Surgery 2012;152:957–64.
54. Viola D, Materazzi G, Valerio I, et al. Prophylactic central compartment lymph node dissection in papillary thyroid carcinoma: clinical implications derived from the first prospective randomized controlled single institution study. J Clin Endocrinol Metab 2015;100:1316–24.
55. Lang B, Ng S, Lau L, et al. A systematic review and meta-analysis of prophylactic central neck dissection on short-term locoregional recurrence in papillary thyroid carcinoma after total thyroidectomy. Thyroid 2013;23:1087–98.
56. Wang T, Cheung K, Farrokhyar F, et al. A meta-analysis of the effect of prophylactic central compartment neck dissection on locoregional recurrence rates in patients with papillary thyroid cancer. Ann Surg Oncol 2013;20:3477–83.
57. Howell G, Nikiforov M, Carty S, et al. BRAF V600E mutation independently predicts central compartment lymph node metastasis is patients with papillary thyroid cancer. Ann Surg Oncol 2013;20:47–52.
58. Xing M, Alzahrani A, Carson K, et al. Association between BRAF V600E mutation and mortality in patients with papillary thyroid cancer. JAMA 2013;309:1493–501.
59. Kim T, Park Y, Lim J, et al. The association of the BRAF V600E mutation with prognostic factors and poor clinical outcome in papillary thyroid cancer: a meta-analysis. Cancer 2012;118:1764–73.
60. Xing M. Prognostic utility of BRAF mutation in papillary thyroid cancer. Mol Cell Endocrinol 2010;321:86–93.
61. Gyorki DE, Untch B, Tuttle R, et al. Prophylactic central neck dissection in differentiated thyroid cancer: an assessment of the evidence. Ann Surg Oncol 2013;20:2285–9.
62. Sugitani I, Fujimoto Y, Yamada K, et al. Prospective outcomes of selective lymph node dissection for papillary thyroid carcinoma based on preoperative ultrasonography. World J Surg 2008;32:2494–502.
63. Leboulleux S, Rubino C, Baudin E, et al. Prognostic factors for persistent or recurrent disease of papillary thyroid carcinoma with neck lymph node metastases and/or tumor extension beyond the thyroid capsule at initial diagnosis. J Clin Endocrinol Metab 2005;90:5723–9.
64. Gemsenjager E, Perren A, Seifert B, et al. Lymph node surgery in papillary thyroid carcinoma. Surgery 2004;197:182–90.
65. Kouvaraki M, Lee J, Shapiro S, et al. Preventable reoperations for persistent and recurrent papillary thyroid carcinoma. Surgery 2004;136:1183–91.
66. Ito Y, Tomodo C, Uruno T, et al. Preoperative ultrasonographic examination for lymph node metastasis: usefulness when designing lymph node dissection for papillary microcarcinoma of the thyroid. World J Surg 2004;28:498–501.

67. Luk L, Milas M, Shindo M. The modified radical neck dissection. VideoEndocrinology, vol. 2;3; Available at: https://www.liebertpub.com/doi/abs/10.1089/ve.2015.0052?id=abstract.pdf&type=media&journalCode=ve. Accessed January 10, 2019.
68. Tuttle R, Haugen B, Perrier N. Updated American Joint Committee on cancer/tumor-node-metastases staging system for differentiated and anaplastic thyroid cancer (eighth edition): what changed and why. Thyroid 2017;26(6):751–6.
69. Sugitani I, Kasai N, Fujimoto Y, et al. A novel classification system for patients with PTC: addition of the new variables of large (3 cm or greater) nodal metastases and reclassification during the follow-up period. Surgery 2004;135:139–48.
70. Adam M, Pura J, Goffredo P, et al. Presence and number of lymph node metastases are associated with compromised survival for patients younger than age 45 years with papillary thyroid cancer. J Clin Oncol 2015;33:2370–5.
71. Torlontano M, Crocetti U, Augello G, et al. Comparative evaluation of the recombinant human thyrotropin-stimulated thyroglobulin levels, 131-I whole-body scintigraphy, and neck ultrasonography in the follow-up of patients with papillary thyroid microcarcinoma who have not undergone radioiodine therapy. J Clin Endocrinol Metab 2006;91:60–3.
72. Pacini F, Molinaro E, Castagna M, et al. Recombinant human thyrotropin-stimulated serum thyroglobulin combined with neck ultrasonography has the highest sensitivity in monitoring differentiated thyroid carcinoma. J Clin Endocrinol Metab 2003;88:3668–73.
73. Spencer C, Fatemi S, Singer P, et al. Serum basal thyroglobulin measured by a second-generation assay correlates with the recombinant human thyrotropin-stimulated thyroglobulin response in patients treated for differentiated thyroid cancer. Thyroid 2010;20:587–95.
74. Bachelot A, Cailleux A, Klain M, et al. Relationship between tumor burden and serum thyroglobulin level in patients with papillary and follicular thyroid carcinoma. Thyroid 2002;12:707–11.
75. Pacini F, Fugazzola L, Lippi F, et al. Detection of thyroglobulin in fine needle aspirates of nonthyroidal neck masses: a clue to the diagnosis of metastatic differentiated thyroid cancer. J Clin Endocrinol Metab 1992;74:1401–4.
76. Torres M, Nobrega Neto S, Rosas R, et al. Thyroglobulin in the washout fluid of lymph-node biopsy: what is its role in the follow-up of differentiated thyroid carcinoma? Thyroid 2014;24:7–18.
77. Frasoldati A, Toschi E, Zini M, et al. Role of thyroglobulin measurement in fine-needle aspiration biopsies of cervical lymph nodes in patients with differentiated thyroid cancer. Thyroid 1999;9:105–11.
78. Boi F, Baghino G, Atzeni F, et al. The diagnostic value for differentiated thyroid carcinoma metastases of thyroglobulin measurement in washout fluid from fine-needle aspiration biopsy of neck lymph nodes is maintained in the presence of circulating anti-Tg antibodies. J Clin Endocrinol Metab 2006;91:1364–9.
79. Baloch Z, Barroeta J, Walsh J, et al. Utility of thyroglobulin measurement in fine-needle aspiration biopsy specimens of lymph nodes in the diagnosis of recurrent thyroid carcinoma. Cytojournal 2008;5:1–8.
80. Ahn J, Lee J, Yi J, et al. Diagnostic accuracy of CT and ultrasonography for evaluating metastatic cervical lymph nodes in patients with thyroid cancer. World J Surg 2008;32:1552–8.

81. Choi J, Kim J, Kwak J, et al. Preoperative staging of papillary thyroid carcinoma: comparison of ultrasound imaging and CT. AJR Am J Roentgenol 2009;193: 871–8.
82. Misra S, Meiyappan S, Heus L, et al. Patients' experiences following locoregional recurrence of thyroid cancer: a qualitative study. J Surg Oncol 2013; 108:47–51.
83. Rondeau G, Fish S, Hann L, et al. Ultrasonographically detected small thyroid bed nodules identified after total thyroidectomy for differentiated thyroid cancer seldom show clinically significant structural progression. Thyroid 2011;21: 845–53.
84. Robenshtok E, Fish S, Bach A, et al. Suspicious cervical lymph nodes detected after thyroidectomy for papillary thyroid cancer usually remain stable over years in properly selected patients. J Clin Endocrinol Metab 2012;97:2706–13.
85. Grant C, Hay I, Gough I, et al. Local recurrence in papillary thyroid carcinoma: is extent of surgical resection important? Surgery 1988;104:954–62.
86. Ito Y, Higashiyama T, Takamura Y, et al. Prognosis of patients with papillary thyroid carcinoma showing postoperative recurrence to the central neck. World J Surg 2011;35:767–72.
87. Uchida H, Imai T, Kikumori T, et al. Long-term results for papillary thyroid carcinoma with local recurrence. Surg Today 2013;43:848–53.
88. Newman K, Black T, Heller G, et al. Differentiated thyroid cancer: determinants of disease progression in patients <21 years of age at diagnosis: a report from the Surgical Discipline Committee of the Children's Cancer Group. Ann Surg 1998;227:533–41.
89. Robie D, Dinauer C, Tuttle R, et al. The impact of initial surgical management on outcome in young patients with differentiated thyroid cancer. J Pediatr Surg 1998;33:1134–8.
90. Rosentahl M, Angelos P, Cooper D, et al. Clinical and professional ethics guidelines for the practice of thyroidology. Thyroid 2013;23:1203–10.
91. Tufano R, Clayman G, Heller K, et al. Management of recurrent/persistent nodal disease in patients with differentiated thyroid cancer: a critical review of the risks and benefits of surgical intervention versus active surveillance. Thyroid 2014;25: 15–27.
92. Phelan E, Kamani D, Shin J, et al. Neural monitored revision thyroid cancer surgery: surgical safety and thyroglobulin response. Otolaryngol Head Neck Surg 2013;149:47–52.
93. Urken M, Milas M, Randolph G, et al. Management of recurrent and persistent metastatic lymph nodes in well-differentiated thyroid cancer: a multifactorial decision-making guide created for the Thyroid Cancer Care Collaborative. Head Neck 2015;37:605–14.
94. Merdad M, Eskander A, Kroeker T, et al. Predictors of level II and Vb neck disease in in metastatic papillary thyroid cancer. Arch Otolaryngol Head Neck Surg 2012;138:1030–3.
95. Al-Saif O, Farrar W, Bloomston M, et al. Long-term efficacy of lymph node reoperation for persistent papillary thyroid cancer. J Clin Endocrinol Metab 2010;95: 2187–94.
96. Yim J, Kim W, Kim E, et al. The outcomes of first reoperation for locoregionally recurrent/persistent papillary thyroid carcinoma in patients who initially underwent total thyroidectomy and remnant ablation. J Clin Endocrinol Metab 2011; 96:2049–56.

97. Kim T, Kim W, Kim E, et al. Serum thyroglobulin levels at the time of 121-I remnant ablation just after thyroidectomy are useful for early prediction of clinical recurrence in low-risk patients with differentiated thyroid carcinoma. J Clin Endocrinol Metab 2005;90:1440–5.
98. Schuff K. Management of recurrent/persistent papillary thyroid carcinoma: efficacy of the surgical option. J Clin Endocrinol Metab 2011;96:2038–9.
99. McCoy K, Yim J, Tublin M, et al. Same-day ultrasound guidance in reoperation for locally recurrent papillary thyroid cancer. Surgery 2007;142:965–72.
100. Hughes D, Laird A, Miller B, et al. Reoperative lymph node dissection for recurrent papillary thyroid cancer and effect on serum thyroglobulin. Ann Surg Oncol 2012;19:2951–7.
101. Roh J, Kim J, Park C. Central compartment reoperation for recurrent/persistent differentiated thyroid cancer: patterns of recurrence, morbidity, and prediction of postoperative hypocalcemia. Ann Surg Oncol 2011;18:1312–8.
102. Shah A. Recurrent differentiated thyroid cancer. Endocr Pract 2012;18:600–3.
103. Palme C, Waseem Z, Raza S, et al. Management and outcome of recurrent well-differentiated thyroid carcinoma. Arch Otolaryngol Head Neck Surg 2004;130:819–24.
104. Clayman G, Agarwal G, Edieken B. Long-term outcome of comprehensive central compartment dissection in patients with recurrent/persistent papillary thyroid carcinoma. Thyroid 2011;21:1309–16.
105. Clayman G, Shellenberge T, Ginsberg L, et al. Approach and safety of comprehensive central compartment dissection in patients with recurrent papillary thyroid carcinoma. Head Neck 2009;31:1153–63.
106. Chao T, Jeng L, Lin J, et al. Reoperative thyroid surgery. World J Surg 1997;21:644–7.
107. Erbil Y, Sari S, Agcoaglu O, et al. Radio-guided excision of metastatic lymph nodes in thyroid carcinoma: a safe technique for previously operated neck compartments. World J Surg 2010;34:2581–8.
108. Alzahrani A, Raef H, Sultan A, et al. Impact of cervical lymph node dissection on serum Tg and the course of disease in Tg-positive, radioactive iodine whole body scan-negative recurrent/persistent papillary thyroid cancer. J Endocrinol Invest 2002;25:526–31.
109. Travagli J, Cailleux A, Ricard M, et al. Combination of radioiodine (131-I) and probe-guided surgery for persistent or recurrent thyroid carcinoma. J Clin Endocrinol Metab 1998;83:2675–80.
110. Lee L, Steward D. Sonographically-directed neck dissection for recurrent thyroid carcinoma. Laryngoscope 2008;118:991–4.
111. Steward D. Update in utility of secondary node dissection for papillary thyroid cancer. J Clin Endocrinol Metab 2012;97:3393–8.
112. Rubello D, Salvatori M, Casara D, et al. 99mTc-sestamibi radio-guided surgery of loco-regional 131-I-negative recurrent thyroid cancer. Eur J Surg Oncol 2007;33:902–6.
113. Sabra M, Grewal R, Tala H, et al. Clinical outcomes following empiric radioiodine therapy in patients with structurally identifiable metastatic follicular cell-derived thyroid carcinoma with negative diagnostic but positive post-therapy 131-I whole body scans. Thyroid 2012;22:877–83.
114. Heilo A, Sigstad E, Fagerlid K, et al. Efficacy of ultrasound-guided percutaneous ethanol injection treatment in patients with a limited number of metastatic cervical lymph nodes from papillary thyroid carcinoma. J Clin Endocrinol Metab 2011;96:2750–5.

115. Hay I, Lee R, Davidge-Pitts C, et al. Long-term outcome of ultrasound-guided percutaneous ethanol ablation of selected "recurrent" neck nodal metastases in 25 patients with TNM stages III or IV papillary thyroid carcinoma previously treated by surgery and 131-I therapy. Surgery 2013;154:1448–54.
116. Park K, Shin J, Han B, et al. Inoperable symptomatic recurrent thyroid cancers: preliminary result of radiofrequency ablation. Ann Surg Oncol 2011;18:2564–8.
117. Baek J, Kim Y, Sung J, et al. Locoregional control of metastatic well-differentiated thyroid cancer by ultrasound-guided radiofrequency ablation. AJR Am J Roentgenol 2011;197:W331–6.
118. Dupuy D, Monchik J, Decrea C, et al. Radiofrequency ablation of regional recurrence from well-differentiated thyroid malignancy. Surgery 2001;130:971–7.
119. Monchik J, Donatin G, Iannuccilli J, et al. Radiofrequency ablation and percutaneous ethanol injection treatment for recurrent local and distant well-differentiated thyroid carcinoma. Ann Surg 2006;244:296–304.
120. Shin J, Baek J, Lee J. Radiofrequency and ethanol ablation for the treatment of recurrent thyroid cancers: current status and challenges. Curr Opin Oncol 2013;25:14–9.
121. Na D, Lee J, Jung S, et al. Radiofrequency ablation of benign thyroid nodules and recurrent thyroid cancers: consensus statement and recommendations. Korean J Radiol 2012;13:117–25.
122. Papini E, Bizzari G, Bianchini A, et al. Percutaneous ultrasound-guided laser ablation is effective for treating selected nodal metastases in papillary thyroid cancer. J Clinc Endocrinol Metab 2013;98:E92–7.
123. Schwartz D, Lobo M, Ang K, et al. Postoperative external beam radiotherapy for differentiated thyroid cancer: outcomes and morbidity with conformal treatment. Int J Radiat Oncol Biol Phys 2009;74:1083–91.
124. Romesser P, Sherman E, Shaha A, et al. External beam radiotherapy with or without concurrent chemotherapy in advanced or recurrent non-anaplastic non-medullary thyroid cancer. J Surg Oncol 2014;110:375–82.

The Role of Surgery in Autoimmune Conditions of the Thyroid

Tong Gan, MD[a], Reese W. Randle, MD[b,*]

KEYWORDS

- Autoimmune thyroiditis • Surgical management • Hashimoto's thyroiditis
- Graves' disease

KEY POINTS

- Hashimoto's thyroiditis is the most common cause of hypothyroidism in the United States and is often treated medically with thyroid replacement therapy. Major surgical indications include suspicion for malignancy and compressive symptoms.
- Graves' disease is the most common cause of hyperthyroidism in the United States. Antithyroid drugs and radioactive iodine are often the first-line therapy; however, surgery has a role in selected cases.
- Surgical management of autoimmune thyroid disease requires specific indications, but is safe in the hands of a high volume surgeon.

INTRODUCTION

Autoimmune conditions of the thyroid are frequent causes of thyroiditis or inflammation of the thyroid. Hashimoto's thyroiditis is the most common cause of hypothyroidism in the United States, whereas Graves' disease is the most common cause of hyperthyroidism. These diseases are diagnosed clinically with a detailed history and physical examination, biochemically using laboratory autoimmune antibody levels, or radiographically with ultrasound and thyroid uptake scans. Although an operation is not always the primary consideration for treatment, certain situations make surgery essential to the management of these 2 diseases.

Disclosure Statement: This research was supported by the Markey Cancer Center Support Grant (NCI P30 CA177558) and T32 NIH Training Grants (T32CA160003).
[a] Department of Surgery, University of Kentucky, 800 Rose Street, MN275, Lexington, KY 40536, USA; [b] Department of Surgery, University of Kentucky, 125 East Maxwell Street, Suite 302, Lexington, KY 40508, USA
* Corresponding author.
E-mail address: Reese.Randle@uky.edu

Surg Clin N Am 99 (2019) 633–648
https://doi.org/10.1016/j.suc.2019.04.005 surgical.theclinics.com

HASHIMOTO'S THYROIDITIS

Overview

Chronic lymphocytic thyroiditis, or Hashimoto's thyroiditis, is the most common cause of diffuse goiter and hypothyroidism in the United States.[1] Struma lymphomatosa was the first characterization of Hashimoto's thyroiditis made by Hakaru Hashimoto, a Japanese physician, in 1912.[2] Later, in the 1950s, the presence of thyroid autoantibodies suggested an autoimmune component of Hashimoto's thyroiditis.[3] A diffuse, lymphocytic inflammatory process characterizes Hashimoto's thyroiditis, and clinical manifestations are variable due to differing amounts of gland destruction. Typically, hypothyroid Hashimoto's thyroiditis is well controlled medically with thyroid hormone replacement for those who develop hypothyroidism, but operative management plays a role in specific cases.

Epidemiology

Hashimoto's thyroiditis is the most common cause of hypothyroidism in developed countries and is diagnosed in approximately 30 to 60 people per 100,000 each year, resulting in a prevalence estimated at about 4%.[4,5] Women are 10 to 20 times more likely to develop Hashimoto's thyroiditis compared with men. In the United States, whites have the highest risk, with 5% of white women developing Hashimoto's thyroiditis.[6,7]

Pathogenesis

The cause of Hashimoto's thyroiditis is not fully understood, but both environmental and genetic factors contribute. Anti-thyroid antibodies, including anti-thyroperoxidase (anti-TPO), anti-thyroglobulin (anti-Tg), and thyroid-stimulating hormone (TSH) stimulation blocking antibody (TSBAb), lead to inflammatory reactions. Hashimoto's thyroiditis starts with gradual atrophy of follicular tissue secondary to infiltration of primarily mature lymphocytic cells.[2,8,9]

Clinical Presentation

The development of hypothyroidism in Hashimoto's thyroiditis is slow and insidious. Nearly 20% of patients eventually present with overt hypothyroidism, and 5% present with an initial, transient hyperthyroidism, otherwise known as Hashitoxicosis from gland destruction releasing thyroxine.[10] In some cases, patients may experience cyclic hyperthyroidism secondary to alternating thyroid stimulating and inhibiting autoantibodies (**Table 1**).[11,12] On physical examination, a firm, diffusely enlarged painless thyroid gland is palpated, although some patients progress toward a small, atrophic gland.[9] Patients may complain of compressive symptoms, such as dysphonia and dysphagia, and rarely, pain.[11]

Diagnosis

Laboratory investigations and imaging help support a clinical diagnosis of Hashimoto's thyroiditis (**Table 2**). Associated antibodies include serum anti-TPO antibody in 70% to 90% of the patients, anti-Tg antibody in 20% to 70% of the patients, and TSBAb in 60% of the patients.[7,13,14] Although not always indicated, an ultrasound is the most useful imaging modality to describe Hashimoto's thyroiditis, demonstrating diffuse heterogeneity, echogenic septations, and hypervascularity (**Fig. 1**).[15,16] Often patients have extensive pseudonodularity. Radioactive iodine uptake scans (RAIU; iodine-123) uptake scans are rarely useful for diagnosis, because uptake is extremely variable.[17]

Any suspicious hypoechoic nodules identified on ultrasound will require fine-needle aspiration (FNA) to rule out malignancy. However, indeterminate biopsy results are

Table 1
Signs and symptoms of hypothyroidism and hyperthyroidism

	Hypothyroidism	Hyperthyroidism
General	Fatigue, weight gain, cold intolerance	Fatigue, increased appetite, weight loss, heat intolerance, increased basal metabolic rate, flushing
Neurologic	Poor memory, depression, psychosis, paresthesias	Mania, anxiety, nervousness, irritability
Head and neck	Hoarseness, neck pain, periorbital edema, hair loss, goiter	Hoarseness, goiter, hair thinning, periorbital edema,[a] eyelid retraction,[a] proptosis,[a] excessive tearing,[a] exophthalmos,[a] ocular dysmotility[a]
Cardiovascular	Bradycardia, peripheral nonpitting edema, pericardial effusion, hyperlipidemia, hypertension	Palpitations, tachycardia, atrial arrhythmia
Pulmonary	Dyspnea, pleural effusion	Shortness of breath
Gastrointestinal	Dysphagia, constipation	Dysphagia, nausea, diarrhea
Genitourinary	Decreased glomerular filtration rate, elevated creatinine, infertility, menstrual irregularities, infertility	Oligomenorrhea, erectile dysfunction
Musculoskeletal	Muscle weakness, muscle cramping, joint pain, ataxia, carpal tunnel syndrome, delayed tendon reflexes	Pretibial myxedema, peripheral tremors, hyperactive deep tendon reflex
Dermatologic	Cool, dry, rough, brittle nails	Warm, moist skin, smooth, pretibial dermopathy,[a] brittle nails

[a] Specific to Graves' disease.

common in patients with Hashimoto's thyroiditis. Cytologically, it can be challenging to distinguish Hashimoto's thyroiditis from Hürthle cell changes, follicular neoplasms, papillary thyroid carcinoma, or thyroid lymphoma.[5,7] Notably, patients with Hashimoto's thyroiditis have an 80 times higher risk of thyroid lymphoma, and 30% of patients with thyroid lymphoma have a history of a rapidly enlarging goiter with compressive symptoms.[18] Because treatment of thyroid lymphoma is vastly different from other thyroid malignancies, this distinction is important.[7] In addition, the development of papillary thyroid cancer is relatively common in patients with Hashimoto's thyroiditis. Although most will not develop thyroid cancer, between 11% and 36% of patients with papillary thyroid cancer have associated Hashimoto's thyroiditis.[19]

Histologically, Hashimoto's thyroiditis specimens will contain follicular cells, Hurthle cells, and lymphocyte infiltration.[1] Follicular epithelial cells have a variable appearance from hyperplastic to atrophic. Nuclei and nucleoli become prominent, and multinuclear giant cells are apparent. Glandular tissue is diffusely infiltrated by lymphocytes, forming germinal centers that cause fibrosis and diminish colloid.[7]

Medical Management

Most patients with Hashimoto's thyroiditis are asymptomatic and require no specific treatment. Those who develop hypothyroidism will receive thyroid hormone replacement, and surgery is rarely indicated.[20] In addition, thyroxine replacement provides suppression of endogenous TSH, thus decreasing growth stimulation of thyroid

Table 2
Diagnosis of Hashimoto's thyroiditis

History and physical examination	• Symptoms consistent with hypothyroidism • May or may not have signs of enlarged palpable goiter, firm or tender gland
Laboratory testing	• Elevated TSH • Decreased serum T4 • Presence of anti-thyroid antibodies ○ Anti-TPO ○ Anti-Tg ○ TSBAb
Ultrasound	• Diffuse type: Diffusely enlarged gland with heterogeneity, echogenic septation, hypervascular, micronodular pattern • Nodular type: Discrete macronodules, either diffuse pattern background or normal parenchyma
FNA	• Suspicious nodules on ultrasound require biopsy to rule out malignancy • On cytology, nodular goitrous follicular cells, Hurthle cells, and lymphocytic infiltration

goiters.[21] However, over-replacing thyroid hormone to suppress TSH below physiologic levels is discouraged as a means to prevent or shrink goiter formation, because it is rarely if ever successful, and medically induced hyperthyroidism carries long-term risks.[22]

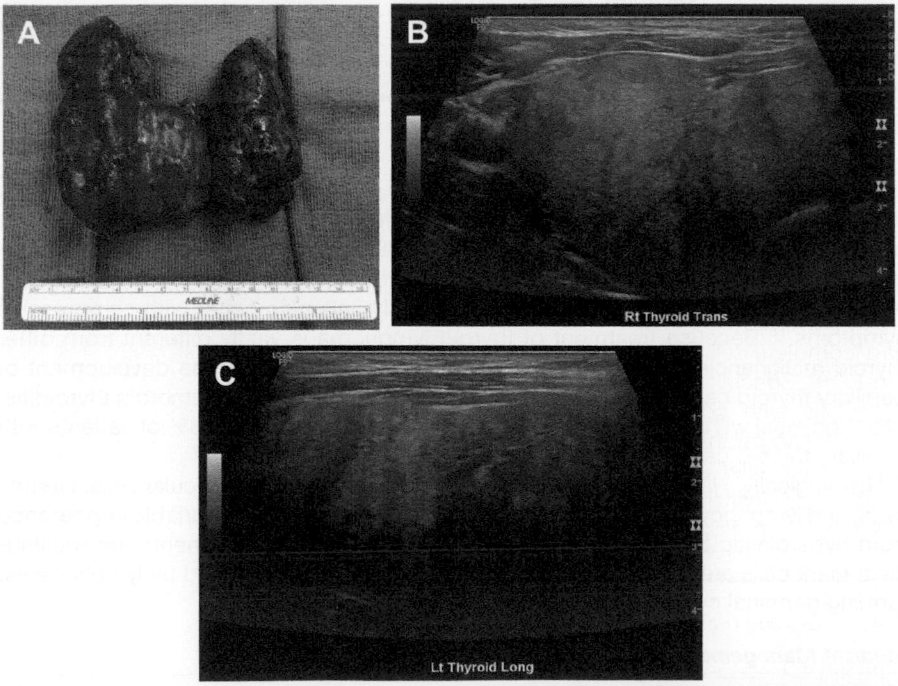

Fig. 1. Hashimoto's thyroiditis. Surgical specimen of enlarged thyroid demonstrating asymmetrical lobes (*A*). Ultrasonography of bilateral lobes preoperatively demonstrates characteristic Hashimoto findings of diffuse heterogeneity, nodularity, and echogenic septations in the transverse (*B*) and longitudinal view (*C*).

Surgical Management

There are several indications for the operative treatment of Hashimoto's thyroiditis (**Table 3**). In general, indications for a partial or total thyroidectomy in patients with Hashimoto's thyroiditis are similar to those without. Cancer, suspicious nodules, or compressive symptoms remain the most common indications for surgery, but there are also a few rare considerations for thyroidectomy that are specific to Hashimoto's thyroiditis.

The most common indication for thyroidectomy when there is confirmed malignancy or high suspicion of malignancy based on FNA cytology, clinical, and sonographic features.[1] Dominant nodules and pseudonodules in Hashimoto's thyroiditis are commonly benign, but nodules may be firm on examination and adherent to adjacent structures, with enlarged lymph nodes mimicking cancer. FNA results may simply demonstrate lymphocytic thyroiditis; however, there may still be a risk of malignancy in this population.[1,23]

The association of Hashimoto's thyroiditis and papillary thyroid cancer is well established.[11,24–29] Those patients with the nodular type of Hashimoto have a 60% increased risk of developing papillary thyroid cancer. In addition, patients with Hashimoto's thyroiditis are more likely to be higher stage at diagnosis when compared with those without Hashimoto's thyroiditis (36% vs 21%). The difficulty in obtaining accurate ultrasounds and quality FNA likely contributes to the delayed diagnosis.[24] The chronic inflammation in patients with Hashimoto's thyroiditis may provide a mutagenic environment, generating a higher risk of disease as evidenced by the higher proportion of multifocal disease (56%).[24,28] For those with nodules and low concern for malignancy, close sonographic follow-up is required to facilitate early diagnosis of papillary thyroid cancer.[24] Once malignancy is confirmed in patients with Hashimoto's thyroiditis, thyroidectomy is recommended due to high risk of multicentricity, difficulty in accurate imaging, and lower accuracy of FNA surveillance.[24,26]

Compressive symptoms secondary to a large goiter is the second most common indication for thyroidectomy in patients with Hashimoto's thyroiditis (**Fig. 2**). Up to 20% of patients with Hashimoto's thyroiditis may experience dysphagia, coughing or choking spells, dyspnea, and hoarseness.[26,29] Because of significant inflammatory and fibrotic changes to the thyroid gland in patients with Hashimoto's thyroiditis, a difficult thyroidectomy may be anticipated. However, thyroidectomy is safe when performed by a high-volume surgeon.[1] After thyroidectomy, 96% of patients had complete relief of symptoms, and nearly all had substantial relief of symptoms.[1,20] Special consideration should be given to patients with Hashimoto's thyroiditis with compressive symptoms without an obviously enlarged thyroid. Fibrosis can be the cause of the compressive symptoms, and these patients may also obtain relief with a thyroidectomy. However, a thorough discussion of risks weighed against the severity of symptoms should precede any plans for operative intervention in this select group.

Table 3
Indications and contraindications of thyroidectomy in Hashimoto's thyroiditis

Indications	Contraindications
• Confirmed malignancy or highly suspicious nodule • Compressive symptoms secondary to large goiter • Cervical pain • Inability to regulate thyroid function medically (rare)	• Inability to tolerate general anesthesia • Confirmed thyroid lymphoma

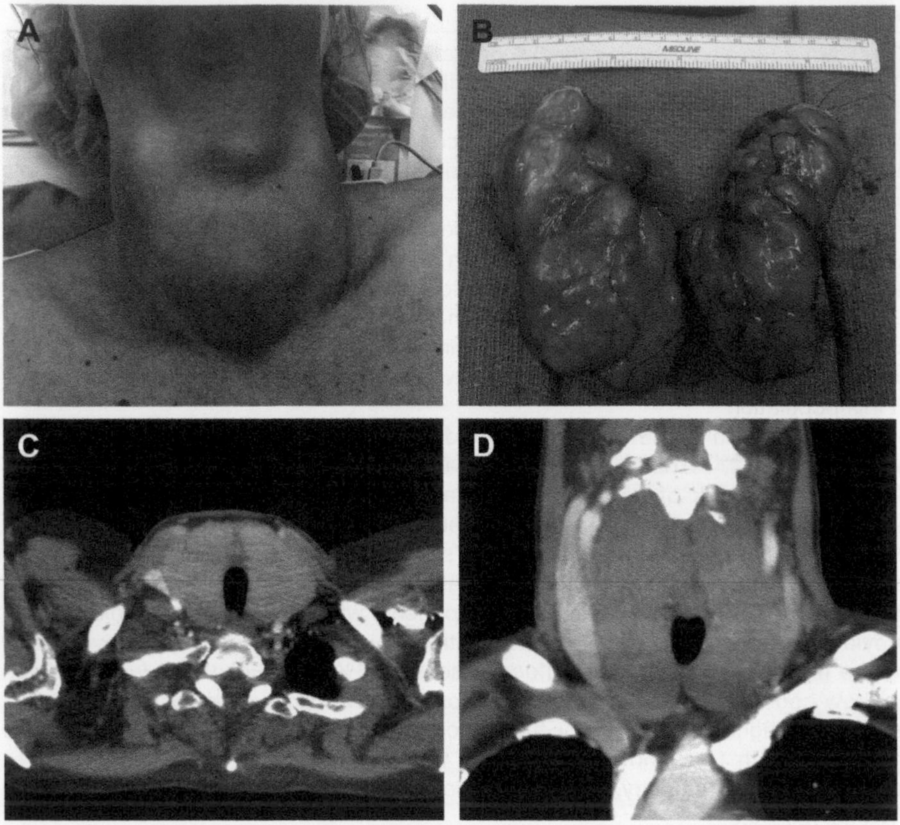

Fig. 2. Fibrosing Hashimoto's thyroiditis. Patient has significant palpable firm goiter (*A*). Patient experienced compressive symptoms, including dysphagia, shortness of breath, and decreased neck mobility. Note bilateral lobes with irregular shape on final specimen (*B*). Computed tomography scan of neck demonstrating significant compression of trachea and esophagus as source of symptoms. Axial view (*C*), coronal view (*D*).

Rarely, total thyroidectomy can be considered for patients with medically refractory disease in the absence of specific compressive symptoms. Some may have large fluctuations in thyroid function severely impacting patient quality of life despite compliant treatment by an endocrinologist. The removal of the thyroid in these patients may facilitate thyroid hormone replacement to a physiologic steady state. Again, in these scenarios, patients must have a clear understanding of the risks and benefits of this intervention.

Lastly, cervical pain is an additional consideration for thyroidectomy in Hashimoto's thyroiditis. The most common cause of cervical pain is trauma, nodular hemorrhage, and subacute thyroiditis, and very rarely is from Hashimoto's thyroiditis. Nonetheless, cervical pain from Hashimoto's thyroiditis can be successfully treated with total thyroidectomy.[24,29,30]

Surgical Risks

Complications of thyroidectomy are more common in patients with Hashimoto's thyroiditis. Surgical dissection of the thyroid gland is more difficult with an enlarged and densely fibrotic gland. Interestingly, the presence of anti-Tg antibodies in

Hashimoto's thyroiditis correlates with the difficulty of thyroidectomy.[31] The most serious complications are recurrent laryngeal nerve injury and hypocalcemia. Nerve injury rates range from 0.8% to 5.1% in this population.[26,32–34] Transient hypocalcemia secondary to hypoparathyroidism from surgical retraction occurs at a more frequent rate in patients with Hashimoto's thyroiditis ranging from 20% to 38% of the time.[1,26,34] In addition the need for parathyroid autotransplantation is described in 4.4% to 6% of cases.[26,35] The most important factor in preventing operative complications is treatment at a high-volume center with a high-volume surgeon.[29]

GRAVES' DISEASE

Overview

Graves' disease is the most common cause of hyperthyroidism in the United States.[36] Aristotle and Xenophon first described the symptoms of Graves' disease in the fifth century BCE when a goiter was linked with signs of exophthalmos. The triad of tachycardia, goiter, and exophthalmos was further characterized in the nineteenth century by Robert James Graves in Ireland as signs of the same disease. Graves' disease was classified as an autoimmune disease when a long-acting thyroid stimulator was identified in 1958 by McKenzie and was confirmed as an autoantibody by Adams in 1965.[37]

Epidemiology

Graves' disease represents up to 80% of hyperthyroid patients.[38] Similarly to Hashimoto's thyroiditis, women have a much higher incidence (0.5 per 1000) compared with men (0.05 per 1000).[37] Peak incidence occurs around 40 to 60 years of age, but it can present much younger.[38] Graves' disease is diagnosed more commonly in smokers and in those with personal and family history of autoimmune diseases.[39] In fact, nearly half of those with Graves' disease have a family history of autoimmune thyroid disease.[12,39,40]

Pathogenesis

Thyrotoxicosis in Graves' disease occurs secondary to thyrotropin receptor antibodies (TRAb), which constitutively stimulate TSH receptors to synthesize excessive thyroxine.[36] Twin studies suggest that 80% of Graves' disease are due to genetic factors, and the other 20% are due to environmental factors.[41]

Clinical Presentation

Patients with Graves' disease can present with the spectrum of subclinical to overt hyperthyroidism (see **Table 1**). Most common signs include tachycardia, atrial arrhythmia, tremor, warm moist skin, hyperreflexia, and pretibial myxedema.[36,37,40] Even patients with mild Graves' disease can experience changes in basal metabolic rate, cardiovascular output, and psychiatric symptoms.[36,42]

Graves' ophthalmopathy occurs in up to 60% of patients with Graves' disease and is associated with high TRAb titers.[12] Clinical signs of Graves' ophthalmopathy include eyelid retraction, proptosis, excessive tearing, exophthalmos, and motility disorders. Most patients have mild symptoms, but up to 5% may experience severe symptoms, including intense pain, corneal ulceration, and compressive optic neuropathy.[43]

Thyroid dermopathy occurs in patients with Graves' disease from the accumulation of glycosaminoglycans in the pretibial area. Although a classic sign of Graves' disease, it only occurs in about 2% to 3% of patients. When it does occur, it usually clusters in patients with Graves' ophthalmopathy with very high TRAb titers.[12]

Diagnosis

Graves' disease can be diagnosed clinically, biochemically, or radiographically (**Table 4**). Signs and symptoms do not necessarily correlate with T3 and free T4 levels, but symptoms of hyperthyroidism, when present, may be the first clue.[36] On physical examination, there is often a palpable smooth, diffusely enlarged goiter. Measurement of serum TSH is the most sensitive laboratory test and should be used as the initial screening test.[36,40] In Graves' disease, expect undetectable TSH and increased T3 and free T4. An ultrasound is often obtained demonstrating classically a diffusely enlarged, heterogeneous, and hypervascular thyroid gland (**Fig. 3**). The combination of hyperthyroidism and extrathyroidal signs, including Graves' ophthalmopathy or thyroid dermopathy, is adequate for the diagnosis of Graves' disease.[37]

Laboratory values and imaging can aid to confirm a diagnosis of Graves' disease, including the measurement of TRAb and the use of radioactive iodine uptake scan. TRAb can stimulate or block the thyrotropin receptors, but thyroid-stimulating immunoglobulin (TSI) is present in up to 90% of patients with Graves' disease. Measuring antibody levels can also help distinguish between exogenous use of thyroid hormone and autoimmune disease. RAIU uptake is increased in both Graves' disease and toxic multinodular goiters, but Graves' disease has a diffusely homogeneous rather than heterogeneous uptake.[37]

Medical Management

Once the diagnosis of Graves' disease and disease severity is confirmed, 3 different treatment regimens can be considered (**Table 5**):

- Anti-thyroid drugs (ATDs)
- Radioactive iodine (RAI, iodine-131)
- Total thyroidectomy

Treatment preferences vary geographically[44]; however, contraindications exist for each treatment modality, and the ultimate treatment selection should be individualized to provide the best outcome for the patient. Patient preference should play a role in the decision-making process after a thorough discussion of the risks and advantages of each option.

ATDs are recommended by 77% of European endocrinologists as the mainstay of Graves' disease treatment.[45] Although it has gained popularity in the United States, ATDs typically serve as a bridge to manage hyperthyroidism in preparation

Table 4
Diagnosis of Graves' disease

History and physical examination	• Symptoms consistent with hyperthyroidism • Periorbital edema, eyelid retraction, proptosis, excessive tearing, exophthalmos, ocular dysmotility • May or may not have signs of a diffusely enlarged goiter, may have a "spongy" gland on palpation
Laboratory testing	• Undetectable TSH • High serum T3/free T4 • Presence of anti-TRAb
Imaging	• Ultrasound demonstrates an enlarged gland with heterogeneous texture. Hypervascularity is commonly identified • RAIU can be used to differentiate toxic multinodular goiter, toxic adenoma, and Graves' disease

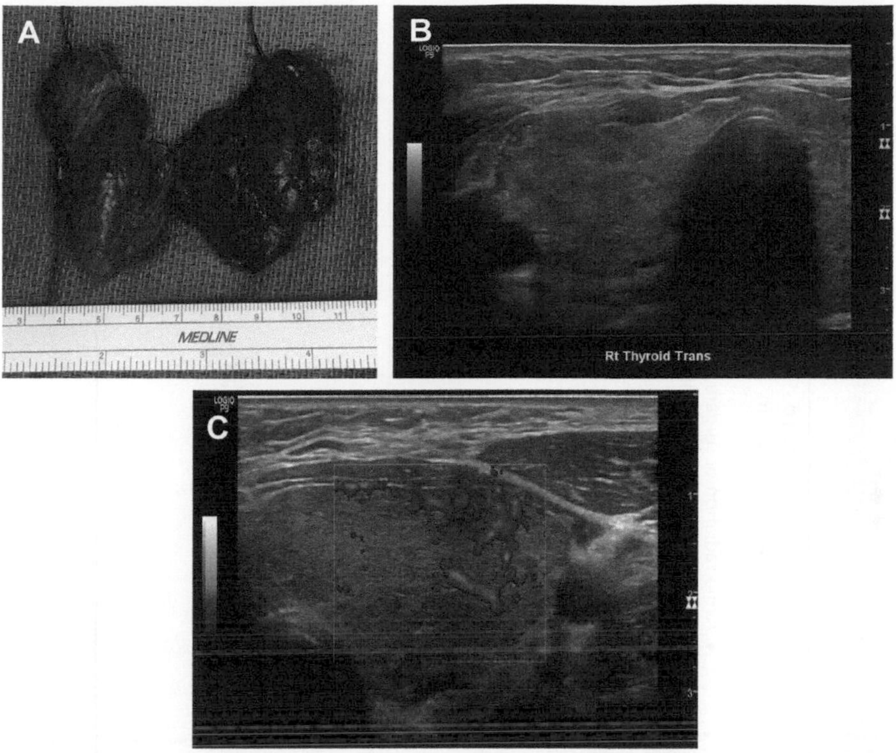

Fig. 3. Graves' disease. Surgical specimen of Graves' disease treated with Lugol solution preoperatively (*A*). Ultrasonography of a thyroid gland with Graves' disease demonstrates diffuse heterogeneity, relative lack of nodularity (*B*) as well as hypervascularity (*C*).

for more definitive treatment with RAI or thyroidectomy.[36,46] The main medication used is Methimazole or its prodrug Carbimazole (only in Europe).[40] Propylthiouracil can be used in pregnant women due to teratogenicity with Methimazole, or for those with an allergic or other adverse reaction to Methimazole. All ATDs inhibit organification of iodine to decrease thyroid hormone production, and Propylthiouracil also inhibits T4 conversion to the active T3. Methimazole is more effective than Propylthiouracil at rapid restoration to euthyroid state and is preferred due to a lower overall risk profile. Both drugs have a small risk of agranulocytosis (0.5%).[37,40] Rarely, ATDs can cause significant hepatic injury requiring monitoring with liver function tests. Most patients who receive ATDs become euthyroid by 6 weeks, and nearly all become euthyroid by 3 months. Remission rates are between 50% and 60% after 1 year of treatment, but do not improve further after 18 months.[37,47]

RAI is recommended by most (70%) US endocrinologists as the primary treatment of Graves' disease as well as relapsed Graves' disease from ATDs.[40,48] RAI, using the iodine 131 isotope, was first developed in the 1930s and provides a definitive treatment option for Graves' disease.[37] About 70% of patients become euthyroid in 4 to 8 weeks, but the full effect of RAI may not occur until up to 6 months.[37] Many patients are not successfully treated with just 1 dose.[12] The dosing of RAI aims to balance the recurrence of hyperthyroidism (5%–25% risk) with the induction of hypothyroidism (20% in the first year, then 3%–5% per year). ATD pretreatment for 4 to 8 weeks before

Table 5
Graves' disease treatment options

Treatment Type	Indications	Contraindications	Advantages	Risks
Anti-thyroid drugs	• Patients with high likelihood of remission (women, mild disease, smaller goiters, negative or low titers of anti-TRAb) • Pregnant (only PTU) • Life-threatening thyroid storm	• Prior major adverse reactions (agranulocytosis, vasculitis, hepatic injury) • Allergy • Liver dysfunction	• Generally well tolerated • Relatively rapid return to euthyroidism • Avoid radiation or surgery • Safe in pregnancy (PTU only)	• Relatively high failure rate • Agranulocytosis • Vasculitis • Hepatic injury
RAI	• Definitive treatment of Graves' disease	• Pregnancy or planning within 6 mo • Lactation or recent lactation • Suspicious nodules or confirmed malignancy • Poor patient compliance • Graves' ophthalmopathy • Smoker • Child	• Avoid surgery • Possible restoration to euthyroidism	• May require repeat doses • Can exacerbate ophthalmopathy • Requires temporary isolation • Possible salivary gland dysfunction • Risk of secondary malignancy
Surgical thyroidectomy	• Confirmed malignancy or highly suspicious nodule • Compressive symptoms • Pronounced Graves' ophthalmopathy • Inability to tolerate anti-thyroid drugs • Low uptake or treatment failure of RAI • Coexisting hyperparathyroidism	• Inability to tolerate general anesthesia • First and third trimester of pregnancy	• Rapid resolution of hyperthyroidism • Safe in pregnancy (second trimester) • Does not require isolation from small children or animals • Safe option for children	• Operative risks: hematoma, nerve injury, hypoparathyroidism • Permanent hypothyroidism

Abbreviation: PTU, propylthiouracil.

RAI is recommended for cardiac patients with severe hyperthyroidism to decrease the risk of thyroid storm.[12]

Absolute contraindications to RAI include pregnancy or planning a pregnancy within 6 months, current or recent lactation, suspicious nodules or thyroid malignancy, and poor compliance. RAI crosses the placenta, causing profound neonatal hypothyroidism, neonatal goiter, and even asphyxia and remains in breast milk 8 weeks after treatment.[36,37,49] Relative contraindications to RAI include Graves' ophthalmopathy (may worsen with treatment) and thyroid storm.[37,40] In addition, smokers can experience an exacerbation of Graves' ophthalmopathy with RAI and may be better served with surgical management. Last, RAI also requires temporary isolation from children and small animals and limited contact with other adults. For some, this limitation renders RAI undesirable.

Surgical Management

Thyroidectomy is growing in popularity as a first-line treatment for Graves' disease. Emil Theodor Kocher developed the subtotal thyroidectomy for Graves' disease to prevent cretinism, which remained the mainstay of treatment for Graves' disease for decades. RAI, first introduced in the 1930s, led to a drastic decrease in surgical management of Graves' disease.[50] When used, however, surgery provides a prompt and definitive treatment of hyperthyroidism.[36] In contrast to Kocher's era, total thyroidectomy is now the operative treatment of choice and is associated with nearly zero risk of relapse. Good candidates for total thyroidectomy for Graves' disease are those with nodules or malignancy, compressive symptoms, pronounced Graves' ophthalmopathy, treatment relapse, or the inability to tolerate ATDs. It is also safe for children and pregnant and nursing women.[36] At some institutions in the United States, surgery is the primary treatment modality for patients with Graves' disease, and this trend is driven by a combination of clinical and social factors.[51]

Large goiters with compressive symptoms (dysphagia, dyspnea, hypophonia) are best treated with total thyroidectomy.[36,52] Goiters with suspicious nodules should have an FNA to evaluate for malignancy. Those with confirmed malignancy or indeterminant nodules should undergo thyroidectomy. With a palpable nodule on examination, the risk of malignancy is 2.3% to 45.8% (mean of 16.9%). With a cold, enlarged thyroid nodule, the malignancy rate is 15% to 20%.[45,53,54] Some consider differentiated thyroid cancer to behave more aggressively in patients with Graves' disease due to the presence of TSI. Women who are pregnant or wish to become pregnant within 6 months who have failed ATD therapy should undergo thyroidectomy, because RAI is contraindicated.[53] There is debate regarding if ATDs are safe in nursing mothers, so women who are breastfeeding or planning to breastfeed should consider thyroidectomy.[55] The second trimester is the optimal time for thyroidectomy because of the higher spontaneous abortion rate with surgery and anesthesia in the first trimester.[56]

Patients younger than age 40 have much lower remission rates with ATD/RAI treatment for Graves' disease. Many endocrinologists prefer thyroidectomy in this population.[57] In children, thyroidectomy is recommended as the first-line therapy.[58] Up to 80% of children fail medical therapy and experience a high rate of recurrence or hypothyroidism with RAI.[53] Patients with moderate to severe Graves' ophthalmopathy should undergo thyroidectomy, because both ATD and RAI may worsen the ophthalmopathy. In addition, thyroidectomy has been demonstrated to improve signs and symptoms of Graves' ophthalmopathy.[36,53,59] This finding may be in part related to the resolution of TRAbs following total thyroidectomy. Last, patient preference is important in the decision for thyroidectomy. Surgical management has relatively faster recovery time, because ATDs and RAI require longer commitment to therapy. Typical length of stay after thyroidectomy is 1 to 3 days, and overall recovery is 1 to 3 weeks. RAI treatment is up to 6 months for maximal effect, and both RAI and ATDs alone have a higher relapse rate.[37,53,57] Patients who elect to have thyroidectomy as the primary treatment of Graves' disease have high levels of satisfaction.[60]

Relative contraindications to surgery include first and third trimester of pregnancy and lack of access to a high-volume surgeon.[36] The preference of RAI treatment over surgery is often due to perceived risks of thyroidectomy. However, with an experienced, high-volume surgeon, the risks are acceptably low. In fact, improved outcomes, lower complication rates, and shorter length of stay are associated with the volume of thyroidectomy performed by the surgeon.[61]

A euthyroid state is ideal preoperatively to prevent thyroid storm at the operation. Pretreatment with ATDs and beta-blockade helps achieve a euthyroid state.[12] In cases whereby patients have contraindications to ATDs, higher doses of beta-blockers can be used alone to help mitigate symptoms. Urgent surgical preparation can be performed within 7 days with a combination of corticosteroids, beta-blockers, and sodium iopanoate.[36] In severe cases, total plasma exchange can remove circulating thyroxine levels and rapidly render a patient euthyroid before surgery. Some surgeons use potassium iodide (Lugol solution or saturated solution of potassium iodide) to decrease hypervascularity of the gland before resection.

Although subtotal thyroidectomy was the preferred operative choice for Graves' disease in the past, the preferred operation is now nearly ubiquitously a total thyroidectomy.[62,63] The universal availability of thyroid hormone replacement has antiquated the need for a thyroid remnant in developed countries, and total thyroidectomy practically eliminates the risk of relapse.[64]

After successful thyroidectomy, there is a need to evaluate for transient hypocalcemia through laboratory testing. Some recommend routine postoperative oral calcium and calcitriol replacement to decrease the development of symptomatic hypocalcemia, allowing for earlier discharge.[65] ATDs need to be stopped immediately after surgery, whereas beta-blockers should be weaned slowly. Thyroxine replacement should be started once the patient is clinically euthyroid. For many patients well blocked before thyroidectomy, thyroid hormone replacement could be safely initiated the day after surgery. For others, delaying the treatment a few days or even a week may be beneficial.

Surgical Risks

Graves' disease is associated with a difficult thyroidectomy and longer operative times.[31,66] Major complications to thyroidectomy in Graves' disease are similar to those for Hashimoto's thyroiditis and include recurrent laryngeal nerve injury, permanent hypoparathyroidism, and postoperative bleeding. In fact, Graves' disease is independently associated with postoperative hematoma, but hematomas occur in less than 1% of patients.[65,67,68] Recurrent laryngeal nerve injury rate ranges from 0% to 3.4%,[57,65,69] and the rate of permanent hypoparathyroidism ranges from 0% to 3.3%.[69,70] In addition, pretreatment with Lugol solution may mitigate some risk of nerve injury and hypoparathyroidism.[71] Again, these complications decrease significantly when thyroidectomy is performed by a high-volume surgeon. Surgeons who perform less than 25 per year have 51% higher complication rates.[72]

SUMMARY

The 2 most common autoimmune diseases of the thyroid in the United States are Hashimoto's thyroiditis and Graves' disease. Pathogenesis of both diseases is heavily contributed by family history and personal history of autoimmune diseases as well as several environmental factors. Patients may experience mild to debilitating symptoms that may become lifelong. Diagnosis requires a combination of clinical, laboratory, and imaging techniques. Although most are managed medically, these diseases are immeasurably complex, and surgical management is required for specific indications. The surgical management of Hashimoto's thyroiditis and Graves' disease will render the patient hypothyroid, but ultimately is able to provide symptomatic relief safely under an experienced surgeon.

REFERENCES

1. Wormer BA, McHenry CR. Hashimoto's thyroiditis: outcome of surgical resection for patients with thyromegaly and compressive symptoms. Am J Surg 2011; 201(3):416–9.
2. Hashimoto H. Zur kenntniss der lymphomatosen veranderung der schilddruse (struma lymphomatosa). Langenberks Arch Klin Chir 1912;97:219–48.
3. Roitt IM, Doniach D, Campbell PN, et al. Auto-antibodies in Hashimoto's disease. Lancet 1956;271(6947):820–1.
4. Mincer DL, Jialal I. Hashimoto thyroiditis. Treasure Island (FL): StatPearls Publishing; 2018.
5. Gayathri B, Kalyani R, Harendra KM, et al. Fine needle aspiration cytology of Hashimoto's thyroiditis - a diagnostic pitfall with review of literature. J Cytol 2011; 28(4):210–3.
6. Dayan CM, Daniels GH. Chronic autoimmune thyroiditis. N Engl J Med 1996; 335(2):99–107.
7. Takami HE, Miyabe R, Kameyama K. Hashimoto's thyroiditis. World J Surg 2008; 32(5):688–92.
8. Pyzik A, Grywalska E, Matyjaszek-Matuszek B, et al. Immune disorders in Hashimoto's thyroiditis: what do we know so far? J Immunol Res 2015;2015:979167.
9. Pearce EN, Farwell AP, Braverman LE. Thyroiditis. N Engl J Med 2003;348(26): 2646–55.
10. Fatourechi V, McConahey WM, Woolner LB. Hyperthyroidism associated with histologic Hashimoto's thyroiditis. Mayo Clin Proc 1971;46(10):682–9.
11. Clark OH, Duh Q-Y, Kebebew E, et al. Textbook of endocrine surgery. 3rd edition. New Delhi (India): Jaypee Brothers Medical Publishers; 2016.
12. Heizmann O, Oertli D. Thyroiditis. In: Randolph GW, editor. Surgery of the thyroid and parathyroid glands. Berlin: Springer Berlin Heidelberg; 2012. p. 153–64.
13. Singer PA. Thyroiditis. Acute, subacute, and chronic. Med Clin North Am 1991; 75(1):61–77.
14. Cho BY, Kim WB, Chung JH, et al. High prevalence and little change in TSH receptor blocking antibody titres with thyroxine and antithyroid drug therapy in patients with non-goitrous autoimmune thyroiditis. Clin Endocrinol 1995;43(4): 465–71.
15. Anderson L, Middleton WD, Teefey SA, et al. Hashimoto thyroiditis: part 1, sonographic analysis of the nodular form of Hashimoto thyroiditis. AJR Am J Roentgenol 2010;195(1):208–15.
16. Oppenheimer CD, Giampoli CE, Montoya CS, et al. Sonographic features of nodular Hashimoto thyroiditis. Ultrasound Q 2016;32(3):271–6.

17. Ramtoola S, Maisey MN, Clarke SE, et al. The thyroid scan in Hashimoto's thyroiditis: the great mimic. Nucl Med Commun 1988;9(9):639–45.
18. Sakorafas GH, Kokkoris P, Farley DR. Primary thyroid lymphoma: diagnostic and therapeutic dilemmas. Surg Oncol 2010;19(4):e124–9.
19. Jankovic B, Le KT, Hershman JM. Clinical review: Hashimoto's thyroiditis and papillary thyroid carcinoma: is there a correlation? J Clin Endocrinol Metab 2013;98(2):474–82.
20. Shimizu K, Nakajima Y, Kitagawa W, et al. Surgical therapy in Hashimoto's thyroiditis. J Nippon Med Sch 2003;70(1):34–9.
21. Thomas CG, Rutledge RG. Surgical intervention in chronic (Hashimoto's) thyroiditis. Ann Surg 1981;193(6):769–76.
22. Cooper DS, Doherty GM, Haugen BR, et al. Revised American Thyroid Association management guidelines for patients with thyroid nodules and differentiated thyroid cancer. Thyroid 2009;19(11):1167–214.
23. Okayasu I, Fujiwara M, Hara Y, et al. Association of chronic lymphocytic thyroiditis and thyroid papillary carcinoma. A study of surgical cases among Japanese, and white and African Americans. Cancer 1995;76(11):2312–8.
24. Consorti F, Loponte M, Milazzo F, et al. Risk of malignancy from thyroid nodular disease as an element of clinical management of patients with Hashimoto's thyroiditis. Eur Surg Res 2010;45(3–4):333–7.
25. Pisanu A, Piu S, Cois A, et al. Coexisting Hashimoto's thyroiditis with differentiated thyroid cancer and benign thyroid diseases: indications for thyroidectomy. Chir Ital 2003;55(3):365–72.
26. Shih ML, Lee JA, Hsieh CB, et al. Thyroidectomy for Hashimoto's thyroiditis: complications and associated cancers. Thyroid 2008;18(7):729–34.
27. Singh B, Shaha AR, Trivedi H, et al. Coexistent Hashimoto's thyroiditis with papillary thyroid carcinoma: impact on presentation, management, and outcome. Surgery 1999;126(6):1070–6.
28. Kebebew E, Treseler PA, Ituarte PH, et al. Coexisting chronic lymphocytic thyroiditis and papillary thyroid cancer revisited. World J Surg 2001;25(5):632–7.
29. Pradeep PV, Ragavan M, Ramakrishna BA, et al. Surgery in Hashimoto's thyroiditis: indications, complications, and associated cancers. J Postgrad Med 2011;57(2):120–2.
30. van Schaik J, Dekkers OM, van der Kleij-Corssmit EP, et al. Surgical treatment for unexplained severe pain of the thyroid gland: report of three cases and concise review of the literature. Case Rep Med 2011;2011:349756.
31. Mok VM, Oltmann SC, Chen H, et al. Identifying predictors of a difficult thyroidectomy. J Surg Res 2014;190(1):157–63.
32. Chiang FY, Wang LF, Huang YF, et al. Recurrent laryngeal nerve palsy after thyroidectomy with routine identification of the recurrent laryngeal nerve. Surgery 2005;137(3):342–7.
33. Burkey SH, van Heerden JA, Thompson GB, et al. Reexploration for symptomatic hematomas after cervical exploration. Surgery 2001;130(6):914–20.
34. Bergamaschi R, Becouarn G, Ronceray J, et al. Morbidity of thyroid surgery. Am J Surg 1998;176(1):71–5.
35. Lo CY. Parathyroid autotransplantation during thyroidectomy. ANZ J Surg 2002;72(12):902–7.
36. Ross DS, Burch HB, Cooper DS, et al. 2016 American Thyroid Association guidelines for diagnosis and management of hyperthyroidism and other causes of thyrotoxicosis. Thyroid 2016;26(10):1343–421.

37. Schussler-Fiorenza CM, Bruns CM, Chen H. The surgical management of Graves' disease. J Surg Res 2006;133(2):207–14.
38. Girgis CM, Champion BL, Wall JR. Current concepts in Graves' disease. Ther Adv Endocrinol Metab 2011;2(3):135–44.
39. Manji N, Carr-Smith JD, Boelaert K, et al. Influences of age, gender, smoking, and family history on autoimmune thyroid disease phenotype. J Clin Endocrinol Metab 2006;91(12):4873–80.
40. Franklyn JA, Boelaert K. Thyrotoxicosis. Lancet 2012;379(9821):1155–66.
41. Brand OJ, Gough SC. Genetics of thyroid autoimmunity and the role of the TSHR. Mol Cell Endocrinol 2010;322(1–2):135–43.
42. Wang Z, Zhang Q, Lu J, et al. Identification of outer membrane porin f protein of Yersinia enterocolitica recognized by antithyrotopin receptor antibodies in Graves' disease and determination of its epitope using mass spectrometry and bioinformatics tools. J Clin Endocrinol Metab 2010;95(8):4012–20.
43. Wiersinga WM, Bartalena L. Epidemiology and prevention of Graves' ophthalmopathy. Thyroid 2002;12(10):855–60.
44. Wartofsky L, Glinoer D, Solomon B, et al. Differences and similarities in the diagnosis and treatment of Graves' disease in Europe, Japan, and the United States. Thyroid 1991;1(2):129–35.
45. Glinoer D, Hesch D, Lagasse R, et al. The management of hyperthyroidism due to Graves' disease in Europe in 1986. Results of an international survey. Acta Endocrinol Suppl (Copenh) 1987;285:3–23.
46. Emiliano AB, Governale L, Parks M, et al. Shifts in propylthiouracil and methimazole prescribing practices: antithyroid drug use in the United States from 1991 to 2008. J Clin Endocrinol Metab 2010;95(5):2227–33.
47. Abraham P, Avenell A, Park CM, et al. A systematic review of drug therapy for Graves' hyperthyroidism. Eur J Endocrinol 2005;153(4):489–98.
48. Solomon B, Glinoer D, Lagasse R, et al. Current trends in the management of Graves' disease. J Clin Endocrinol Metab 1990;70(6):1518–24.
49. Levetan C, Wartofsky L. A clinical guide to the management of Graves' disease with radioactive iodine. Endocr Pract 1995;1(3):205–12.
50. Rivkees SA, Sklar C, Freemark M. The management of Graves' disease in children, with special emphasis on radioiodine treatment. J Clin Endocrinol Metab 1998;83(11):3767–76.
51. Elfenbein DM, Schneider DF, Havlena J, et al. Clinical and socioeconomic factors influence treatment decisions in Graves' disease. Ann Surg Oncol 2015;22(4):1196–9.
52. Falk SA. Surgical treatment of hyperthyroidism. In: Falk SA, editor. Thyroid disease: endocrinology, surgery, nuclear medicine, andradiotherapy. Philadelphia: Lippincott-Raven; 1997. p. 319–40.
53. Alsanea O, Clark OH. Treatment of Graves' disease: the advantages of surgery. Endocrinol Metab Clin North Am 2000;29(2):321–37.
54. Kraimps JL, Bouin-Pineau MH, Mathonnet M, et al. Multicentre study of thyroid nodules in patients with Graves' disease. Br J Surg 2000;87(8):1111–3.
55. Mandel SJ, Cooper DS. The use of antithyroid drugs in pregnancy and lactation. J Clin Endocrinol Metab 2001;86(6):2354–9.
56. Masiukiewicz US, Burrow GN. Hyperthyroidism in pregnancy: diagnosis and treatment. Thyroid 1999;9(7):647–52.
57. Patwardhan NA, Moront M, Rao S, et al. Surgery still has a role in Graves' hyperthyroidism. Surgery 1993;114(6):1108–13.

58. Allahabadia A, Daykin J, Holder RL, et al. Age and gender predict the outcome of treatment for Graves' hyperthyroidism. J Clin Endocrinol Metab 2000;85(3):1038–42.
59. Lowery AJ, Kerin MJ. Graves' ophthalmopathy: the case for thyroid surgery. Surgeon 2009;7(5):290–6.
60. Grodski S, Stalberg P, Robinson BG, et al. Surgery versus radioiodine therapy as definitive management for graves' disease: the role of patient preference. Thyroid 2007;17(2):157–60.
61. Sosa JA, Mehta PJ, Wang TS, et al. A population-based study of outcomes from thyroidectomy in aging Americans: at what cost? J Am Coll Surg 2008;206(6):1097–105.
62. Barakate MS, Agarwal G, Reeve TS, et al. Total thyroidectomy is now the preferred option for the surgical management of Graves' disease. ANZ J Surg 2002;72(5):321–4.
63. Liu J, Bargren A, Schaefer S, et al. Total thyroidectomy: a safe and effective treatment for Graves' disease. J Surg Res 2011;168(1):1–4.
64. Palit TK, Miller CC, Miltenburg DM. The efficacy of thyroidectomy for Graves' disease: a meta-analysis. J Surg Res 2000;90(2):161–5.
65. Röher HD, Goretzki PE, Hellmann P, et al. Complications in thyroid surgery. Incidence and therapy. Chirurg 1999;70(9):999–1010.
66. Schneider DF, Mazeh H, Oltmann SC, et al. Novel thyroidectomy difficulty scale correlates with operative times. World J Surg 2014;38(8):1984–9.
67. Campbell MJ, McCoy KL, Shen WT, et al. A multi-institutional international study of risk factors for hematoma after thyroidectomy. Surgery 2013;154(6):1283–9 [discussion: 1289–91].
68. Abbas G, Dubner S, Heller KS. Re-operation for bleeding after thyroidectomy and parathyroidectomy. Head Neck 2001;23(7):544–6.
69. Kasuga Y, Sugenoya A, Kobayashi S, et al. Clinical evaluation of the response to surgical treatment of Graves' disease. Surg Gynecol Obstet 1990;170(4):327–30.
70. Sugrue D, McEvoy M, Feely J, et al. Hyperthyroidism in the land of Graves: results of treatment by surgery, radio-iodine and carbimazole in 837 cases. Q J Med 1980;49(193):51–61.
71. Randle RW, Bates MF, Long KL, et al. Impact of potassium iodide on thyroidectomy for Graves' disease: implications for safety and operative difficulty. Surgery 2018;163(1):68–72.
72. Sosa JA, Bowman HM, Tielsch JM, et al. The importance of surgeon experience for clinical and economic outcomes from thyroidectomy. Ann Surg 1998;228(3):320–30.

Diagnosis and Evaluation of Primary Hyperparathyroidism

Nikita N. Machado, MD[a,b], Scott M. Wilhelm, MD[c,*]

KEYWORDS

- Primary hyperparathyroidism • Epidemiology • Diagnosis • Parathyroid localization
- Surveillance

KEY POINTS

- Primary hyperparathyroidism (PHPT) is a biochemical diagnosis with hallmarks of hypercalcemia with an increased/inappropriately high (nonsuppressed) parathyroid hormone level.
- Although there are iatrogenic or environmental causes of PHPT (ionizing radiation, medications and so forth), the disease is mostly sporadic.
- Although rare, a genetic source of PHPT should be considering in the setting of young patients, aged less than 45 years, family history of PHPT or accompanying endocrine disorders, as well as multigland disease.
- Although preoperative imaging is helpful in preoperative planning, negative imaging does not preclude referral of patients for operative consideration.
- Parathyroidectomy remains the only established cure for PHPT.

INTRODUCTION AND EPIDEMIOLOGY

Primary hyperparathyroidism (PHPT) is a result of autonomous production of parathyroid hormone (PTH) from 1 or more abnormal parathyroid glands. The hallmarks of the diagnosis are hypercalcemia with an increased/inappropriately high (nonsuppressed) PTH level, although a small percentage of patients present with normocalcemia.[1]

Although the clinical presentations of this disease vary from subtle changes to disabling symptoms that affect patient quality of life, some patients have asymptomatic PHPT, without disease-specific symptoms.

Disclosure: The authors have nothing to disclose.
[a] Department of Surgery, University Hospitals Conneaut, Suite 203, 158 West Main Road, Conneaut, OH 44030, USA; [b] Case Western Reserve University, Cleveland, OH, USA; [c] Department of Surgery, Endocrine Surgery, Case Western Reserve University, University Hospitals Cleveland, 11100 Euclid Avenue, Cleveland, OH 44106, USA
* Corresponding author.
E-mail address: scott.wilhelm@uhhospitals.org
; @machado_nikita (N.N.M.)

Surg Clin N Am 99 (2019) 649–666
https://doi.org/10.1016/j.suc.2019.04.006 surgical.theclinics.com

PHPT is a common endocrine disorder, owing in part to a surge in incidental diagnoses from routine laboratory testing. Prevalence is thought to be 1 to 7 cases per 1000 adults, whereas the estimated incidence between 1998 and 2010 was approximately 50 per 100,000 person-years.[2,3] However, the disease still remains vastly underdiagnosed because of the large proportion of asymptomatic patients. The reported incidence is likely to be even higher.[4]

PHPT is more common in patients more than the age of 50 to 65 years, but can occur at any age, including childhood. There is a 2:1 to 3:1 preponderance of disease in women, which may in part be caused by menopause resulting in increased bone resorption, which can unmask parathyroid dysfunction.

Population studies have shown that the incidence of hyperparathyroidism is highest in the African American population, followed by white, Asian, Hispanic and other races.[3]

CAUSE

Although studies have assessed multiple possible causes for PHPT, most cases are sporadic. Genetic syndromes and prior radiation exposure account for a small number of cases. Factors known to be associated with the development of PHPT are listed here.

Iatrogenic/Environmental Causes

Radiation exposure

Head and neck irradiation has been associated with PHPT with a latency period from exposure to disease expression of about 20 to 40 years. This association was seen in populations with environmental radiation exposure such as Hiroshima [5] and the nuclear power plant accident in Chernobyl, as well as patients who received radiation for benign or malignant conditions (eg, acne, thymic irradiation for sudden infant death syndrome, or mantle irradiation for lymphoma).[6] The relative risk (RR) for the development of PHPT from radiation exposure is dose dependent, RR $\approx$ 5 to 10 at 1 Gy.[6] The probability of PHPT at this degree of exposure is still low, being less than 1% at 35 years and close to 5% at 50 years of follow-up. Studies have shown that prior radiation exposure does not increase the chance of parathyroid hyperplasia versus single-gland disease, and a minimally invasive operative approach is still an option.[7,8]

Radioactive iodine therapy

Although most case reports and case series suggest an association between radioactive iodine therapy for thyroid disease and the development of PHPT, it is still rare.[9]

Medication-associated primary hyperparathyroidism

Thiazides These diuretics reduce urinary calcium excretion and can cause mild hypercalcemia (up to 11.5 mg/dL). They are not a direct cause of PHPT but may unmask underlying PHPT, which is more likely when the hypercalcemia persists even after stopping the medication, or if the initial serum concentration is greater than 12 mg/dL.

Lithium This medication increases both total serum and ionized calcium levels as well as PTH levels within weeks, but they usually still remain within normal ranges. Lithium can also induce a persistent defect in calcium-PTH regulation resulting in a slightly increased PTH level and increase in gland volume despite normocalcemia.[10] This increase can be seen in up to 15% of long-term lithium users.[1]

Genetic/Chromosomal Abnormalities

Cells in abnormal parathyroid tissue tend to be monoclonal in adenomas and carcinomas. Abnormal proto-oncogenes and tumor suppressor genes form a basis for the development of parathyroid tumors. These abnormal genes include gain-of-function mutations (eg, cyclin D1/PRAD1 gene in sporadic tumors and rearranged during transfection [RET] in familial tumors) as well as loss-of-function tumors (multiple endocrine neoplasia type 1 [MEN-1] or CDC73 in sporadic and familial tumors).[11]

Familial hyperparathyroidism

Although these are rare causes of PHPT, the most common cause of familial hyperparathyroidism is MEN-1 syndrome. Other commonly associated conditions are familial isolated PHPT, familial hyperparathyroidism–jaw tumor syndrome and MEN-2A.

Multiple endocrine neoplasia type 1 This syndrome is inherited in an autosomal dominant (AD) fashion, with a prevalence of 2 to 3 per 100,000 and a predisposition for endocrine tumors of the pancreas, pituitary, and parathyroid glands. PHPT is the most common manifestation of MEN-1, seen in ~90% of patients by the age of 25 years, and essentially 100% by the age of 50 years. It presents as multigland hyperplasia, and is associated with the MEN-1 (menin) gene.[12]

Multiple endocrine neoplasia type 2A Inherited in an AD manner, this comprises an increased incidence of parathyroid tumors, pheochromocytoma, and medullary thyroid cancer. This syndrome usually presents in adulthood. PHPT occurs in 20% to 30% of cases. It is usually mild and asymptomatic, except for a small proportion of patients who may present with renal stones caused by hypercalciuria. Age of onset of PHPT in these patients is usually late 30s, long after the onset of medullary thyroid cancer. Gland involvement ranges from an adenoma to multigland hyperplasia. MEN-2A is associated with the RET proto-oncogene, localized on chromosome 10.[13]

Multiple endocrine neoplasia type 4 Initially identified as an autosomal recessive disorder in rats, MEN-4 was noted to be a mutation in the CDKN1B gene (encodes the cell cycle inhibitor p27). Affected animals developed multiple endocrine tumors, with overlapping features of MEN-1 and MEN-2. However, they did not show any mutations in MEN-1 or RET proto-oncogene.

This condition was later observed in patients who showed MEN-like phenotypes but were RET and MEN-1 negative. This condition was labeled MEN-4. More studies are being performed to better understand the syndrome and its phenotypic manifestations.[14]

Hyperparathyroidism–jaw tumor syndrome Initially described in 1958, it is inherited as an AD trait. Patients are affected by fibro-osseous tumors of the mandible and/or maxilla (ossifying fibromas), as well as Wilms tumor, papillary renal carcinoma, polycystic kidney disease, renal cysts, and PHPT. In greater than 95% of cases, PHPT is the first manifestation of the disease, with an aggressive behavior and a significantly higher incidence of parathyroid carcinoma (10%–15%). PHPT in these patients tends to be more aggressive, with severe hypercalcemia and possibly hypercalcemic crisis. This condition is associated with an altered function in the HRPT2 gene (which codes for the protein parafibromin).[15]

Familial isolated hyperparathyroidism Familial isolated hyperparathyroidism is a rare AD inherited disorder that presents with either single-gland or multigland disease, in the absence of other endocrine disorders. A variety of germline mutations have been observed in these patients (including MEN1, CaSR, and HRPT2).[16]

Some patients with presumed sporadic PHPT have a familial form of hyperparathyroidism. In a study of 86 younger patients (<45 years) with nonsyndromic PHPT, genetic testing showed mutations in susceptibility genes in 9.3% of cases (MEN1, calcium sensing receptor [CASR] and HRPT2).[17]

ROLE OF GENETIC TESTING

Because of the possibility of a genetic component in 10% to 15% cases of PHPT, certain triggers should result in further genetic evaluation. The algorithm presented later is a modification of the Consensus Statement of the Fourth International Workshop on Primary Hyperparathyroidism (**Fig. 1**).[13,18,19]

PARATHYROID INVOLVEMENT IN PRIMARY HYPERPARATHYROIDISM

The number of glands involved in PHPT is variable and can take several forms.

Adenoma

Single adenomas are the most common cause of PHPT (80%–85% of patients). Double adenomas may be found in up to 5%.[20,21] Double adenomas tend to occur in an embryologic fashion with both abnormal glands developing from the same branchial pouch.[22] Adenomas tend to be well encapsulated and are composed primarily of chief cells. A small subgroup is composed of oxyphil cells, which tend to be larger.

Glandular Hyperplasia

Multigland disease, involving all 4 parathyroid glands, is noted in 5% to 15% of cases of PHPT. It is more commonly seen in familial disorders like MEN-I or MEN-IIA or in familial HPT, but can be seen in PHPT.

Carcinoma

Parathyroid cancer represents the rarest cause of PHPT (1%). Severe hypercalcemia, PTH levels greater than 500 pg/ml, and patient age greater than 70 years may be preoperative clues to a diagnosis of parathyroid cancer. Cancer diagnosis is made intraoperatively, with the finding of local/extracapsular invasion as well as possible spread to lymph nodes. Distant metastases are rare.[23]

CLINICAL PRESENTATION OF PRIMARY HYPERPARATHYROIDISM

The most common manifestation of PHPT is asymptomatic hypercalcemia detected during routine biochemical testing. Patients are often diagnosed before the onset of the classic "bones, stones, abdominal moans, and psychic groans," which are more common in developing nations. These symptoms may overlap with those of hypercalcemia from other causes, which underscores the importance of definitive laboratory diagnosis.

In the United States, around 80% of cases are identified through biochemical screening. Most patients show stable calcium and PTH levels, although they can increase over time (<5% of cases). The mean serum concentration is less than 1 mg/dL

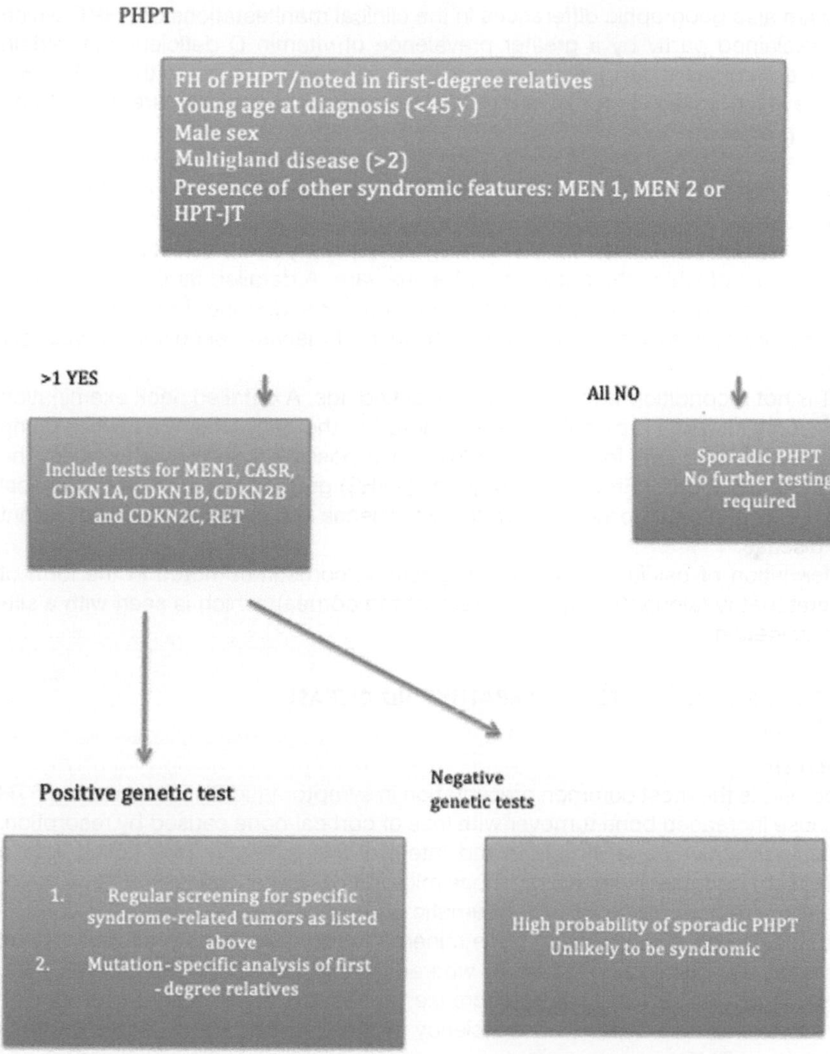

Fig. 1. Approach to genetic testing in patients with PHPT. FH, family history.

more than the upper limit of the normal range (8.5–10.5 mg/dL). Significantly higher calcium levels (around 15 mg/dL) should raise a strong suspicion of parathyroid carcinoma.

Of the patients that are considered to have asymptomatic PHPT, many admit to nonspecific symptoms such as fatigue, weakness, decreased appetite, mild depression, and cognitive slowing if carefully questioned.[24] These patients may or may not go on to develop classic symptoms of PHPT, including peptic ulcer disease, nephrocalcinosis, pathologic fractures, and clinical depression.

The signs and symptoms are a combination of the effects of increased PTH secretion as well as hypercalcemia. Both bone disease and nephrolithiasis are directly attributable to increased PTH levels, whereas anorexia, constipation, polydipsia, polyuria, and nausea are related more to hypercalcemia.

There are also geographic differences in the clinical manifestations of PHPT, which can be explained partly by a greater prevalence of vitamin D deficiency in certain regions. A concomitant deficiency in vitamin D is common in patients with PHPT. However, there is a predilection for severe clinical disease in countries where hypovitaminosis D is prevalent.

Studies show that patients with combined vitamin D deficiency and HPT have more clinically significant disease (including larger gland size, higher PTH concentration, increased osteoclastic activity, and a higher incidence of pathologic fractures).[25,26]

Evaluation of PHPT begins with a detailed patient history. Careful history taking may elicit symptoms of which the patient may be unaware. A detailed family and medication history, focusing on parathyroid disease and other endocrine disorders, may uncover a history suggestive of syndromic parathyroid disease, especially in younger patients.

PHPT is not a condition with classic physical findings. A detailed neck examination is often inconclusive. If a palpable mass is noted in the neck, it is worthwhile doing further evaluation to look for thyroid nodules or a possible parathyroid cancer. The American Association of Endocrine Surgeons (AAES) guidelines recommend cervical ultrasonography in order to localize parathyroid disease and to assess for concomitant thyroid disease.[1]

The formation of calcium phosphate deposits is sometimes noted in the form of band keratopathy (along the exposed areas of the cornea), which is seen with a slit-lamp examination.

SPECIFIC SYMPTOMS RELATED TO PARATHYROID DISEASE

Skeletal Symptoms

Osteoporosis

Osteoporosis is the most common presentation in symptomatic PHPT. Increased PTH levels cause increased bone turnover with loss of cortical bone caused by resorption. However, trabecular bone structure and integrity are generally maintained with a possible slight periosteal expansion. These microarchitectural changes in bone structure result in a higher propensity for traumatic and pathologic fractures.[27]

Most studies show a decreased bone mineral density (BMD) in cortical sites (long bone shafts; eg, distal radius, femur), whereas trabecular bone sites (pelvis, ribs, vertebrae, and skull) show a slight decrease or possibly an increase in BMD. The frequent coexistence of vitamin D deficiency in these patients may also contribute to a decreased BMD.

The World Health Organization defines osteopenia from a dual energy x-ray absorptiometry scan with a T score greater than 1.0 to 2.5 standard deviations (SD) less than the mean, whereas osteoporosis occurs when the BMD is more than 2.5 SD less than the mean.

Epidemiologic studies show that most patients have an increased risk of both spine and nonspine fractures in untreated patients even up to 10 years before the point of diagnosis.[28]

Fractures

The overall standardized fracture risk is significantly increased in patients with PHPT, with a 2-fold to 3-fold increase in the risk of vertebral, distal forearm, and pelvic fractures.

Some studies show an increased fracture risk.[29] This increased risk is slightly more complicated in postmenopausal women who are already at risk because of estrogen deficiency. In such patients, fracture risk may be caused by a multitude of factors.

The skeletal effects of normocalcemic PHPT, although not yet fully characterized, may be different from the hypercalcemic variant.[30]

Osteitis fibrosa cystica

This is now a rare event because most cases are diagnosed at a much earlier point in the clinical presentation.

The true incidence of osteitis fibrosa cystica is currently less than 5% of cases. It occurs more typically in patients with severe disease and those with parathyroid carcinoma.

It clinically manifests as bone pain and radiographically as subperiosteal bone resorption on the radial aspect of the middle phalanges, tapering of the distal clavicles and a so-called salt-and-pepper appearance of the skull, bone cysts, and brown tumors of the long bones.[31]

Brown tumors arise from increased osteoclastic activity and consist of collections of admixed osteoclasts and fibrous tissue with poorly mineralized woven bone. The brown discoloration arises from hemosiderin deposition.

Nephrolithiasis

At present, the most common complication of PHPT is nephrolithiasis, affecting 15% to 20% of newly diagnosed patients.[32,33] Nephrocalcinosis (deposition of calcium salts within the parenchyma of the kidney) is much less common, with an unclear incidence.

Most stones associated with PHPT tend to be calcium oxalate; however, a slightly alkaline urine may favor the precipitation of calcium phosphate stones. Other contributing factors include hypercalciuria, high animal protein intake, dehydration, and a high serum calcitriol concentration (caused by PTH stimulation of the renal hydroxylation of vitamin D).[34]

Neuromuscular Symptoms

Patients with PHPT often endorse easy fatigability and weakness. In patients who are more severely affected, symptoms can be improved after surgery, as shown by Chou and colleagues.[35] Larger-scale studies are pending at this time.

Neurocognitive Symptoms

The symptoms commonly associated with PHPT are lethargy, depressed mood, psychosis, decreased social interaction, as well as cognitive dysfunction. The prevalence of these symptoms is hard to estimate given their subjective nature as well as variations in the instruments used to assess their severity. There are several randomized trials that have shown benefit for parathyroidectomy to correct these symptoms, which many times the patients consider the most debilitating in their daily lives. Three randomized clinical trials showed neurocognitive benefits of surgery versus observation with varying response patterns.[36–38]

At present, AAES recommends parathyroidectomy for patients with neurocognitive and/or neuropsychiatric symptoms that are attributable to PHPT.

Cardiovascular

PHPT may be associated with hypertension, arrhythmias, ventricular hypertrophy, as well as vascular/valvular calcification, which has been shown to date in observational studies.[39,40] It is uncertain whether normocalcemic HPT has a similar cardiometabolic effect, although initial data suggest an association with hypertension.

Gastrointestinal

Gastrointestinal symptoms are less common; however, a thorough history in patients that seem to be asymptomatic may reveal a variety of complaints. The most common are constipation, heartburn, and loss of appetite (seen in 15%–30% of cases). Vague abdominal pain is seen in up to 30% of patients[41] and is thought to be caused by gut atony from sustained hypercalcemia.

There seems to be an association between PHPT and peptic ulcer disease; however, most studies on this subject were performed before the advent of proton pump inhibitors.

The incidence of acute pancreatitis in patients with PHPT ranges from 1% to 10% in retrospective series,[42] although this seems to be related more to hypercalcemia.

Parathyroid Crisis

Parathyroid crisis is a rare phenomenon, estimated at about 1% to 2% in long-term studies of untreated patients with mild PHPT.[43]

It is characterized by severe hypercalcemia (>15 mg/dL) and an increased incidence of central nervous system dysfunction.[44]

The mechanism for the development of parathyroid crisis is unknown but may be related to severe illness, volume depletion, or infarction of a parathyroid adenoma.[45]

NORMOCALCEMIC PRIMARY HYPERPARATHYROIDISM

In 2009, an international panel described a new phenotype of PHPT, characterized by normal serum calcium, and increased PTH levels. This diagnosis requires certain criteria to be met, including normal ionized calcium level and the absence of any secondary causes for hyperparathyroidism.[46]

A study by Lowe and colleagues[30] showed that 40% of the patients developed progressive hyperparathyroid disease during a period ranging from 1 to 8 years. Nineteen percent of these patients developed hypercalcemia eventually; however, a significant number of them developed worsening symptoms, including osteoporosis, kidney stones, and fractures despite persistent normocalcemia.

No studies to date show data regarding how many of these patients go on to become hypercalcemic if given a longer period of time. The understanding now is that this subset of patients is not simply an early form of PHPT but a unique phenotype of disease.

LABORATORY TESTING

The diagnosis of PHPT is a biochemical one.

A serum calcium level and PTH level are always required for the initial diagnosis. Given that patients with PHPT are usually hypercalcemic but occasionally have normal total/ionized calcium levels, multiple calcium measurements may be needed.

It is also important to correct for the serum albumin level.

$$\text{Corrected calcium} = \text{serum calcium} + 0.8 \times (4 - \text{serum albumin})$$

Vitamin D levels should be obtained as a part of the diagnostic work-up. This information is essential because a coexisting vitamin D deficiency may result in a lower serum calcium level, causing diagnostic uncertainty. It has also been observed that patients with PHPT with vitamin D deficiency seem to have a more severe disease presentation than those without.[47]

In the case of normocalcemic PHPT, an ionized calcium level is necessary to establish the diagnosis. Also, before confirming the diagnosis, all other causes of secondary increase of PTH level must be ruled out.

Hypercalcemia associated with nonparathyroid disorders is distinguished by a suppressed PTH level.

Differential Diagnosis for Primary Hyperparathyroidism

Discussion of secondary and tertiary hyperparathyroidism is beyond the scope of this article but must be entertained when establishing the diagnosis of PHPT.

Differential Diagnosis for Hypercalcemia

When attempting to diagnose a patient with PHPT, which is one of the most common causes of hypercalcemia, other common cause of hypercalcemia must be excluded:

1. Increased bone resorption: all types of HPT as well as thyrotoxicosis.
2. Increased calcium absorption: chronic kidney disease, milk-alkali syndrome, hypervitaminosis D.
3. Malignancy (primary bone tumors such as multiple myeloma; bony metastases from other primary tumors, such as breast, prostate) or hypercalcemia of malignancy that can lead to the production of PTH-related protein).
4. Familial hypocalciuric hypercalcemia (FHH): a 24-hour urinary calcium level is required to distinguish PHPT from FHH, which is an AD disorder of the renal CASR. This diagnosis should be considered in patients with long-standing hypercalcemia, urinary calcium level less than 100 mg/24 h, and a calcium/creatinine ratio less than 0.01 (detailed supplement in AAES guidelines).[1]The AAES strongly recommends obtaining both a 24-hour urinary calcium level and creatinine level in these patients.[1]
5. Miscellaneous causes: lithium, thiazides, pheochromocytoma, adrenal insufficiency, rhabdomyolysis, and theophylline toxicity.

Other Laboratory Abnormalities

Hypophosphatemia

Phosphate levels may be in the lower half of the normal range in most patients with mild forms of disease; however, they are significantly lower in severe PHPT because of increased phosphate excretion after proximal tubule reabsorption.

1,25-Dihydroxyvitamin D

Patients with PHPT convert more 25-hydroxyvitamin D to 1,25-dihydroxyvitamin D (ie, calcitriol) than the normal population, causing serum levels to be at the upper limits of normal or increased.

Magnesium levels

Magnesium excretion tends to be slightly increased, and a few patients have mild hypomagnesemia.

Anemia

A normocytic, normochromic anemia may be seen in severe cases of PHPT. This condition is thought to be caused by marrow fibrosis, at least in part, and responds to parathyroidectomy.[48]

Acid-base balance

The effect of PTH on decreasing proximal tubule bicarbonate absorption is counterbalanced by alkali liberation from osteoclastic activity in bone. Therefore, metabolic acidosis is unusual in patients with PHPT unless they have underlying renal disease or significantly high PTH levels.

LOCALIZATION STUDIES

Once the diagnosis of PHPT has been confirmed, there is a role for localization techniques in order to identify suitable candidates for a minimally invasive, targeted parathyroidectomy. Imaging studies are unnecessary to make the diagnosis, and can sometimes complicate decision making with false-positive or false-negative results. In addition, a negative localization test does not exclude/refute the diagnosis of PHPT. However, it should make clinicians more suspicious for multigland disease as the cause of PHPT.

In those cases in which patients are candidates for surgery but have negative/discordant imaging results, referral to a parathyroid surgeon for evaluation is appropriate.[1]

Localization studies are also of value in patients with persistent/recurrent disease, especially those who require a remedial exploration.[49]

The goal of localizing imaging, in conjunction with intraoperative PTH monitoring, is to minimize surgical dissection, reduce the risk of recurrent nerve injury, and to identify both coexisting thyroid disorder and ectopic parathyroid tissue, which would alter operative management.

The type of localization study performed depends also on the available radiologic expertise in the institution. The commonly used localization studies are discussed here.

Ultrasonography

One of the most commonly used modalities for localization, ultrasonography is highly sensitive in experienced hands and is noninvasive.

The study is operator dependent, as shown by the sensitivity for identification of enlarged parathyroid glands ranging from 72% to 89%.[50]

Many high-volume institutions strongly recommend surgeon-performed ultrasonography scans, and studies show a comparable degree of sensitivity for localizing adenomas compared with radiologist-performed ultrasonography scans (77%–87%).[51,52]

Ultrasonography is also able to identify concomitant thyroid disorder, an important advantage given that the incidence of associated thyroid disorder is about 20% to 30%.[53] This ability allows surgeons to perform preoperative fine-needle aspiration for tissue diagnosis, as well as the possible diagnosis of an intrathyroidal parathyroid adenoma.

Sestamibi Scintigraphy

Technetium-99m methoxyisobutylisonitrite (MIBI), or 99m-Tc sestamibi, was initially used for cardiac scintigraphy, in which it was noted to concentrate in parathyroid adenomas. The physiology behind this is a dual uptake in both the thyroid and parathyroid glands with residual retention in the oxyphilic parathyroid tissue.[54] Repeat planar images are obtained soon after injection and again at around 2 hours to identify areas of retained tracer.

A negative study does not rule out the diagnosis of PHPT, because false-negatives are seen in 12% to 25% of cases,[55] and this holds true especially for small glands in the superior position, as for those with a paucity of oxyphil cells.[56]

In addition, sestamibi scans can be misleading in the case of parathyroid hyperplasia, multiple adenomas, and underlying thyroid disease.

Significant thyroid disease can lead to both false-positive and false-negative scintigraphy.[57] Medications such as calcium channel blockers also induce a false-negative result in these tests, because of their interference with the uptake of isotope by parathyroid tissue.[58]

Scintigraphy alone provides little helpful anatomic detail, and therefore is sometimes combined with three-dimensional (3D) imaging (single-photon emission computed tomography [SPECT]), thyroid subtraction scans, or fusion with computed tomography (CT), as described here.[59]

Single-photon Emission Computed Tomography

Sestamibi- SPECT is a 3D sestamibi scan that provides higher-resolution imaging. These images show both the depth of the parathyroid glands and their relationship to thyroid tissue. They also help identify ectopic glands, which allows surgeons to adopt a minimally invasive approach.[60,61]

SPECT imaging reduces the risk of missing multiglandular disease compared with scintigraphy alone; however, there is still a possibility of unrecognized multiglandular disease (ranging from 7%-16%).[62] Therefore, most experts recommend the addition of routine intraoperative PTH monitoring and 4-gland exploration in cases that are not straightforward.

Single-photon Emission Computed Tomography and Computed Tomography Fusion

SPECT-CT also allows the ability to distinguish parathyroid adenomas from other anatomic landmarks more clearly.[63] A study evaluating 30 patients with multigland disease showed that SPECT-CT predicted the location of all abnormal glands in 46% of cases (compared with 37% for CT alone and 13% for SPECT alone).[59]

Subtraction Thyroid Scan

Despite the addition of SPECT, some abnormal parathyroid glands are not easily distinguished from other tissue. A subtraction thyroid scan can be obtained if needed by using dual radiotracers (dual-isotope scintigraphy).

It involves the use of technetium plus 123-I or 99m-Tc pertechnetate (thallium) to allow for selective imaging of the thyroid gland.

The physiologic basis for this is that 99m-Tc sestamibi (MIBI) shows the parathyroid gland, whereas thallium is taken up by both thyroid and parathyroid glands.[64] The technetium image is then subtracted from the thallium image to distinguish thyroid and parathyroid tissue. This technique can also be applied to 123-I.[65]

Four-dimensional Computed Tomography

These scans take advantage of rapid contrast uptake and washout by parathyroid adenomas in order to accurately localize the lesions. The primary issue with four-dimensional (4D) CT is the significantly higher radiation dose required for these images (>50-fold higher than sestamibi alone), which implies that they should be used with caution in younger patients. This issue is caused by the additional radiation leading to a cumulative age-dependent risk of developing thyroid cancer.[66]

The main role of 4D CT is in the reoperative setting when initial sestamibi imaging is negative. A study of 45 patients who had undergone a prior neck exploration showed that 4D CT had 88% sensitivity for abnormal parathyroid glands (compared with 54% for sestamibi SPECT and 21% for neck ultrasonography).[67]

MRI

MRI does not play a significant role in parathyroid imaging. MRI currently finds its role mostly in cases in which a noninvasive method is required without iodinated contrast or exposure to ionizing radiation (eg, during pregnancy).[68]

Parathyroid adenomas on MRI show intermediate to low signal intensity on T1 imaging and high intensity on T2 imaging. This pattern may prove confusing in the setting of enlarged cervical lymph nodes, which also have similar characteristics. The reported sensitivity of MRI for abnormal parathyroid tissue ranges from 40% to 85%.[69,70]

PET and Computed Tomography

The combination of 11C-methionine PET and CT uses 11C-methionine as a radiotracer to identify pathologic parathyroid glands.[71] A prospective study that included 102 patients undergoing parathyroidectomy for PHPT found that the methionine-PET-CT scan accurately localized single adenomas in 85% of patients, with a positive predictive value of 93%.[72]

Invasive Localization

Procedures such as selective venous or arterial sampling are reserved for those cases in which patients are undergoing reoperation for persistent PHPT, and all noninvasive imaging studies have been inconclusive. Procedural risks include contrast anaphylaxis, acute renal failure, groin hematoma from access sites, and stroke. These procedures require an experienced interventional radiologist and are not as commonly done now because of the vast improvement in scanning techniques.

Selective venous sampling

Selective venous sampling is the more commonly used invasive modality, and it shows a 1.5-fold to 2-fold increase in PTH levels obtained from representative cervical vein drainage locations (inferior, middle, superior thyroid, thymic, and vertebral veins) compared with peripheral veins in patients with PHPT.[73]

Selective arteriography

Selective arteriography is performed by combining selective transarterial hypocalcemic stimulation with nonselective venous sampling. Both baseline and timed superior vena cava samplings are taken after injection with sodium citrate to induce hypocalcemia. At the same time, arteriography is performed. The test is considered positive if the PTH level increases to 1.4 times the baseline or if a blush in noted on arteriography.[74]

WHEN IMAGING STUDIES ARE NEGATIVE

Nonlocalizing imaging studies should not preclude surgery, especially for patients with biochemically confirmed disease who meet operative criteria; this is a key point in the management of PHPT. Despite negative imaging, patients who meet biochemical criteria for PHPT and are symptomatic warrant referral to an endocrinologist or surgeon to determine whether they are candidates for parathyroidectomy. Because high-quality parathyroid imaging is generally a by-product of both an interest in the disease and case experience, the AAES guidelines have suggested that imaging should be deferred to an expert clinician to decide which imaging studies to perform based on the expert's knowledge of regional capabilities.

ROLE OF SURVEILLANCE IN PRIMARY HYPERPARATHYROIDISM

Patients with PHPT who are diagnosed incidentally and are asymptomatic or do not yet meet criteria for surgery can be monitored periodically for disease progression until they do. In addition, there may be patients who are poor surgical candidates who may be better served by observation and medical management of their hypercalcemia. Measurements of annual serum calcium level, creatinine level, and estimated glomerular filtration rate as well as bone density (hip, spine, and forearm) every 1 to 2 years is sufficient.[60] Although some studies recommend confirmation of the absence of nephrocalcinosis or silent nephrolithiasis (by ultrasonography or CT) at the time of initial evaluation, routine monitoring with serial imaging is not recommended.[75] However, if after initial evaluation patients develop symptoms consistent with development of renal stones, repeat imaging is indicated. Patients with asymptomatic normocalcemic PHPT can continue to be monitored similarly to their hypercalcemic counterparts.

INDICATIONS FOR PARATHYROIDECTOMY

Although the complete management of PHPT is beyond the scope of this article, the National Institutes of Health (NIH) consensus conference (last updated in 2013) makes note of certain groups of patients that may be referred for a parathyroidectomy. This recommendation pertains more to patients who are clinically asymptomatic (as discussed earlier with regard to presentation).

However, surgery may be offered to any patient with PHPT regardless of the presence of symptoms, because parathyroidectomy is the only definitive treatment of this disease (**Box 1**).

Although PHPT may or may not have an adverse effect on long-term mortality, it is likely that parathyroidectomy results in both subjective and objective benefits even in currently asymptomatic disease. Furthermore, at least a quarter of these patients eventually require surgery (even though no current accurate predictive model exists to identify those patients before the onset of complications).[76,77] The NIH consensus and AAES guidelines propose that patients with PHPT benefit from a symptomatic, metabolic, and survival standpoint after surgery, and referral to an experienced endocrine surgeon is appropriate.[78]

Box 1 **National Institutes of Health consensus conference recommendations**
Increased serum calcium level greater than 1 mg/dL above baseline
History of an episode of life-threatening hypercalcemia
Creatinine clearance reduced by 30% with age-matched normal patients
Markedly increased 24-hour urine calcium level (>400 mg/d)
Nephrolithiasis or nephrocalcinosis
Age less than 50 years
Osteitis fibrosa cystica
Osteoporosis (defined as bone mass >2 SD less than controls matched for age, gender, ethnic group)
Symptomatic disease

SUMMARY

PHPT is a common endocrine disorder that has a broad spectrum of disease presentation from asymptomatic to debilitating multiorgan disease. At present, surgical intervention is the only adequate treatment of this disease, which is seen in approximately 100,000 individuals each year. The diagnosis of the disease is biochemical and, once that diagnosis is made, referral to an appropriate expert for management and treatment is appropriate. Appropriate diagnosis along with preoperative imaging and the use of intraoperative parathyroid monitoring by an experienced surgeon can result in up to a 98% lifelong cure rate.

REFERENCES

1. Wilhelm SM, Wang TS, Ruan DT, et al. The American Association of Endocrine Surgeons guidelines for definitive management of primary hyperparathyroidism. JAMA Surg 2016;151(10):959–68.
2. Griebeler ML, Kearns AE, Ryu E, et al. Secular trends in the incidence of primary hyperparathyroidism over five decades (1965–2010). Bone 2015;73:1–7.
3. Yeh MW, Ituarte PHG, Zhou HC, et al. Incidence and prevalence of primary hyperparathyroidism in a racially mixed population. J Clin Endocrinol Metab 2013; 98(3):1122–9.
4. Dombrowsky A, Borg B, Xie R, et al. Why is hyperparathyroidism underdiagnosed and undertreated in older adults? Clin Med Insights Endocrinol Diabetes 2018; 11. 1179551418815916.
5. Fujiwara S, Sposto R, Ezaki H, et al. Hyperparathyroidism among atomic bomb survivors in Hiroshima. Radiat Res 1992;130(3):372–8. Available at: http://www.ncbi.nlm.nih.gov/pubmed/1594765. Accessed December 9, 2018.
6. Schneider AB, Gierlowski TC, Shore-Freedman E, et al. Dose-response relationships for radiation-induced hyperparathyroidism. J Clin Endocrinol Metab 1995; 80(1):254–7.
7. Tezelman S, Rodriguez JM, Shen W, et al. Primary hyperparathyroidism in patients who have received radiation therapy and in patients who have not received radiation therapy. J Am Coll Surg 1995;180(1):81–7. Available at: http://www.ncbi.nlm.nih.gov/pubmed/8000660. Accessed December 9, 2018.
8. Woll M, Sippel RS, Chen H. Does previous head and neck irradiation increase the chance of multigland disease in patients with hyperparathyroidism? Ann Surg Oncol 2011;18(8):2240–4.
9. Colaço SM, Si M, Reiff E, et al. Hyperparathyroidism after radioactive iodine therapy. Am J Surg 2007;194(3):323–7.
10. Mallette LE, Khouri K, Zengotita H, et al. Lithium treatment increases intact and midregion parathyroid hormone and parathyroid volume. J Clin Endocrinol Metab 1989;68(3):654–60.
11. Westin G, Björklund P, Akerström G. Molecular genetics of parathyroid disease. World J Surg 2009;33(11):2224–33.
12. Agarwal SK, Kester MB, Debelenko LV, et al. Germline mutations of the MEN1 gene in familial multiple endocrine neoplasia type 1 and related states. Hum Mol Genet 1997;6(7):1169–75. Available at: http://www.ncbi.nlm.nih.gov/pubmed/9215689. Accessed December 9, 2018.
13. Marini F, Cianferotti L, Giusti F, et al. Molecular genetics in primary hyperparathyroidism: The role of genetic tests in differential diagnosis, disease prevention strategy, and therapeutic planning. A 2017 update. Clin Cases Miner Bone Metab 2017;14(1):60–70.

14. Lee M, Pellegata NS. Multiple endocrine neoplasia type 4. Frontiers of hormone research, vol. 41, 2013. p. 63–78. https://doi.org/10.1159/000345670.
15. Marx SJ, Simonds WF, Agarwal SK, et al. Hyperparathyroidism in hereditary syndromes: special expressions and special managements. J Bone Miner Res 2002;17(Suppl 2):N37–43. Available at: http://www.ncbi.nlm.nih.gov/pubmed/12412776. Accessed December 9, 2018.
16. Simonds WF, Robbins CM, Agarwal SK, et al. Familial isolated hyperparathyroidism is rarely caused by germline mutation in HRPT2, the gene for the hyperparathyroidism-jaw tumor syndrome. J Clin Endocrinol Metab 2004;89(1):96–102.
17. Starker LF, Akerström T, Long WD, et al. Frequent germ-line mutations of the MEN1, CASR, and HRPT2/CDC73 genes in young patients with clinically nonfamilial primary hyperparathyroidism. Horm Cancer 2012;3(1–2):44–51.
18. Lakis M El, Nockel PJ, Guan B, et al. Discussion. J Am Coll Surg 2017;225(1):75–6.
19. Eastell R, Brandi ML, Costa AG, et al. Diagnosis of asymptomatic primary hyperparathyroidism: proceedings of the fourth international workshop. J Clin Endocrinol Metab 2014;99(10):3570–9.
20. Bartsch D, Nies C, Hasse C, et al. Clinical and surgical aspects of double adenoma in patients with primary hyperparathyroidism. Br J Surg 1995;82(7):926–9. Available at: http://www.ncbi.nlm.nih.gov/pubmed/7648110. Accessed December 9, 2018.
21. Ruda JM, Hollenbeak CS, Stack BC. A systematic review of the diagnosis and treatment of primary hyperparathyroidism from 1995 to 2003. Otolaryngol Head Neck Surg 2005;132(3):359–72.
22. Tezelman S, Shen W, Shaver JK, et al. Double parathyroid adenomas. Clinical and biochemical characteristics before and after parathyroidectomy. Ann Surg 1993;218(3):300–7 [discussion: 307–9]. Available at: http://www.ncbi.nlm.nih.gov/pubmed/8103983. Accessed December 9, 2018.
23. Wynne AG, van Heerden J, Carney JA, et al. Parathyroid carcinoma: clinical and pathologic features in 43 patients. Medicine 1992;71(4):197–205. Available at: http://www.ncbi.nlm.nih.gov/pubmed/1518393. Accessed December 9, 2018.
24. Clark OH. "Asymptomatic" primary hyperparathyroidism: is parathyroidectomy indicated? Surgery 1994;116(6):947–53.
25. Nuti R, Merlotti D, Gennari L. Vitamin D deficiency and primary hyperparathyroidism. J Endocrinol Invest 2011;34(7 Suppl):45–9. Available at: http://www.ncbi.nlm.nih.gov/pubmed/21985980. Accessed December 9, 2018.
26. Minisola S, Pepe J, Scillitani A, et al. Explaining geographical variation in the presentation of primary hyperparathyroidism. Lancet Diabetes Endocrinol 2016;4(8):641–3.
27. Mazzuoli GF, D'Erasmo E, Pisani D. Primary hyperparathyroidism and osteoporosis. Aging (Milano) 1998;10(3):225–31. Available at: http://www.ncbi.nlm.nih.gov/pubmed/9801732. Accessed December 9, 2018.
28. Mosekilde L. Primary hyperparathyroidism and the skeleton. Clin Endocrinol (Oxf) 2008;69(1):1–19.
29. Khosla S, Melton J. Fracture risk in primary hyperparathyroidism. J Bone Miner Res 2002;17(Suppl 2):N103–7. Available at: http://www.ncbi.nlm.nih.gov/pubmed/12412786. Accessed December 9, 2018.
30. Lowe H, McMahon DJ, Rubin MR, et al. Normocalcemic primary hyperparathyroidism: further characterization of a new clinical phenotype. J Clin Endocrinol Metab 2007;92(8):3001–5.

31. Misiorowski W, Czajka-Oraniec I, Kochman M, et al. Osteitis fibrosa cystica—a forgotten radiological feature of primary hyperparathyroidism. Endocrine 2017; 58(2):380–5.
32. Parks J, Coe F, Favus M. Hyperparathyroidism in nephrolithiasis. Arch Intern Med 1980;140(11):1479–81. Available at: http://www.ncbi.nlm.nih.gov/pubmed/7436644. Accessed December 9, 2018.
33. Peacock M. Primary hyperparathyroidism and the kidney: biochemical and clinical spectrum. J Bone Miner Res 2002;17(Suppl 2):N87–94. Available at: http://www.ncbi.nlm.nih.gov/pubmed/12412783. Accessed December 9, 2018.
34. Silverberg SJ, Shane E, Jacobs TP, et al. Nephrolithiasis and bone involvement in primary hyperparathyroidism. Am J Med 1990;89(3):327–34. Available at: http://www.ncbi.nlm.nih.gov/pubmed/2393037. Accessed December 9, 2018.
35. Chou FF, Sheen-Chen SM, Leong CP. Neuromuscular recovery after parathyroidectomy in primary hyperparathyroidism. Surgery 1995;117(1):18–25. Available at: http://www.ncbi.nlm.nih.gov/pubmed/7809831. Accessed December 9, 2018.
36. Rao DS, Phillips ER, Divine GW, et al. Randomized controlled clinical trial of surgery *versus* no surgery in patients with mild asymptomatic primary hyperparathyroidism. J Clin Endocrinol Metab 2004;89(11):5415–22.
37. Ambrogini E, Cetani F, Cianferotti L, et al. Surgery or surveillance for mild asymptomatic primary hyperparathyroidism: a prospective, randomized clinical trial. J Clin Endocrinol Metab 2007;92(8):3114–21.
38. Sheldon DG, Lee FT, Neil NJ, et al. Surgical treatment of hyperparathyroidism improves health-related quality of life. Arch Surg 2002;137(9):1022–6 [discussion 1026–8]. Available at: http://www.ncbi.nlm.nih.gov/pubmed/12215152. Accessed December 9, 2018.
39. Walker MD, Silverberg SJ. Cardiovascular aspects of primary hyperparathyroidism. J Endocrinol Invest 2008;31(10):925–31.
40. Lind L, Hvarfner A, Palmér M, et al. Hypertension in primary hyperparathyroidism in relation to histopathology. Eur J Surg 1991;157(8):457–9. Available at: http://www.ncbi.nlm.nih.gov/pubmed/1681931. Accessed December 9, 2018.
41. Abboud B, Daher R, Boujaoude J. Digestive manifestations of parathyroid disorders. World J Gastroenterol 2011;17(36):4063–6.
42. Carnaille B, Oudar C, Pattou F, et al. Pancreatitis and primary hyperparathyroidism: forty cases. Aust N Z J Surg 1998;68(2):117–9. http://www.ncbi.nlm.nih.gov/pubmed/9494002. Accessed December 9, 2018.
43. Corlew DS, Bryda SL, Bradley EL, et al. Observations on the course of untreated primary hyperparathyroidism. Surgery 1985;98(6):1064–71. Available at: http://www.ncbi.nlm.nih.gov/pubmed/3878002. Accessed December 9, 2018.
44. Bondeson AG, Bondeson L, Thompson NW. Clinicopathological peculiarities in parathyroid disease with hypercalcaemic crisis. Eur J Surg 1993;159(11–12):613–7. Available at: http://www.ncbi.nlm.nih.gov/pubmed/8130303. Accessed December 9, 2018.
45. Fitzpatrick LA, Bilezikian JP. Acute primary hyperparathyroidism. Am J Med 1987;82(2):275–82. Available at: http://www.ncbi.nlm.nih.gov/pubmed/3812520. Accessed December 9, 2018.
46. Manuscript A, Hyperparathyroidism NP. NIH Public Access. 2014;16(1):33–9.
47. Silverberg SJ. Vitamin D deficiency and primary hyperparathyroidism. J Bone Miner Res 2007;22(S2):V100–4.
48. Boxer M, Ellman L, Geller R, et al. Anemia in primary hyperparathyroidism. Arch Intern Med 1977;137(5):588–93. Available at: http://www.ncbi.nlm.nih.gov/pubmed/857757. Accessed December 9, 2018.

49. Silverberg SJ, Fuleihan GE, Rosen CJ. Official reprint from UpToDate ® www.uptodate.com ©2018 UpToDate, Inc. and/or its affiliates. All Rights Reserved. Preoperative localization for parathyroid surgery in patients with primary hyperparathyroidism. 2018:1–19.
50. Haber RS, Kim CK, Inabnet WB. Ultrasonography for preoperative localization of enlarged parathyroid glands in primary hyperparathyroidism: comparison with (99m)technetium sestamibi scintigraphy. Clin Endocrinol (Oxf) 2002;57(2): 241–9. Available at: http://www.ncbi.nlm.nih.gov/pubmed/12153604. Accessed December 9, 2018.
51. Solorzano CC, Carneiro-Pla DM, Irvin GL. Surgeon-performed ultrasonography as the initial and only localizing study in sporadic primary hyperparathyroidism. J Am Coll Surg 2006;202(1):18–24.
52. Siperstein A, Berber E, Barbosa GF, et al. Predicting the success of limited exploration for primary hyperparathyroidism using ultrasound, sestamibi, and intraoperative parathyroid hormone: analysis of 1158 cases. Ann Surg 2008;248(3): 420–8.
53. Bentrem DJ, Angelos P, Talamonti MS, et al. Is preoperative investigation of the thyroid justified in patients undergoing parathyroidectomy for hyperparathyroidism? Thyroid 2002;12(12):1109–12.
54. Palestro CJ, Tomas MB, Tronco GG. Radionuclide imaging of the parathyroid glands. Semin Nucl Med 2005;35(4):266–76.
55. Chiu B, Sturgeon C, Angelos P. What is the link between nonlocalizing sestamibi scans, multigland disease, and persistent hypercalcemia? A study of 401 consecutive patients undergoing parathyroidectomy. Surgery 2006;140(3): 418–22.
56. Stephen AE, Roth SI, Fardo DW, et al. Predictors of an accurate preoperative sestamibi scan for single-gland parathyroid adenomas. Arch Surg 2007;142(4): 381–6. Available at: http://www.ncbi.nlm.nih.gov/pubmed/17441292. Accessed December 9, 2018.
57. Gómez-Ramírez J, Sancho-Insenser JJ, Pereira JA, et al. Impact of thyroid nodular disease on 99mTc-sestamibi scintigraphy in patients with primary hyperparathyroidism. Langenbecks Arch Surg 2010;395(7):929–33.
58. Friedman K, Somervell H, Patel P, et al. Effect of calcium channel blockers on the sensitivity of preoperative 99mTc-MIBI SPECT for hyperparathyroidism. Surgery 2004;136(6):1199–204.
59. Wimmer G, Profanter C, Kovacs P, et al. CT-MIBI-SPECT image fusion predicts multiglandular disease in hyperparathyroidism. Langenbecks Arch Surg 2010; 395(1):73–80.
60. Pappu S, Donovan P, Cheng D, et al. Sestamibi scans are not all created equally. Arch Surg 2005;140(4):383–6. Available at: http://www.ncbi.nlm.nih.gov/pubmed/15841562. Accessed December 9, 2018.
61. Schachter PP, Issa N, Shimonov M, et al. Early, postinjection MIBI-SPECT as the only preoperative localizing study for minimally invasive parathyroidectomy. Arch Surg 2004;139(4):433–7.
62. Sharma J, Mazzaglia P, Milas M, et al. Radionuclide imaging for hyperparathyroidism (HPT): which is the best technetium-99m sestamibi modality? Surgery 2006;140(6):856–63 [discussion: 863–5].
63. Lavely WC, Goetze S, Friedman KP, et al. Comparison of SPECT/CT, SPECT, and planar imaging with single- and dual-phase (99m)Tc-sestamibi parathyroid scintigraphy. J Nucl Med 2007;48(7):1084–9.

64. Singh N, Krishna BA. Role of radionuclide scintigraphy in the detection of parathyroid adenoma. Indian J Cancer 2007;44(1):12–6. Available at: http://www.ncbi.nlm.nih.gov/pubmed/17401219. Accessed December 9, 2018.
65. McBiles M, Lambert AT, Cote MG, et al. Sestamibi parathyroid imaging. Semin Nucl Med 1995;25(3):221–34. Available at: http://www.ncbi.nlm.nih.gov/pubmed/7570042. Accessed December 9, 2018.
66. Mahajan A, Starker LF, Ghita M, et al. Parathyroid four-dimensional computed tomography: evaluation of radiation dose exposure during preoperative localization of parathyroid tumors in primary hyperparathyroidism. World J Surg 2012;36(6):1335–9.
67. Mortenson MM, Evans DB, Lee JE, et al. Parathyroid exploration in the reoperative neck: improved preoperative localization with 4D-computed tomography. J Am Coll Surg 2008;206(5):888–95 [discussion: 895–6].
68. Gotway MB, Reddy GP, Webb WR, et al. Comparison between MR imaging and 99mTc MIBI scintigraphy in the evaluation of recurrent of persistent hyperparathyroidism. Radiology 2001;218(3):783–90.
69. Lopez Hänninen E, Vogl TJ, Steinmüller T, et al. Preoperative contrast-enhanced MRI of the parathyroid glands in hyperparathyroidism. Invest Radiol 2000;35(7):426–30. Available at: http://www.ncbi.nlm.nih.gov/pubmed/10901104. Accessed December 9, 2018.
70. Wakamatsu H, Noguchi S, Yamashita H, et al. Parathyroid scintigraphy with 99mTc-MIBI and 123I subtraction: a comparison with magnetic resonance imaging and ultrasonography. Nucl Med Commun 2003;24(7):755–62.
71. Weber T, Cammerer G, Schick C, et al. C-11 methionine positron emission tomography/computed tomography localizes parathyroid adenomas in primary hyperparathyroidism. Horm Metab Res 2010;42(3):209–14.
72. Weber T, Maier-Funk C, Ohlhauser D, et al. Accurate preoperative localization of parathyroid adenomas with C-11 methionine PET/CT. Ann Surg 2013;257(6):1124–8.
73. Lebastchi AH, Aruny JE, Donovan PI, et al. Real-time super selective venous sampling in remedial parathyroid surgery. J Am Coll Surg 2015;220(6):994–1000.
74. Powell AC, Alexander HR, Chang R, et al. Reoperation for parathyroid adenoma: a contemporary experience. Surgery 2009;146(6):1144–55.
75. Mollerup CL, Vestergaard P, Frøkjaer VG, et al. Risk of renal stone events in primary hyperparathyroidism before and after parathyroid surgery: controlled retrospective follow up study. BMJ 2002;325(7368):807. Available at: http://www.ncbi.nlm.nih.gov/pubmed/12376441. Accessed December 9, 2018.
76. Silverberg SJ, Shane E, Jacobs TP, et al. A 10-year prospective study of primary hyperparathyroidism with or without parathyroid surgery. N Engl J Med 1999;341(17):1249–55.
77. Lafferty FW, Hubay CA. Primary hyperparathyroidism. Arch Intern Med 1989;149(4):789.
78. Bilezikian JP, Brandi ML, Eastell R, et al. Guidelines for the management of asymptomatic primary hyperparathyroidism: summary statement from the Fourth International Workshop. J Clin Endocrinol Metab 2014;99(10):3561–9.

Who Benefits from Treatment of Primary Hyperparathyroidism?

Catherine Y. Zhu, MD*, Dalena T. Nguyen, MPH,
Michael W. Yeh, MD

KEYWORDS

- Asymptomatic primary hyperparathyroidism • Parathyroidectomy
- Parathyroid hormone • Endocrine • Hypercalcemia

KEY POINTS

- Parathyroidectomy (PTx) is the most effective treatment for patients with primary hyperparathyroidism (PHPT), but commonly underutilized.
- Emerging evidence suggests asymptomatic patients treated with PTx benefit from fracture risk reduction, regardless of whether consensus criteria are met.
- PTx is a safe surgical procedure and is a cost effective treatment option.
- PHPT is frequently undiagnosed in patients with hypercalcemia, and subsequently undertreated.
- Currently, it is uncertain whether PTx confers similar benefits in fracture risk reduction to patients with normocalcemic PHPT, and medical management may be more appropriate as first-line therapy.

INTRODUCTION

Primary hyperparathyroidism (PHPT) is a common endocrine disorder caused by excessive secretion of parathyroid hormone (PTH), either from a single parathyroid adenoma (80% of cases) or from multigland hyperplasia (15%–20% of cases).[1] PHPT is characterized by hypercalcemia and elevated or inappropriately normal levels of PTH, with highest prevalence found among women (3:1) and African American populations.[2,3] With the advent of the multichannel autoanalyzer in the 1970s and implementation of routine testing of calcium levels, the clinical presentation of PHPT has radically shifted from the symptomatic disease classically represented as "stones, bones, and psychiatric moans" to the diagnosis of an asymptomatic condition

Disclosure Statement: The authors have nothing to disclose.
Section of Endocrine Surgery, Department of Surgery, UCLA David Geffen School of Medicine, 10833 Le Conte Avenue, CHS 72-182, Los Angeles, CA 90095, USA
* Corresponding author.
E-mail address: CatherineZhu@mednet.ucla.edu

Surg Clin N Am 99 (2019) 667–679
https://doi.org/10.1016/j.suc.2019.04.007 **surgical.theclinics.com**
0039-6109/19/

triggered by incidentally discovered hypercalcemia. Accordingly, the incidence of PHPT has grown, with as much as a tripling in prevalence from 1995 to 2010 in some parts of the country.[2]

Although the biochemical features of classic PHPT (elevated serum calcium and elevated PTH) have been known for many decades, variants of PHPT, such as normohormonal and normocalcemic PHPT, have recently been gaining recognition. Patients with normohormonal PHPT have elevated serum calcium levels and inappropriately normal (ie, nonsuppressed) PTH levels. Patients with normocalcemic PHPT have normal serum calcium levels and elevated PTH levels detected after all causes of secondary hyperparathyroidism have been excluded. Although patients with normohormonal PHPT should be managed in the same manner as patients with classic PHPT, patients with the normohormonal variant often go unmonitored and are infrequently referred to surgery due to missed or delayed recognition of the diagnosis.[2] When left untreated, PHPT can insidiously manifest as hypercalciuria, nephrolithiasis, and loss of bone density, which may further progress into renal impairment and fragility fractures.[4–7] The natural history of normocalcemic PHPT, the most biochemically mild form of PHPT, remains to be defined at this time.

MANAGEMENT STRATEGIES

Parathyroidectomy remains the only definitive treatment for PHPT. Observation may be preferred for patients who are poor surgical candidates or those who refuse surgical treatment.[8,9] Surveillance guidelines suggest an annual assessment of serum calcium, serum creatinine, and estimated glomerular filtration rate; bone mineral density (BMD) with dual-energy X-ray absorptiometry (DXA) every 1 to 2 years; and vertebral fracture assessments and abdominal imaging for nephrolithiasis or nephrocalcinosis, if clinically suspected.

Some medications have been used for the purposes of normalizing serum calcium (cinacalcet) and urinary calcium excretion (hydrochlorothiazide) or increasing BMD to reduce fracture risk (hormone replacement therapy, bisphosphonates).[1,10–12] However, no single drug has the potential to deliver the outcomes equal to that of surgical treatment. Bisphosphonate treatment improves BMD but may not actually diminish fracture risk.[13] Cinacalcet decreases serum calcium and PTH levels, but appears to have no significant beneficial impact on BMD.[14]

In 1990, an international workshop acknowledged the rising incidence of PHPT, and invited a diverse panel of experts, including endocrinologists, surgeons, radiologists, epidemiologists, and primary health providers, to produce a set of criteria to determine when surgical treatment should be indicated.[15] Since its initial publication, the consensus statement for asymptomatic PHPT has undergone several revisions, in 2002, 2009, and 2013, incorporating new evidence-based recommendations with each iteration (**Table 1**).[8,16,17] In all versions, PTx is recommended in patients with severe hypercalcemia, osteoporosis, and for those 50 years old or younger.[8] However, PTx recommendation based on renal and skeletal criteria have undergone progressive modifications. Notably, the most recent recommendations included the presence of subclinical vertebral fractures, high-risk urinary biochemical stones, and renal imaging demonstrating nephrocalcinosis or nephrolithiasis as surgical criteria.

In comparison, the surgical criteria put forth by the American Association of Endocrine Surgeons (AAES) are less restrictive.[9] Unlike the Workshop statement, the AAES panel recommends consideration of neurocognitive symptoms attributable to PHPT or other nontraditional symptoms such as muscle weakness and abnormal sleep patterns when offering surgical intervention to patients.

Table 1
Consensus guidelines and subsequent revisions over time

Criterion Category	1990	2002	2008	2013
Ca^{2+} (>upper limit of normal)	1–1.6 mg/dL (0.25–0.4 mmol/L)	1.0 mg/dL (0.25 mmol/L)	1.0 mg/dL (0.25 mmol/L)	1.0 mg/dL (0.25 mmol/L)
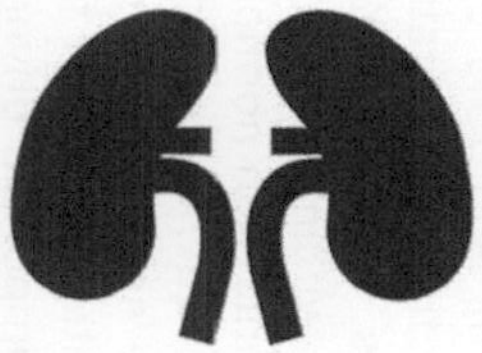	eGFR decreased >30% from expected 24-h urine calcium >400 mg/d (>10 mmol/d)	eGFR decreased >30% from expected. 24-h urine calcium >400 mg/d (>10 mmol/d)	eGFR <60 mL/min	Creatinine clearance <60 mL/min. 24-h urine calcium >400 mg/d (>10 mmol/d) and increased calcium-containing stone risk by complete stone risk profile. +Nephrolithiasis/nephrocalcinosis by radiograph, ultrasound, or CT
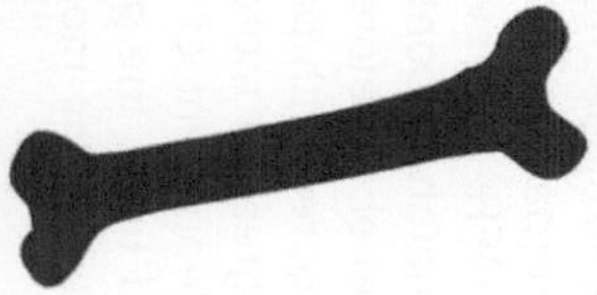	Z-score by DXA <−2.0, unspecified site	T-score by DXA <−2.5, any site	T-score by DXA <−2.5, any site + Previous fragility fracture	T-score by DXA <−2.5, lumbar spine, total hip, femoral neck, or distal radius + Vertebral fracture by radiograph, CT, MRI, or VFA
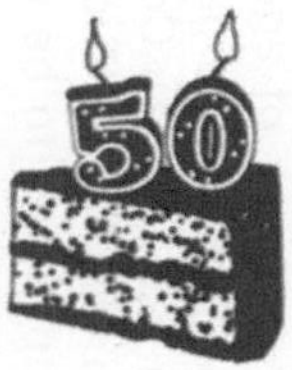	Age <50 y	Age <50 y	Age <50 y	Age <50 y

The most recent revision in 2013 recommended surgical treatment when imaging provided evidence of nephrolithiasis, nephrocalcinosis or vertebral fractures, which might otherwise be clinically silent.

Abbreviations: CT, computed tomography; DXA, dual-energy X-ray absorptiometry; eGFR, estimated glomerular filtration rate; MRI, magnetic resonance imaging; VFA, vertebral fracture assessment.

EFFECTS OF PRIMARY HYPERPARATHYROIDISM ON END-ORGAN SYSTEMS

The main organ systems classically affected by PHPT are the renal and skeletal systems. Nephrolithiasis is one of the most common sequelae of PHPT.[8] The percentage of patients with clinically apparent nephrolithiasis is approximately 20%, whereas only 9% of the general population is afflicted.[18–20] Data on clinically silent nephrolithiasis are limited, but in a recent study of 271 patients with surgically proven PHPT, renal sonograms revealed the presence of kidney stones in 7% of patients, fourfold greater than age-matched control patients without PHPT.[21] Even after surgical intervention, patients with PHPT have an increased risk for stone formation, as much as 27 times the risk, compared with controls, and this elevated risk profile may persist more than 10 years after surgery.[22] Hypercalciuria, defined variably as urinary calcium excretion exceeding 4 mg/kg per day or urinary calcium excretion exceeding 250 mg/d in women and 300 mg/d in men, is also a potential manifestation of PHPT and further increases the risk for kidney stones. Less commonly, renal features of PHPT manifest as nephrocalcinosis, a diffuse calcification of the renal parenchyma. Renal impairment has also long been associated with PHPT, such that one of the long-standing consensus criteria for PTx has been to recommend surgery in patients with renal dysfunction equivalent to chronic kidney disease stage 3.

Progressive bone loss and fragility fractures are feared consequences of this endocrine disorder. BMD assessment in patients with PHPT is essential, as diminished BMD confers an increased risk of fracture. Patients exhibit BMD decline with greater frequency at cortical bone sites, such as the distal third of the radius and the femoral neck. In the observation arm of a cohort of patients with PHPT followed for 15 years, BMD decreased in the distal radius and femoral neck in 35% and 10% of patients, respectively.[23] Although the distal radius is most commonly affected in PHPT, it is not as commonly tested, with only 45% of DXA scans evaluating the distal radius in patients with PHPT.[24] Thus, the true prevalence of osteopenia and osteoporosis in PHPT is likely underestimated.

Assadipour and colleagues[19] performed a population-level study of 9485 patients with PHPT to determine first, the proportion of patients with preexisting end-organ effects at the time of biochemical diagnosis, and second, the likelihood of progression to end-organ effects after establishment of the biochemical diagnosis; 35% of patients exhibited preexisting effects, of whom 59% had osteoporosis, 21% had nephrolithiasis, and 7% had hypercalciuria. In the remaining patients who did not present with end-organ effects, 29% ultimately progressed within 5 years. Of those who progressed, 36% developed osteoporosis. Half of the patients at initial diagnosis also had impaired renal function, defined as glomerular filtration rate (GFR) between 30 and 60 mL/min (those with GFR <30 at the time of diagnosis were excluded to avoid contamination of the cohort by patients with secondary hyperparathyroidism), and 15% of patients who progressed had a decrease in GFR. However, the interpretation of these data is limited by the lack of age-matched controls. Overall, 62% of the initial study cohort developed end-organ effects before or within 5 years of diagnosis, meeting criteria for PTx (**Fig. 1**). Compared with patients with normohormonal PHPT, patients with classic PHPT progressed more frequently to end-organ effects. Progression appeared to be independent of the severity of hypercalcemia. Rather, duration of disease appeared to be the greater risk factor for progression, suggesting life expectancy should be the more important driver of clinical decision-making.

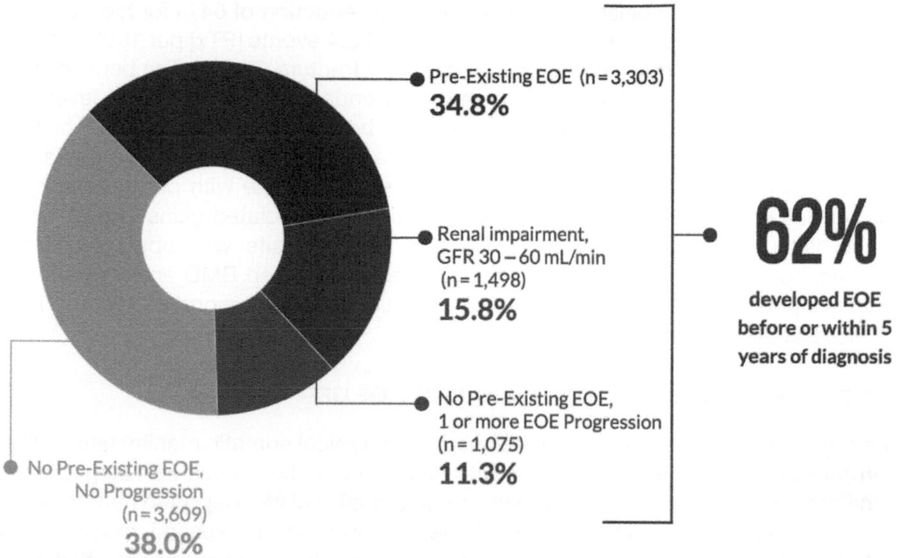

Fig. 1. End-organ effects (EOE) of PHPT at the time of biochemical diagnosis and progression over time. Thirty-five percent of patients have evidence of preexisting EOE at diagnosis. Sixteen percent of patients had preexisting or developed renal impairment within 5 years. Eleven percent of patients without preexisting EOE developed progression. Overall, 62% developed EOE before or within 5 years of diagnosis and meet criteria for PTx.

CLINICAL EFFECTIVENESS OF SURGICAL INTERVENTION

When considering definitive treatment for asymptomatic PHPT, clinicians and patients must weigh the benefits against the risks of surgery. In the hands of experienced surgeons, PTx delivers a high cure rate, with rates greater than 95% reported. High rates of cure are independent of operative technique.[25] Risks of complications are low with fewer than 1% of patients affected by each of persistent vocal cord paralysis, postoperative bleeding, postoperative infection, and permanent hypocalcemia.[25,26] Operative mortality in PTx for PHPT is exceedingly low. The risk for failed parathyroidectomy requiring reoperation is approximately 2%.[27]

Parathyroidectomy confers many benefits for patients who have both end-organ manifestations of the disease and mild asymptomatic disease at diagnosis. One of the major beneficial effects of PTx in the kidney is the reduction of stone formation. PTx decreases stone recurrence in patients with preoperative stone events.[28] Randomized controlled trials have also demonstrated decreased incidence of nephrolithiasis in patients with asymptomatic PHPT when treated with PTx compared with medical observation.[29,30] PTx may also diminish the progression of renal impairment after surgery,[31] although supporting data are limited.

For patients who choose not to undergo surgery or cannot tolerate an operation due to medical comorbidities, clinicians commonly turn to medical treatment with bisphosphonates to mitigate the effects of PHPT on the skeletal system. However, a retrospective analysis of 6272 patients with PHPT demonstrated that although PTx was associated with reduced fracture risk compared with patients who were observed, bisphosphonate treatment was associated with increased fracture risk.[13] This finding regarding bisphosphonates must be interpreted with caution because the prevalence of osteoporosis was higher among bisphosphate-treated patients in this study. PTx was associated with a relative risk reduction of 64% for hip fractures (55.9 fracture events [observation] compared with 20.4 events [PTx] per 1000 patients at 10 years) and 24% relative risk reduction for any fracture (**Fig. 2**). The beneficial effect of PTx on fracture risk was observed independent of baseline BMD level and whether patients satisfied consensus criteria. In both the PTx and bisphosphonate treatment arms, transient increases in BMD were observed, followed by decreasing trends in BMD over time in all treatment groups, compatible with progressive age-related BMD decline. Interestingly, although the PTx-associated gains in BMD were concordant with a reduction in fracture risk, the opposite was observed in the bisphosphonate treatment group. This discordance between BMD and fracture risk supports prior studies suggesting that BMD gains with antiresorptive therapy may not accurately reflect fracture risk.[32]

EFFECT OF PARATHYROIDECTOMY ON QUALITY OF LIFE

Although renal and skeletal manifestations are the typical somatic manifestations that warrant surgical intervention, patients with PHPT frequently consult with surgeons for significant concerns of diminished health-related quality of life. Reported neuropsychiatric disturbances typically include fatigue, drowsiness, depressed mood, sleep disturbance, and cognitive dysfunction. For decades, clinicians have noticed these ailments afflicting their patients with greater frequency than the general population, and recent studies have supported this finding. The argument has been made that most patients with "asymptomatic" PHPT are hardly asymptomatic at all, once neuropsychiatric complaints are considered.[33,34] In a prospective multicenter study, preoperative rates of moderate and severe depression, anxiety, and suicidal ideation, established by validated psychological tests, were found to be higher in patients with PHPT compared with controls.[35] At 12-month follow-up, PTx reduced these psychiatric disturbances. Postoperatively, patients were noted to have improvement in both physical and mental health scores, an effect that was not seen in the control group. Pasieka and colleagues[36] followed quality-of-life measures in patients with PHPT who had undergone PTx and control patients who had undergone

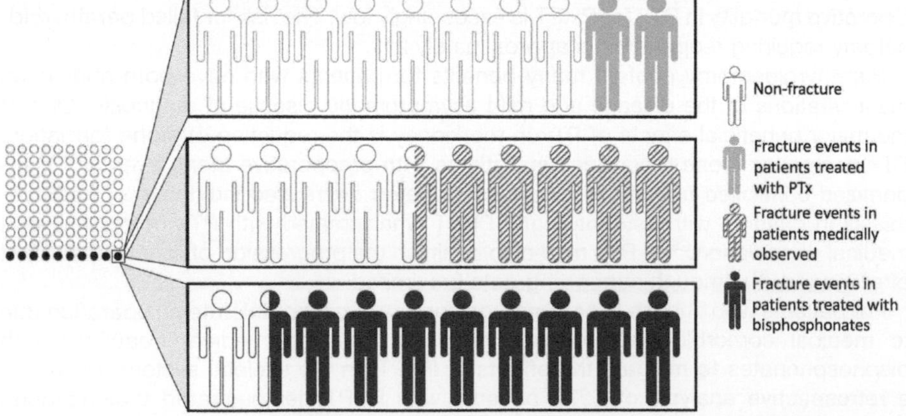

Fig. 2. Risk reduction for hip fractures. In patients followed for fracture over 10 years, the absolute risk for hip fracture was 20.4 events per 1000 patients who had parathyroidectomy (*blue*), 55.9 events per 1000 patients who were observed (*striped*), and 85.5 events per 1000 patients treated with bisphosphonates (*red*).

thyroidectomy over a period of 10 years. Although the patients with PHPT demonstrated higher rates of subjective complaints preoperatively, after surgery there was no difference in symptoms between the PTx group and control group. This effect was sustained at 10 years, indicating a long-lasting benefit of PTx.

The various iterations of the International Workshop statement have not included these neuropsychiatric symptoms as part of their indications for intervention, citing inconsistencies in the reported improvements after surgery and subsequent unpredictability in determining who would benefit from PTx.[8] However, it is the recommendation of the AAES guidelines to offer surgical intervention to patients who present with these symptoms on the basis of several randomized control trials that did demonstrate a benefit in surgery over observation.[29,37,38]

PARATHYROIDECTOMY IS COST-EFFECTIVE

Several reports have evaluated the cost-effectiveness of PTx in patients with asymptomatic PHPT. These studies have focused on patients who do not meet consensus criteria for surgery, typically patients age $\geq$50 with biochemically mild disease (serum calcium <1 mg/dL above normal).

Zanocco and colleagues[39] performed a cost-effectiveness analysis comparing observation, pharmacologic management with calcimimetics, and surgical management for patients with PHPT who do not meet consensus indications for PTx. In this report, PTx was found to be more cost-effective than competing strategies by a narrow margin. Of note, the analysis was based on the assumption that PTx provides an improvement in health-related quality of life in patients with otherwise asymptomatic PHPT. Observation was found to be the least costly, but also least effective. Finally, treatment with cinacalcet was not found to be cost-effective. A 10-year follow-up horizon was assumed for this analysis, based on an observational study by Silverberg and colleagues,[40] which found progression of disease in one-fourth of asymptomatic patients within 10 years.

The age criterion of younger than 50 years for surgical candidacy has remained unchanged throughout all iterations of the Workshop statement, despite limited evidence to support it.[41] When considering age at diagnosis in cost-effectiveness analysis, PTx remains a cost-effective strategy for patients with asymptomatic PHPT at ages well beyond 50.[42] Assuming an otherwise healthy patient with no prior history of neck surgery, outpatient PTx is cost-effective in patients with a predicted life expectancy of 5 years, and inpatient PTx is cost-effective in patients with a predicted life expectancy of 6.5 years. In elderly patients with asymptomatic PHPT who are good operative candidates and have at least 5 years of life expectancy, PTx should be recommended. Conversely, medical observation is more cost-effective for patients with short life expectancy. Thus in our practice, we consider biological age and perioperative risk factors more than chronologic age.

A revised analysis was performed by Zanocco and colleagues[43] in 2016, incorporating fracture risk reduction into the model. The investigators reported an estimated cost of $6487 for PTx associated with an effectiveness of 17.54 quality-adjusted life years (QALYs). In comparison, observation was $1721 more costly than PTx and resulted in a loss of 0.19 QALYs (**Fig. 3**). This revised cost-effectiveness analysis identified PTx as the dominant strategy for patients younger than 70 years. The investigators concluded that operative management at the time of diagnosis should be the recommendation, as it simultaneously increased quality-adjusted life expectancy while decreasing costs in comparison with observation.

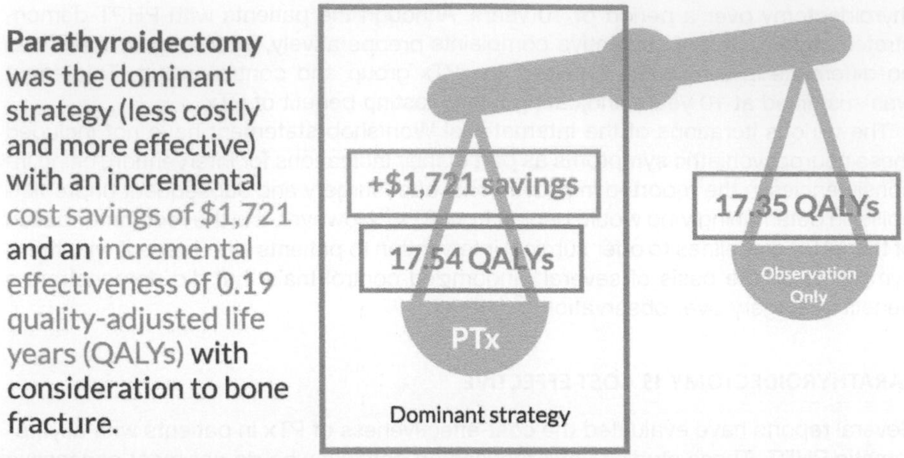
Parathyroidectomy was the dominant strategy (less costly and more effective) with an incremental cost savings of $1,721 and an incremental effectiveness of 0.19 quality-adjusted life years (QALYs) with consideration to bone fracture.
+$1,721 savings
17.54 QALYs
PTx
17.35 QALYs
Observation Only
Dominant strategy

Fig. 3. Cost-effectiveness of PTx compared with observation, when incorporating fracture risk reduction into analysis model.

PRIMARY HYPERPARATHYROIDISM IS UNDERDIAGNOSED AND UNDERTREATED

The path that leads patients with PHPT to appropriate treatment first hinges on correct identification and diagnosis of the disorder. PHPT likely accounts for the vast majority of instances of chronic hypercalcemia seen in routine laboratory testing.[2] In a study of 15,234 patients with at least 2 documented high serum calcium levels, 87% of patients were subsequently found to have normal or high PTH levels (**Fig. 4**). Thus, it is critical that evaluation for PHPT be part of the standard workup for hypercalcemia. Several population-based studies have reported on the incomplete workup of hypercalcemia and subsequent underdiagnosis of PHPT.[44,45] Press and colleagues[44] performed a review of the electronic medical record of all patients with hypercalcemia within the Cleveland Clinic primary care system over a period of 2 years, finding only 32% of patients had PTH levels measured.

Nearly 30 years have passed since the publication of consensus criteria to help clinicians determine when PTx may be appropriate; however, recent studies have demonstrated that PHPT is an undertreated condition despite the presence of these

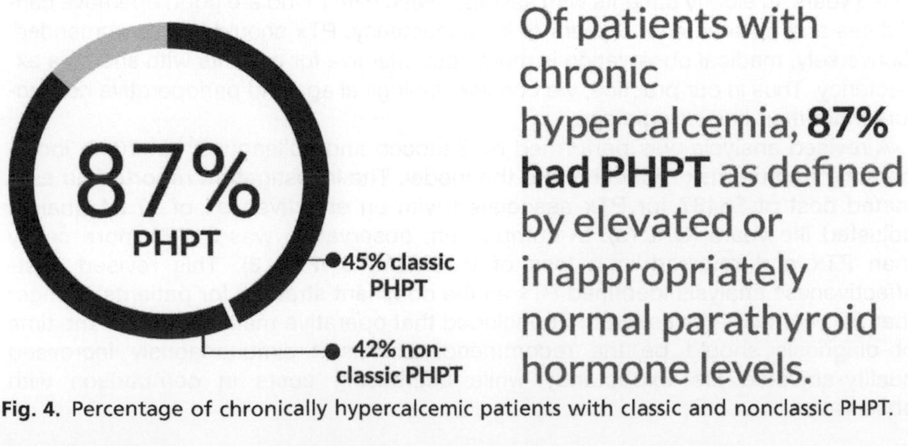
87%
PHPT
45% classic PHPT
42% non-classic PHPT
Of patients with chronic hypercalcemia, 87% had PHPT as defined by elevated or inappropriately normal parathyroid hormone levels.

Fig. 4. Percentage of chronically hypercalcemic patients with classic and nonclassic PHPT.

guidelines. In a study of a community-based patient population of 3388 patients with PHPT, only 28% were treated with PTx.[46] Although all symptomatic patients are recommended to receive curative treatment, only 51% of the symptomatic cohort underwent PTx in this study. Furthermore, fewer than half of asymptomatic patients who met at least one consensus criterion underwent surgery. The low rate of surgery was not explained by preoperative risk factors, as most patients had no significant comorbidities. The guidelines did appear to influence the decision for surgery on asymptomatic patients, because patients who met at least 1 criterion were twice as likely to undergo PTx compared with those who met none.

A similar study was then performed on an academic health system, with the hypothesis that adherence to consensus recommendations may be greater in this environment.[47] The findings did not support this premise: although 40% of patients satisfied 1 or more criteria, only 17% underwent surgery, suggesting that the rate of adherence to the consensus recommendations was no better at the academic health care system level than in community-based practice. The investigators noted that patients evaluated by an endocrinologist were more likely to be referred for surgery, but fewer than half of patients were seen by endocrinologists.

The inappropriate use of localization studies to select patients for surgery represents yet another barrier to surgical treatment. Wu and colleagues[48] found that a negative sestamibi scan resulted in a reduction in surgical referrals and a reduction in frequency of operation, even after evaluation by a surgeon. This improper usage of the sestamibi scan as a diagnostic tool is an independent negative predictor of PTx, even in symptomatic patients. Multigland disease, small parathyroid adenomas, and concomitant thyroid disease are all potential contributors to a negative scan.[49] The sestamibi scan sees its greatest benefit in reoperative cases and patients with ectopic glands. Its use should be limited to the role of preoperative localization and should not influence the referring physician's decision to make a surgical referral or a surgeon's decision to operate.

The previously mentioned points demonstrate multiple opportunities in which we might educate clinicians in the diagnosis and treatment of PHPT. For patients who have an abnormal serum calcium greater than 10.5 mg/dL, a repeat level should be obtained to verify the abnormal result. A second elevated serum calcium should then prompt a biochemical evaluation for PHPT and BMD testing if PHPT is confirmed. In addition to the consensus criteria, other factors, such as quality-of-life indicators, perioperative risk factors, and patient life expectancy, should be considered when making the decision for surgery. Finally, negative imaging should not deter physicians from surgical referral or intervention.

MANAGEMENT OF NORMOCALCEMIC PRIMARY HYPERPARATHYROIDISM

The 2009 revision of the consensus statement by the Third International Workshop formally recognized a new clinical phenotype, normocalcemic PHPT.[17] Current understanding of the clinical manifestations, rates of disease progression, and health outcomes of normocalcemic PHPT remains in its infancy. It is uncertain whether patients who undergo PTx for normocalcemic PHPT are conferred the same benefit in fracture risk reduction. In studies of the biochemical outcomes of patients who are surgically treated for normocalcemic PHPT, persistently elevated PTH after surgery is common, affecting 25% to 46% of patients.[50,51] This phenomenon has been observed even after histologic confirmation of subtotal parathyroid resection. Only patients whose PTH levels normalize postoperatively appear to have BMD improvement.[51] Retrospective studies investigating normocalcemic PHPT are also subject to significant biases, such as ascertainment bias. Patients are not commonly identified with this diagnosis, as PTH is infrequently checked in the absence of hypercalcemia. At the current time, there are not sufficient data to make strong recommendations in the treatment of normocalcemic PHPT, and practices vary even at high-volume institutions.

IN SUMMARY: WHO BENEFITS FROM TREATMENT OF PRIMARY HYPERPARATHYROIDISM?

Patients who would most benefit from PTx are those who would avoid an adverse health outcome related to PHPT while experiencing limited perioperative risk. No controversy exists for symptomatic patients (those with nephrolithiasis or overt skeletal symptoms), who should almost all undergo PTx. The area of debate surrounds identifying which patients with asymptomatic disease may benefit from PTx.

In this article, we have discussed how PTx improves BMD and reduces fracture risk in patients with PHPT. The fracture risk reduction is observed not only in patients with osteoporosis, but also in patients with osteopenia. Furthermore, patients who underwent PTx experienced reduced fracture risk reduction regardless of whether they fulfilled consensus criteria for surgery. Approximately two-thirds of patients with PHPT exhibit end-organ effects either at the time of diagnosis or within 5 years. Last, although controversial, existing data suggest patients with otherwise clinically silent PHPT have diminished health-related quality of life relative to those without PHPT, which may improve after PTx. Given these considerations and the low perioperative risk associated with PTx, surgical treatment is the dominant management strategy when health-related quality of life is considered in cost-effectiveness analyses.

In summary, most patients with PHPT benefit from surgical treatment, whether or not they meet consensus criteria. Benefits due to fracture risk reduction, health-related quality-of-life improvements, and prevention/mitigation of disease progression have been recently demonstrated in the literature. Patients without significant medical comorbidities and with a reasonable life expectancy should be considered for curative treatment.

REFERENCES

1. Walker MD, Silverberg SJ. Primary hyperparathyroidism. Nat Rev Endocrinol 2017;14:115.
2. Yeh MW, Ituarte PH, Zhou HC, et al. Incidence and prevalence of primary hyperparathyroidism in a racially mixed population. J Clin Endocrinol Metab 2013;98(3):1122–9.
3. Gasser RW. Clinical aspects of primary hyperparathyroidism: clinical manifestations, diagnosis, and therapy. Wien Med Wochenschr 2013;163(17–18):397–402.
4. Rejnmark L, Vestergaard P, Mosekilde L. Nephrolithiasis and renal calcifications in primary hyperparathyroidism. J Clin Endocrinol Metab 2011;96(8):2377–85.
5. Viccica G, Cetani F, Vignali E, et al. Impact of vitamin D deficiency on the clinical and biochemical phenotype in women with sporadic primary hyperparathyroidism. Endocrine 2017;55(1):256–65.
6. Walker MD, Cong E, Lee JA, et al. Vitamin D in primary hyperparathyroidism: effects on clinical, biochemical, and densitometric presentation. J Clin Endocrinol Metab 2015;100(9):3443–51.
7. Yamashita H, Noguchi S, Uchino S, et al. Vitamin D status in Japanese patients with hyperparathyroidism: seasonal changes and effect on clinical presentation. World J Surg 2002;26(8):937–41.

8. Bilezikian JP, Brandi ML, Eastell R, et al. Guidelines for the management of asymptomatic primary hyperparathyroidism: summary statement from the Fourth International Workshop. J Clin Endocrinol Metab 2014;99(10):3561–9.
9. Wilhelm SM, Wang TS, Ruan DT, et al. The American Association of Endocrine Surgeons guidelines for definitive management of primary hyperparathyroidism. JAMA Surg 2016;151(10):959–68.
10. Grey AB, Stapleton JP, Evans MC, et al. Effect of hormone replacement therapy on bone mineral density in postmenopausal women with mild primary hyperparathyroidism. A randomized, controlled trial. Ann Intern Med 1996;125(5):360–8.
11. Marcocci C, Bollerslev J, Khan AA, et al. Medical management of primary hyperparathyroidism: proceedings of the fourth International Workshop on the Management of Asymptomatic Primary Hyperparathyroidism. J Clin Endocrinol Metab 2014;99(10):3607–18.
12. Tsvetov G, Hirsch D, Shimon I, et al. Thiazide treatment in primary hyperparathyroidism-a new indication for an old medication? J Clin Endocrinol Metab 2017;102(4):1270–6.
13. Yeh MW, Zhou H, Adams AL, et al. The relationship of parathyroidectomy and bisphosphonates with fracture risk in primary hyperparathyroidism: an observational study. Ann Intern Med 2016;164(11):715–23.
14. Peacock M, Bilezikian JP, Klassen PS, et al. Cinacalcet hydrochloride maintains long-term normocalcemia in patients with primary hyperparathyroidism. J Clin Endocrinol Metab 2005;90(1):135–41.
15. Diagnosis and management of asymptomatic primary hyperparathyroidism. National Institutes of Health Consensus Development Conference. October 29-31, 1990. Consens Statement 1990;8(7):1–18.
16. Bilezikian JP, Potts JT Jr, Fuleihan Gel H, et al. Summary statement from a workshop on asymptomatic primary hyperparathyroidism: a perspective for the 21st century. J Clin Endocrinol Metab 2002;87(12):5353–61.
17. Silverberg SJ, Lewiecki EM, Mosekilde L, et al. Presentation of asymptomatic primary hyperparathyroidism: proceedings of the third international workshop. J Clin Endocrinol Metab 2009;94(2):351–65.
18. Silverberg SJ, Shane E, Jacobs TP, et al. Nephrolithiasis and bone involvement in primary hyperparathyroidism. Am J Med 1990;89(3):327–34.
19. Assadipour Y, Zhou H, Kuo EJ, et al. End-organ effects of primary hyperparathyroidism: a population-based study. Surgery 2019;165(1):99–104.
20. Scales CD Jr, Smith AC, Hanley JM, et al. Prevalence of kidney stones in the United States. Eur Urol 2012;62(1):160–5.
21. Suh JM, Cronan JJ, Monchik JM. Primary hyperparathyroidism: is there an increased prevalence of renal stone disease? AJR Am J Roentgenol 2008;191(3):908–11.
22. Mollerup CL, Vestergaard P, Frøkjær VG, et al. Risk of renal stone events in primary hyperparathyroidism before and after parathyroid surgery: controlled retrospective follow up study. BMJ 2002;325(7368):807.
23. Rubin MR, Bilezikian JP, McMahon DJ, et al. The natural history of primary hyperparathyroidism with or without parathyroid surgery after 15 years. J Clin Endocrinol Metab 2008;93(9):3462–70.
24. Wood K, Dhital S, Chen H, et al. What is the utility of distal forearm DXA in primary hyperparathyroidism? Oncologist 2012;17(3):322–5.
25. Singh Ospina NM, Rodriguez-Gutierrez R, Maraka S, et al. Outcomes of parathyroidectomy in patients with primary hyperparathyroidism: a systematic review and meta-analysis. World J Surg 2016;40(10):2359–77.

26. van Heerden JA, Grant CS. Surgical treatment of primary hyperparathyroidism: an institutional perspective. World J Surg 1991;15(6):688–92.
27. Zheng F, Zhou H, Li N, et al. Skeletal effects of failed parathyroidectomy. Surgery 2018;163(1):17–21.
28. Deaconson TF, Wilson SD, Jacob L Jr. The effect of parathyroidectomy on the recurrence of nephrolithiasis. Surgery 1987;102(6):910–3.
29. Rao DS, Phillips ER, Divine GW, et al. Randomized controlled clinical trial of surgery versus no surgery in patients with mild asymptomatic primary hyperparathyroidism. J Clin Endocrinol Metab 2004;89(11):5415–22.
30. Bollerslev J, Jansson S, Mollerup CL, et al. Medical observation, compared with parathyroidectomy, for asymptomatic primary hyperparathyroidism: a prospective, randomized trial. J Clin Endocrinol Metab 2007;92(5):1687–92.
31. Nair CG, Babu M, Jacob P, et al. Renal dysfunction in primary hyperparathyroidism; effect of parathyroidectomy: a retrospective cohort study. Int J Surg 2016;36:383–7.
32. Cefalu CA. Is bone mineral density predictive of fracture risk reduction? Curr Med Res Opin 2004;20(3):341–9.
33. Chan AK, Duh QY, Katz MH, et al. Clinical manifestations of primary hyperparathyroidism before and after parathyroidectomy. A case-control study. Ann Surg 1995;222(3):402–14.
34. Eigelberger MS, Cheah WK, Ituarte PHG, et al. The NIH criteria for parathyroidectomy in asymptomatic primary hyperparathyroidism: are they too limited? Ann Surg 2004;239(4):528–35.
35. Weber T, Eberle J, Messelhäuser U, et al. Parathyroidectomy, elevated depression scores, and suicidal ideation in patients with primary hyperparathyroidism: results of a prospective multicenter study. JAMA Surg 2013;148(2):109–15.
36. Pasieka JL, Parsons L, Jones J. The long-term benefit of parathyroidectomy in primary hyperparathyroidism: a 10-year prospective surgical outcome study. Surgery 2009;146(6):1006–13.
37. Sheldon DG, Lee FT, Neil NJ, et al. Surgical treatment of hyperparathyroidism improves health-related quality of life. Arch Surg 2002;137(9):1022–8.
38. Ambrogini E, Cetani F, Cianferotti L, et al. Surgery or surveillance for mild asymptomatic primary hyperparathyroidism: a prospective, randomized clinical trial. J Clin Endocrinol Metab 2007;92(8):3114–21.
39. Zanocco K, Angelos P, Sturgeon C. Cost-effectiveness analysis of parathyroidectomy for asymptomatic primary hyperparathyroidism. Surgery 2006;140(6):874–82.
40. Silverberg SJ, Shane E, Jacobs TP, et al. A 10-year prospective study of primary hyperparathyroidism with or without parathyroid surgery. N Engl J Med 1999;341(17):1249–55.
41. Silverberg SJ, Brown I, Bilezikian JP. Age as a criterion for surgery in primary hyperparathyroidism. Am J Med 2002;113(8):681–4.
42. Zanocco K, Sturgeon C. How should age at diagnosis impact treatment strategy in asymptomatic primary hyperparathyroidism? A cost-effectiveness analysis. Surgery 2008;144(2):290–8.
43. Zanocco KA, Wu JX, Yeh MW. Parathyroidectomy for asymptomatic primary hyperparathyroidism: a revised cost-effectiveness analysis incorporating fracture risk reduction. Surgery 2017;161(1):16–24.
44. Press DM, Siperstein AE, Berber E, et al. The prevalence of undiagnosed and unrecognized primary hyperparathyroidism: a population-based analysis from the electronic medical record. Surgery 2013;154(6):1232–8.

45. Balentine CJ, Xie R, Kirklin JK, et al. Failure to diagnose hyperparathyroidism in 10,432 patients with hypercalcemia: opportunities for system-level intervention to increase surgical referrals and cure. Ann Surg 2017;266(4):632–40.
46. Yeh MW, Wiseman JE, Ituarte PHG, et al. Surgery for primary hyperparathyroidism: are the consensus guidelines being followed? Ann Surg 2012;255(6): 1179–83.
47. Kuo EJ, Al-Alusi MA, Du L, et al. Surgery for primary hyperparathyroidism: adherence to consensus guidelines in an academic health system. Ann Surg 2019; 269(1):158–62.
48. Wu S, Hwang SS, Haigh PI. Influence of a negative sestamibi scan on the decision for parathyroid operation by the endocrinologist and surgeon. Surgery 2017; 161(1):35–43.
49. Civelek AC, Ozalp E, Donovan P, et al. Prospective evaluation of delayed technetium-99m sestamibi SPECT scintigraphy for preoperative localization of primary hyperparathyroidism. Surgery 2002;131(2):149–57.
50. Wade TJ, Yen TWF, Amin AL, et al. Surgical management of normocalcemic primary hyperparathyroidism. World J Surg 2012;36(4):761–6.
51. Sho S, Kuo EJ, Chen AC, et al. Biochemical and skeletal outcomes of parathyroidectomy for normocalcemic (incipient) primary hyperparathyroidism. Ann Surg Oncol 2019;26(2):539–46.

Intraoperative Decision Making in Parathyroid Surgery

Dylan S. Jason, MD[a], Courtney J. Balentine, MD, MPH[a,b,*]

KEYWORDS

• Parathyroid gland • Parathyroid surgery • Decision making • Operation

KEY POINTS

- Variable anatomy of the parathyroid glands can complicate parathyroidectomy.
- A systematic and consistent approach to identifying ectopic parathyroids is essential to locating missing glands.
- Surgeons who wish to perform parathyroidectomy should be comfortable with the preoperative and intraoperative use of ultrasound because this can help guide surgery and localize missing glands.
- Management of secondary and familial hyperparathyroidism differs from primary disease.

INTRODUCTION

The operative management of hyperparathyroidism poses many challenges even to experienced surgeons. The purpose of this article is to guide surgeons through these difficult decisions that occur during parathyroidectomy for primary, secondary, and familial disease.[1,2]

NORMAL PARATHYROID ANATOMY

A normal parathyroid is approximately 3 mm × 3 mm × 3 mm (the size of a grain of rice) and yellow-brown in color. The gland typically weighs approximately 40 mg to 60 mg and is normally situated in the posterolateral capsule of the thyroid. Embryologically, the parathyroid glands are derived from the third and fourth pouches between the branchial arches that arise during the fourth to fifth weeks of development. The

Disclosure Statement: The authors have nothing to disclose.
[a] Department of Surgery, The University of Texas Southwestern Medical Center, 5323 Harry Hines Boulevard, E6.104B, Dallas, TX 75390, USA; [b] VA North Texas Health Care System, 4500 S Lancaster Rd, Dallas, TX 75216, USA
* Corresponding author. VA North Texas Health Care System, 4500 S Lancaster Rd, Dallas, TX 75216.
E-mail address: courtney.balentine@utsouthwestern.edu

Surg Clin N Am 99 (2019) 681–691
https://doi.org/10.1016/j.suc.2019.04.008
0039-6109/19/Published by Elsevier Inc.

upper glands arise from the lower or fourth pouch, whereas the lower glands develop from the higher or third pouch and descend lower into the neck as the embryo matures. Because the upper glands travel a shorter distance during embryologic development, they are more consistent in their location and usually are found near the intersection of the inferior thyroid artery and the recurrent laryngeal nerve (RLN) (**Fig. 1**). The lower parathyroid typically is found near the inferior pole of the thyroid or within the thyrothymic ligament (the parathyroid is derived from the dorsal portion of the third pouch, whereas the thymus develops from the ventral portion).

Common ectopic locations for superior parathyroid glands include above the level of the thyroid cartilage or in the retroesophageal or paraesophageal spaces, because these are the areas traversed during embryo maturation (**Fig. 2**). Due to its different embryologic origin, there is more variation in the ectopic location of an inferior gland. Lower glands can be found cranial to the superior pole of the thyroid, inside the carotid sheath, in the upper mediastinum/thymus, and even in the chest. Additionally, both superior and inferior parathyroid glands may be found within the thyroid.

The development of the parathyroid glands can illustrate why the ectopic glands appear in the location that they do. The inferior parathyroid arises from the third pharyngeal pouch and initially descends with the thymus thus their ectopic locations can be anywhere along the track of descent. The superior glands arise from the fourth pharyngeal pouch and have a much shorter length of descent. The RLN is the most important landmark in delineating the superior gland from the inferior. If a coronal plane is made along the path of the RLN, the superior gland would be located more dorsal and the inferior more ventral. The superior gland can be found deep in the neck in the retrophryngeal and retrolaryngeal space and even as deep as the posterior mediastinum. As discussed previously, above the inferior gland can be more variable in its ectopic locations because the descent of the thymus is anywhere from the angle of the mandible to the pericardium.

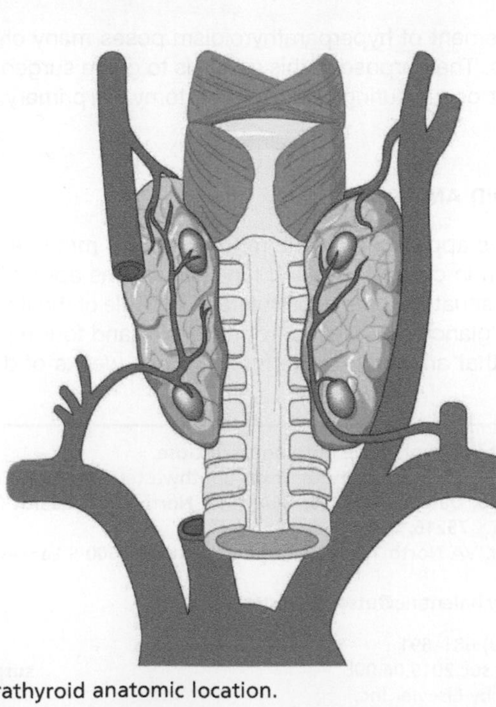

Fig. 1. Normal parathyroid anatomic location.

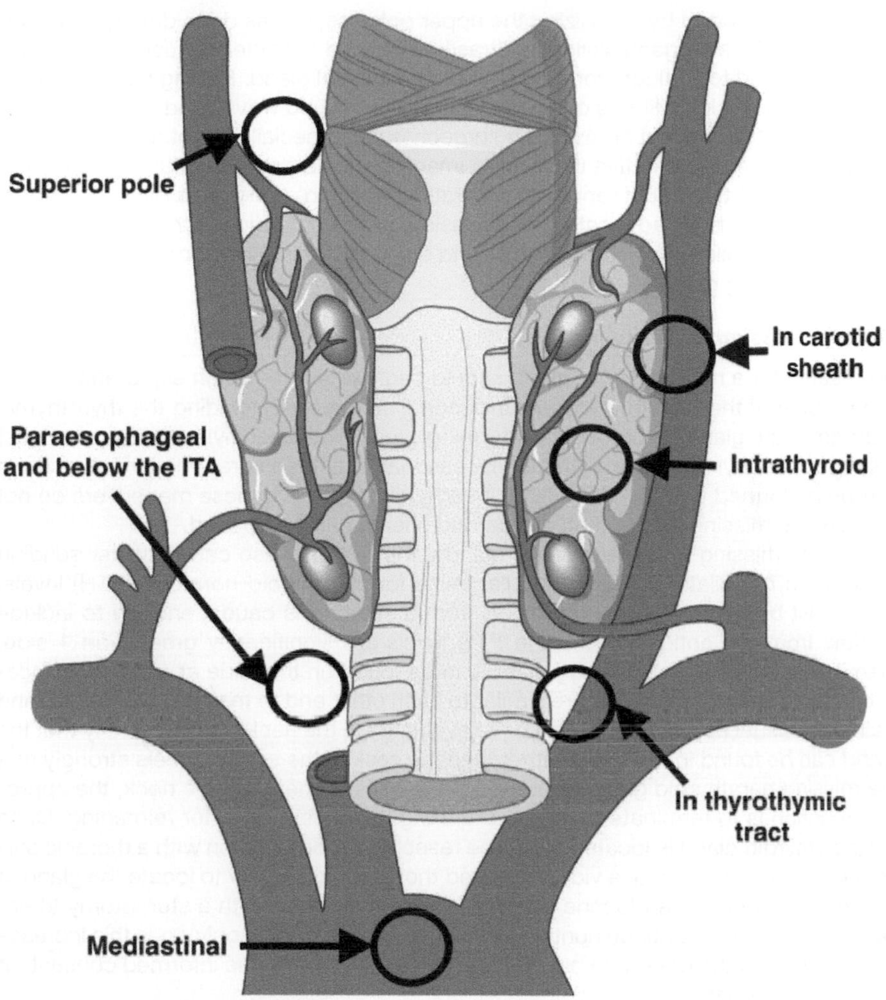

Fig. 2. Locations of ectopic parathyroid glands. ITA, inferior thyroid artery.

LOCATING AN ECTOPIC PARATHYROID

When searching for a missing parathyroid, it is important to make sure that the thyroid is fully mobilized from its surrounding soft tissue attachments so that an adequate view of the neck is obtained. It often may be found that a gland hiding on the true posterior surface of the thyroid can be found simply by doing a little more dissection so the gland can be fully rolled medially. Beyond these basic measures, it is important to follow a systematic approach for identifying an ectopic upper or lower gland.

Finding a Missing Upper Gland

A systematic search for an upper gland may begin by fully exploring the tracheoesophageal groove with palpation and by gently dissecting the tissue plane. The surgeon also should take care to check the retropharyngeal space and to make sure that the gland has not dropped below the inferior pole of the thyroid in a deeper than usual plane. The search for an undescended ectopic upper gland above the thyroid cartilage also may be assisted by mobilizing the upper pole vessels, as done during a thyroidectomy. Finally, a surgeon skilled in ultrasound should consider the use of intraoperative ultrasound to evaluate for a possible intrathyroidal gland. Putting some saline or water into the neck facilitates conduction of the ultrasound waves and makes it easier to explore all the relevant areas. If the surgeon is not especially adept at ultrasound, a re-review of the preoperative ultrasound imaging should prove helpful to see if there are any nodules that could represent a parathyroid gland. Although a blind lobectomy traditionally may been advocated for a missing gland not found in other locations, the absence of any likely targets on ultrasound suggests that a lobectomy likely will not yield the missing gland.

Finding a Missing Lower Gland

The search for a missing lower gland should begin with a thorough exploration of the inferior pole of the thyroid and the surrounding soft tissue, including the thyrothymic ligament. If the gland is not found, performing a formal cervical thymectomy (or at least pulling up the thymus for examination is reasonable) and an intraoperative ultrasound can be performed to see if there is an intrathyroidal gland. If these maneuvers do not uncover the missing gland, then the carotid sheath can be opened.

For both missing upper and lower glands, the surgeon also can consider sending blood from the bilateral internal jugular veins for parathyroid hormone (PTH) levels. Care must be taken to draw the blood from a site that is caudal enough to include outflow from the entire neck. If the PTH levels are significantly greater on 1 side, then it suggests that the missing gland can be found on that side at an ectopic location. If the bilateral PTH levels are similar to each other and to the peripheral level, and if all of the usual ectopic sites have been evaluated in the neck, then it is likely that the gland can be found in the chest rather than the neck. If the surgeon feels strongly that the missing parathyroid gland is located in the chest rather than the neck, the appropriate action is to terminate the case and bring the patient back for reimaging. Once the parathyroid gland is located, it can be resected in combination with a thoracic surgery colleague who can use video-assisted thorascopic surgery to locate the gland. It is imperative that the endocrine surgeon does not proceed with a sternotomy to access the chest and continue hunting for the missing gland. Not only does this increase the morbidity of the operation but also it is rarely included on the informed consent for parathyroid surgery.

The authors also emphasize that asking for help from a more experienced colleague should not be considered a source of shame and is preferable to continuing an increasingly frustrating dissection for an interminable period of time. A fresh set of eyes and a new set of fingers often can uncover a gland that is missed by the original surgeon, and having help from a colleague can spare a patient the morbidity of a prolonged operation and increasing destruction of surrounding tissue.

CONFIRMING THAT PARATHYROID TISSUE HAS BEEN RESECTED

Experienced surgeons typically are adept at identifying parathyroids by visual inspection alone, but there may be times when there is not complete certainty as to whether or not a piece of tissue is parathyroid (vs thyroid nodule, lymph node, and so forth). Although there is no role for routine frozen section to confirm tissue diagnosis, this modality may be helpful in cases of uncertainty.

If intraoperative PRH monitoring is available, the surgeon can aspirate some of the relevant tissue with a fine needle, mix the aspirate with saline, and send it to the laboratory for rapid analysis. A PRH level in the thousands confirms that the right tissue has been found. This technique generally is preferable to frozen section because it does not require resenting a piece of the gland and potentially impairing its function.

Some surgeons take advantage of the parathyroid glands' affinity for technetium Tc 99m (the same tracer used for sestamibi imaging) to confirm that parathyroid tissue is being removed. Patients are injected with technetium Tc 99m 1 hour to 2 hours prior surgery. Intraoperatively, a handheld gamma probe is held against the thyroid to establish a background or baseline level. When the surgeon is prepared to ligate the parathyroid pedicle or after the gland is removed, the probe can be held against the gland to check the gamma count. An ex vivo radiation count greater than 20% of the background signal is considered evidence of a parathyroid gland.[3] This method can be effective even in the setting of nonlocalizing preoperative imaging,[4] for hyperplastic glands,[5] and for ectopic glands.[6] The gamma probe is not necessarily helpful in finding a missing gland unless it is far enough away from the thyroid to avoid the noise of the background signal. This technique is helpful primarily to confirm that the resected tissue is parathyroid in origin.

MANAGING 4-GLAND HYPERPLASIA

A majority of parathyroid disease is due to a single adenoma, but surgeons still encounter patients with 4-gland hyperplasia. In these cases, it is important to remove all abnormal parathyroid tissue while leaving enough remnant parathyroid to maintain normal calcium homeostasis. If all glands are hyperplastic, then, depending on the relative size of each gland and the drop in intraoperative PTH levels (discussed later), the patient may undergo resection of 3 or 3.5 glands. Whenever a parathyroid gland is manipulated, there is the potential for temporary and permanent injury to that gland, and this is why clear identification of all 4 glands as well as care not to damage them during dissection is important. Consequently, it is important to balance the need for intraoperative cure with the risk of permanent postoperative hypocalcemia and hypoparathyroidism. In general, the smallest or least abnormal gland is selected to be the remnant, although there is some preference for choosing an inferior gland when possible. Importantly, the decision regarding which gland to leave and which glands to resect should be made only after all 4 glands are clearly identified, even though there may be a temptation to remove 1 or more glands that clearly appear abnormal. By waiting to resect parathyroids until after all glands are identified, the surgeon ensures that the remaining gland is the most normal appearing and also avoids missing an adenoma that appears in the setting of slightly plump-appearing glands that could be mistaken for hyperplasia.

If a surgeon decides that a 3.5-gland excision is needed, a clip is placed across the distal portion of the remnant gland before that segment of the gland is excised. It is important to understand where the pedicle is located for the gland so that this is preserved and only the distal portion is removed. The remnant may be tagged with a suture to aid in its identification if reoperation becomes necessary, but care must be taken not to disrupt the vascular supply. Typically, a remnant of approximately 30 mg to 50 mg of tissue is adequate to maintain calcium homeostasis. The creation of the remnant should be done prior to resecting any of the other glands so that the remnant can be examined to ensure it remains viable.

There are several potential options that can reduce the risk of permanent hypocalcemia after resection of 3 or 3.5 parathyroids. When the hospital has the capacity to cryopreserve resected parathyroid tissue, it may be helpful to save a fragment of each resected parathyroid for potential reimplantation. Alternately, if the hospital does not maintain cryopreservation facilities, it may be helpful to keep a fragment of each resected parathyroid on ice at the time of surgery and to check the change in intraoperative PTH levels. If the final level is detectable, then the fragments on ice can be either thrown away or sent to pathology. If the final level is not detectable and there is concern for permanent hypoparathyroidism, then the gland fragments can be reimplanted on the same day of surgery. This does not prevent temporary hypoparathyroidism but likely avoids a permanent hormone deficiency.

DETERMINING WHEN A PATIENT IS CURED

If a surgeon wishes to perform a unilateral (also called focused or minimally invasive) parathyroidectomy rather than a bilateral exploration, then utilizing intraoperative PRH monitoring is necessary to verify that the operation is complete and no abnormal glands remain. A common practice is to obtain a predissection level (preferably after induction of anesthesia and intubation) and then look for a drop in intraoperative PTH to confirm that all abnormal parathyroid tissue has been removed. PTH has a half-life of less than 5 minutes, which means that postexcision levels can be reliably checked in the operating room without undue extension of operative time.

There is significant variation in how surgeons approach the postresection timing and frequency for intraoperative PTH monitoring. Practices include a single check at 10 minutes to 15 minutes postexcision or after the trend by taking levels at 5 minutes, 10 minutes, and 15 minutes after excision. The authors' bias is to check multiple levels to observe the trend and avoid missing a rebound in PTH levels that signals an inadequate resection.[7,8]

There also is ongoing debate about what change in PTH level during surgery constitutes an intraoperative cure. Most surgeons either wait for a 50% drop in intraoperative PTH levels or they wait for a 50% drop and a normal/low normal value, although a mix of criteria have been proposed and tested.[9] Data on which strategy is superior remain somewhat murky, and surgeons need to balance the relative accuracy of different interpretive rules versus the rates of unnecessary bilateral exploration.[9,10]

Several randomized trials have demonstrated that a unilateral neck exploration guided by preoperative imaging and intraoperative PTH monitoring offers equivalent cure rates with fewer complications than routine bilateral neck exploration.[11] Retrospective studies from high-volume referral centers have suggested, however, that unilateral exploration frequently leaves behind abnormal glands that could eventually contribute to recurrence.[12] The difficulty in identifying the optimal strategy is complicated by relatively short follow-up times from randomized trials that would miss recurrence 10 years or more after surgery. Similarly, retrospective studies showing a higher incidence of abnormal glands found on bilateral compared with unilateral exploration do not definitively demonstrate that unilateral exploration leads to higher recurrence rates. Surgeons who look at 4 glands may find reasons to convince themselves to remove a borderline abnormal gland in addition to an obvious adenoma, but there is no way to demonstrate that the second gland was truly pathologic or that it eventually would become abnormal enough to cause recurrence.

Advocates of unilateral exploration argue that subsequent exploration of the contralateral side in the event of recurrence can be performed with minimal morbidity and that a vast majority of patients (>85% to 90%) experience a long-term cure with unilateral exploration. Advocates of routine bilateral exploration continue to argue that the only effective way to determine whether a gland is abnormal is to have it evaluated by an experienced surgeon and that complication rates for reoperative surgery are still higher than for the initial operation. In the absence of a trial with sufficient long-term follow-up that compares the 2 methods, this debate is likely to continue.[12–14]

MANAGING A DEVASCULARIZED NORMAL PARATHYROID GLAND

Due to their diminutive blood supply and fragile nature, it is remarkably easy to devascularize a normal parathyroid gland. Thus, the phrase, "to treat each parathyroid gland as carefully as if it were the last," was coined. If parathyroid function cannot be preserved, then the patient may suffer from permanent hypoparathyroidism, which would cause lifelong dependency on calcium and calcitriol supplementation. The most reliable method to preserve parathyroid function when it is noted that a normal parathyroid gland has been devascularized is autotransplantation,[15] and graft viability can exceed 90% when performed immediately.[16]

Once a gland appears devascularized, there are methods to determine if the gland may be viable. Piercing the capsule with a needle or incising the capsule with scissors or scalpel will, hopefully, illicit immediate brisk red oozing that indicates continued arterial profusion.[17] This should be done with caution, however, because the attempt to confirm perfusion may itself cause injury. If it is decided that parathyroid autotransplantation should be conducted, the surgeon should be confident that the tissue is indeed parathyroid. An experienced surgeon may be able to confidently identify the tissue, but if there is any concern, then any of the approaches, discussed previously, can be used.[18]

Some centers are also utilizing autofluorescence to determine gland viability. The most commonly used method is indocyanine green (ICG) angiography to detect vascular inflow into remnant parathyroids (or glands left behind after thyroidectomy). If there is concern for viability, 25 mg of ICG is injected and a measurement system is used (most commonly a pinpoint endoscopic system). The intensity of the color, which is determined by the viewing mode, correlates with the level of vascularization. The more intense the color, the better the blood flow. ICG has a half-life of 3 minutes to 4 minutes and can be redosed to a maximum safe dose of 5 mg/kg/d.[19] A recent randomized controlled trial using ICG angiography after thyroidectomy found that no patients with well-perfused parathyroid glands after thyroid surgery showed evidence of postoperative hypocalcemia and did not require calcium supplementation.[20]

An alternative approach uses laser speckle contrast imaging to assess parathyroid viability.[21] This approach relies on differences in the interference pattern of light on the surface of tissue with and without vascular inflow. A preliminary validation study demonstrated that viable and nonviable glands can be differentiated using a 785-nm light source in combination with a near-infrared camera to provide real-time feedback on a gland's perfusion status.[21]

These promising new techniques may help remove many of the subjective aspects of determining whether parathyroid glands are fully viable, and eliminate some uncertainty from intraoperative decision- making.

If the surgeon decides a gland is not viable and needs to be autotransplanted, there are several possible locations that could be used. The forearm is a reasonable site when there is concern for recurrence of hyperparathyroidism. Placing a gland in the forearm makes it easier to localize abnormal PTH production because levels adjacent to the implantation site can be compared with peripheral PTH levels to confirm localization. Removing the reimplanted tissue at a later date, however, is not a simple endeavor. Typically, the gland is minced and then inserted into the muscular tissue of the forearm after gentle creation of a pocket with blunt dissection. The implantation site is then closed with a silk suture and further marked with clips. Alternately, there is evidence that simply reimplanting the parathyroid into the subcutaneous tissue rather than muscle also results in a functional gland.[22]

Alternatively, the surgeon can reimplant the parathyroid into the chest muscle or subcutaneous tissue or into the sternocleidomastoid muscle using a similar technique as that discussed previously. The main disadvantage of using the neck for reimplantation is having to deal with scar tissue from the original neck operation if the disease recurs.

SECONDARY HYPERPARATHYROIDISM

Unlike with primary hyperparathyroidism, patients with renal failure develop hyperparathyroidism due to peripheral resistance to PTH. As a result, all 4 parathyroids (and any rests of parathyroid tissue in the thymus) begin to hypertrophy. The treatment of secondary hyperparathyroidism begins with medical management to control calcium, PTH, and phosphate levels.[23] When medical management fails or is not tolerated, then it is reasonable to proceed with parathyroidectomy.

Surgeons managing secondary hyperparathyroidism typically choose between 2 options: subtotal parathyroidectomy or total parathyroidectomy with reimplantation (although there are some advocates for total parathyroidectomy without autotransplantation). A subtotal resection may result in less severe postoperative hypocalcemia but carries a slightly higher risk of recurrence compared with total parathyroidectomy with autotransplantation.[24] Patients who receive total parathyroidectomy with autotransplantation require higher doses of calcium and calcitriol to manage the lack of PTH until the grafted tissue begins producing adequate amounts of hormone. Regardless of which procedure is chosen, a bilateral thymectomy is recommended to remove any rests of parathyroid, and patients need to be monitored for recurrence that increases over time.

FAMILIAL HYPERPARATHYROIDISM

Preoperative work-up of patients with possible genetic cause of their hyperparathyroidism should focus on the diagnosis of the type of genetic disorder. For patients with multiple endocrine neoplasia type 1, a subtotal parathyroidectomy or a total parathyroidectomy with reimplantation should be performed. Given the high rate of recurrence with this disease, it is important to resist the urge to resect only a single gland even if 1 gland appears significantly more abnormal than the others. Additionally, a thymectomy should be performed to remove any ectopic parathyroid tissue and the surgeon should consider cryopreserving parathyroid tissue in the event that reoperation renders the patient hypoparathyroid.

For patients with multiple endocrine neoplasia type 2A, a less aggressive approach is reasonable because hyperparathyroidism in this group tends to be milder than type 1 and may often be due to a single adenoma rather than hyperplasia.

PARATHYROID CANCER

Parathyroid a rare entity that accounts for less than 1% of operations for primary hyperparathyroidism.[25] Parathyroid cancer classically presents with a palpable gland in the setting of a markedly elevated calcium and PTH.[26] Cancer patients also are more likely to have had complications related to their hyperparathyroidism (kidney stones and bone disease) although up to 10% may be nonfunctioning.[27] Parathyroid carcinoma frequently has gross invasion of the thyroid and surrounding structures, and this may be visible on preoperative ultrasound along with an irregular border in the presence of abnormal lymph nodes. Fine-needle aspiration generally is not recommended because the features may be confused with thyroid neoplasms and could seed the biopsy tract.

Intraoperatively, any evidence of invasion into surrounding structures strongly suggests the presence of parathyroid cancer, as does discoloration (white or gray color) compared with a normal parathyroid. If the surgeon encounters a parathyroid carcinoma, the treatment is en bloc resection while avoiding disruption of the tumor capsule. There is some debate over the role for prophylactic central neck dissection and removal of the ipsilateral remaining parathyroid.[28] Advocates argue that parathyroid cancer is an aggressive disease with no effective adjuvant therapy. Therefore, an aggressive surgical resection on the affected side is the only possibility for cure.

INTRAOPERATIVE NERVE INJURY

Injury to the RLN is one of the most feared complications of parathyroid surgery. Injury rates vary considerably depending on the method of detection, but nerve injury has been reported in less than 1% of initial operations in the hands of experienced surgeons. Injury to the RLN results in poor voice quality and an increased risk of aspiration. Every effort should be made to repair an RLN transection if identified intraoperatively, because immediate repair may improve voice quality.[29]

Several techniques exist for the repair of a transected nerve including gluing, microsuture, and grafting.[29] A repair using 3 to 4 interrupted small-diameter sutures is appropriate for a nerve that can be brought together without undue tension. If the cut edges cannot be brought together, an interposition graft, usually of ipsilateral ansa cervicalis, can be used. A major factor in success of nerve repair is surgeon experience with microsurgical nerve repair. If the operative surgeon is not comfortable with nerve repair, then the authors strongly recommend an intraoperative consult to a specialist with experience in nerve repair.

SUMMARY

Parathyroid surgery can be extremely rewarding when patients experience a rapid improvement in symptoms. There are many phases of the operation, however, that can stress even the most experienced surgeons. A thoughtful approach to intraoperative decision making during parathyroidectomy can lead to improved outcomes for patients and contentment for surgeons.

REFERENCES

1. Delbridge LW, Dolan SJ, Hop TT, et al. Minimally invasive parathyroidectomy: 50 consecutive cases. Med J Aust 2000;172(9):418–22.
2. Smit PC, Borel Rinkes IH, van Dalen A, et al. Direct, minimally invasive adenomectomy for primary hyperparathyroidism: An alternative to conventional neck exploration? Ann Surg 2000;231(4):559–65.
3. Murphy C, Norman J. The 20% rule: a simple, instantaneous radioactivity measurement defines cure and allows elimination of frozen sections and hormone assays during parathyroidectomy. Surgery 1999;126(6):1023–8 [discussion: 1028–9].
4. Chen H, Sippel RS, Schaefer S. The effectiveness of radioguided parathyroidectomy in patients with negative technetium tc 99m-sestamibi scans. Arch Surg 2009;144(7):643–8.
5. Chen H, Mack E, Starling JR. Radioguided parathyroidectomy is equally effective for both adenomatous and hyperplastic glands. Ann Surg 2003;238(3):332–7 [discussion: 337–8].
6. Weigel TL, Murphy J, Kabbani L, et al. Radioguided thoracoscopic mediastinal parathyroidectomy with intraoperative parathyroid hormone testing. Ann Thorac Surg 2005;80(4):1262–5.

7. Irvin GL 3rd, Prudhomme DL, Deriso GT, et al. A new approach to parathyroidectomy. Ann Surg 1994;219(5):574–9 [discussion: 579–81].
8. Carneiro DM, Solorzano CC, Nader MC, et al. Comparison of intraoperative iPTH assay (QPTH) criteria in guiding parathyroidectomy: which criterion is the most accurate? Surgery 2003;134(6):973–9 [discussion: 979–81].
9. Patel KN, Caso R. Intraoperative parathyroid hormone monitoring: optimal utilization. Surg Oncol Clin N Am 2016;25(1):91–101.
10. Chen H, Pruhs Z, Starling JR, et al. Intraoperative parathyroid hormone testing improves cure rates in patients undergoing minimally invasive parathyroidectomy. Surgery 2005;138(4):583–7 [discussion: 587–90].
11. Schneider DF, Mazeh H, Chen H, et al. Predictors of recurrence in primary hyperparathyroidism: an analysis of 1386 cases. Ann Surg 2014;259(3):563–8.
12. Lou I, Balentine C, Clarkson S, et al. How long should we follow patients after apparently curative parathyroidectomy? Surgery 2017;161(1):54–61.
13. Norman J, Lopez J, Politz D. Abandoning unilateral parathyroidectomy: why we reversed our position after 15,000 parathyroid operations. J Am Coll Surg 2012;214(3):260–9.
14. Norman J, Politz D. 5,000 parathyroid operations without frozen section or PTH assays: measuring individual parathyroid gland hormone production in real time. Ann Surg Oncol 2009;16(3):656–66.
15. Testini M, Rosato L, Avenia N, et al. The impact of single parathyroid gland autotransplantation during thyroid surgery on postoperative hypoparathyroidism: a multicenter study. Transplant Proc 2007;39(1):225–30.
16. Wagner PK, Seesko HG, Rothmund M. Replantation of cryopreserved human parathyroid tissue. World J Surg 1991;15(6):751–5.
17. Promberger R, Ott J, Kober F, et al. Intra- and postoperative parathyroid hormone-kinetics do not advocate for autotransplantation of discolored parathyroid glands during thyroidectomy. Thyroid 2010;20(12):1371–5.
18. Shaha AR, Burnett C, Jaffe BM. Parathyroid autotransplantation during thyroid surgery. J Surg Oncol 1991;46(1):21–4.
19. Vidal Fortuny J, Sadowski SM, Belfontali V, et al. Indocyanine green angiography in subtotal parathyroidectomy: technique for the function of the parathyroid remnant. J Am Coll Surg 2016;223(5):e43–9.
20. Vidal Fortuny J, Sadowski SM, Belfontali V, et al. Randomized clinical trial of intraoperative parathyroid gland angiography with indocyanine green fluorescence predicting parathyroid function after thyroid surgery. Br J Surg 2018;105(4):350–7.
21. Mannoh EA, Thomas G, Solórzano CC, et al. Intraoperative assessment of parathyroid viability using laser speckle contrast imaging. Sci Rep 2017;7(1):14798.
22. Cavallaro G, Iorio O, Centanni M, et al. Parathyroid reimplantation in forearm subcutaneous tissue during thyroidectomy: a simple and effective way to avoid hypoparathyroidism. World J Surg 2015;39(8):1936–42.
23. Kidney Disease: Improving Global Outcomes (KDIGO) CKD-MBD Update Work Group. KDIGO 2017 clinical practice guideline update for the diagnosis, evaluation, prevention, and treatment of chronic kidney disease-mineral and bone disorder (CKD-MBD). Kidney Int Suppl (2011) 2017;7(1):1–59.
24. Rothmund M, Wagner PK, Schark C. Subtotal parathyroidectomy versus total parathyroidectomy and autotransplantation in secondary hyperparathyroidism: a randomized trial. World J Surg 1991;15(6):745–50.
25. Mohebati A, Shaha A, Shah J. Parathyroid carcinoma: challenges in diagnosis and treatment. Hematol Oncol Clin North Am 2012;26(6):1221–38.

26. Dudney WC, Bodenner D, Stack BC Jr. Parathyroid carcinoma. Otolaryngol Clin North Am 2010;43(2):441–53, xi.
27. Gao WC, Ruan CP, Zhang JC, et al. Nonfunctional parathyroid carcinoma. J Cancer Res Clin Oncol 2010;136(7):969–74.
28. Hsu KT, Sippel RS, Chen H, et al. Is central lymph node dissection necessary for parathyroid carcinoma? Surgery 2014;156(6):1336–41 [discussion: 1341].
29. Paniello RC. Laryngeal reinnervation. Otolaryngol Clin North Am 2004;37(1): 161–81, vii-viii.

Surgical Management of Multiple Endocrine Neoplasia 1 and Multiple Endocrine Neoplasia 2

Colleen M. Kiernan, MD, MPH*, Elizabeth G. Grubbs, MD

KEYWORDS

- Multiple endocrine neoplasia type 1 • Multiple endocrine neoplasia type 2
- Surgical management • Parathyroid • Pancreas • Medullary thyroid carcinoma
- Pheochromocytoma

KEY POINTS

- Multiple endocrine neoplasia (MEN) encompasses a group of rare hereditary disorders of the endocrine system, which are typically characterized by the occurrence of tumors involving 2 or more endocrine glands in the same patient or kindred.
- The overall goal in any surgery for tumors associated with MEN1 or MEN2 is to treat the disease while minimizing the complications and the physiologic effects and the impact on quality of life that occurs with the loss of hormones produced by the target organ.
- Because of the known risk of recurrence of disease in all tumors associated with MEN1 and MEN2, routine surveillance and thoughtful consideration of the timing and extent of reoperative surgery are necessary.

INTRODUCTION

The term multiple endocrine neoplasia (MEN) encompasses a group of rare hereditary disorders of the endocrine system, which are typically characterized by the occurrence of tumors involving 2 or more endocrine glands in the same patient or kindred. This article focuses on the surgical management of the tumors commonly encountered in patients with MEN1 or MEN2 syndrome. Specifically, it discusses the management of disease after the patient has met indications for operative intervention and the decision has been made to proceed to the operating room. Thus, this article provides a thoughtful discussion of preoperative planning, the goals of surgery, the

---

Disclosure Statement: The authors have no financial disclosures.
Department of Surgical Oncology, The University of Texas MD Anderson Cancer Center, 1400 Pressler Street, FCT 17.6000, Houston, TX 77030, USA
* Corresponding author.
E-mail address: CMKiernan@mdanderson.org

Surg Clin N Am 99 (2019) 693–709
https://doi.org/10.1016/j.suc.2019.04.015 surgical.theclinics.com

extent of surgery, intraoperative considerations, and the management of recurrent disease.

MULTIPLE ENDOCRINE NEOPLASIA TYPE 1

MEN1 is an autosomal-dominant disorder that occurs because of mutations of the MEN-1 tumor suppressor gene MENIN on chromosome 11q13.[1–3] The syndrome most commonly manifests with endocrine tumors of the parathyroid, pancreas, and duodenum and anterior pituitary.[1] However, multiple other tumors have also been associated with the syndrome, including adrenal cortical tumors, pheochromocytomas, bronchopulmonary, gastric and thymic neuroendocrine tumors, lipomas, collagenomas, angiofibromas, and meningiomas. **Table 1** demonstrates the tumors associated with MEN1 syndrome and the associated penetrance.

This section focuses on the preoperative planning, goals of surgery, extent of surgery, intraoperative considerations, and management of recurrent disease for hyperparathyroidism (HPT), enteropancreatic neuroendocrine tumors (EP-NETs), including the most commonly encountered nonfunctional, gastrin, and insulin-producing pancreatic neuroendocrine tumors (PNETs).

Hyperparathyroidism

Primary HPT is the most commonly experienced endocrinopathy in patients with MEN1 occurring in approximately 95% of those affected and is commonly the presenting disease process.[1–3] HPT in MEN1 is associated with multigland hyperplasia and an increased incidence of supernumerary or ectopic glands. Symptoms are

Table 1
Tumors associated with multiple endocrine neoplasia 1 syndrome and the estimated disease penetrance

Tumor	Penetrance, %
Parathyroid tumors	90
EP-NETs	30–70
Nonfunctioning	20–55
Gastrinoma	40
Insulinoma	10
Glucagonoma	<1
VIPoma	<1
Pituitary adenoma	30–40
Prolactinoma	20
Somatotropinoma	10
Corticotropinoma	5
Nonfunctioning	5
Associated tumors	
Adrenal cortical tumor	40
Pheochromocytoma	<1
Bronchopulmonary neuroendocrine tumor	2
Thymic neuroendocrine tumor	2
Gastric neuroendocrine tumor	10
Lipoma	30
Angiofibroma	85
Collagenoma	70
Meningioma	8

similar to those experienced in patients with sporadic HPT. However, when compared with sporadic HPT, the hypercalcemia is commonly mild, occurs at an early age of onset, with a greater reduction in bone mineral density and at an equal ratio in male and female patients.[1–3]

SURGICAL MANAGEMENT

The indications for surgery are similar to those described for sporadic adenomas causing HPT (**Box 1**); however, earlier intervention is often considered to reduce the effects of prolonged unopposed parathyroid hormone (PTH) even before symptoms or hypercalcemia occurs.[4] It has been shown that both bone mineral density loss and decreased kidney function can occur early on in disease progression even though patients may be asymptomatic or have mild hypercalcemia.[5,6]

The goals of surgery are to achieve and maintain eucalcemia for the longest time possible, to avoid iatrogenic hypoparathyroidism and the associated life altering hypocalcemia, to avoid operative complications, and to minimize the need for, but to facilitate the ease of, future surgery for recurrent disease.[7]

Because all parathyroid glands are affected in MEN1, surgical management requires removal of all abnormal tissue using an open bilateral exploration.[3] However, debate remains over the most appropriate operation, that is, subtotal parathyroidectomy (extirpation of 3.5 glands) or total parathyroidectomy with or without autotransplantation to achieve this goal.

The decision to perform a subtotal parathyroidectomy or a total parathyroidectomy with autotransplantation should be made with the risk of recurrent or persistent disease and the risk of permanent hypoparathyroidism in mind. In the largest series published to date, Pieterman and colleagues[8] demonstrated that among 73 patients with MEN1-related HPT who underwent parathyroidectomy, there were similar rates of persistent or recurrent disease between subtotal parathyroidectomy (17%) and total parathyroidectomy with autotransplantation (19%), but a significantly higher risk of permanent hypoparathyroidism in the total parathyroidectomy group (66% vs 39%).

Before proceeding to the operating room, preoperative imaging should be considered. The authors recommend routine performance of preoperative ultrasound of the neck to evaluate the thyroid gland for any concomitant pathologic condition that should be addressed at the time of parathyroidectomy. For the index operative procedure, use of additional localizing imaging, such as 4-dimensional (4D) computed tomography (CT) or sestamibi study, is not essential given that a 4-gland exploration will be performed. However, performance of such cross-sectional imaging to evaluate for intrathoracic or ectopic glands is reasonable.

Box 1
Indications for parathyroidectomy in setting of multiple endocrine neoplasia 1

Indications for parathyroidectomy in patients with MEN1

Symptomatic HPT

Serum calcium >1 mg/dL above normal regardless of whether symptoms are present or absent

Renal involvement: nephrolithiasis on renal imaging, nephrocalcinosis, hypercalciuria with increased stone risk, impaired renal function (glomerular filtration rate <60 mL/min)

HPT and evidence of osteoporosis, fragility fracture, or vertebral compression fracture

Age less than 50 with biochemical evidence of HPT regardless of symptoms

Intraoperatively, it is the authors' practice to perform a 4-gland exploration and a 3.5-gland parathyroidectomy with bilateral cervical thymectomy leaving the remnant gland in situ. The choice of which gland to leave as a remnant is made based on visualization of the smallest or most normal-appearing gland after frozen section biopsy confirms it is in fact parathyroid tissue. A secondary goal is to choose a remnant that will be the least complicated to address upon reoperation, if necessary. The chosen remnant is usually an inferior gland; superior glands are often located near the laryngeal insertion of the recurrent laryngeal nerve and thus more concerning to redissect. The goal is to leave a remnant 1.5 to 2 times the size of a normal parathyroid gland or approximately 40 to 60 mg of parathyroid tissue.[7] This practice, in the authors' experience, has resulted in lower rates of recurrence or persistence when compared with less than subtotal parathyroidectomy while conferring a lower risk of permanent hypoparathyroidism than total parathyroidectomy with cryopreservation and autotransplantation of a small remnant portion of gland in the forearm.[4] Cervical thymectomy is performed to remove any ectopic or supranumerary parathyroid tissue present in the thymus and to decrease the risk of developing thymic carcinoid. If, at the conclusion of the case, the remnant does not appear vascularly intact, an autograft of a 40-mg piece of parathyroid may be placed in a pocket fashioned in the brachioradialis muscle of the nondominant arm. This pocket should be closed with a clip and Prolene so that it may be located on future imaging and at the time of potential future debulking. Sterile cryopreservation of the removed gland may also be performed in case implantation is necessary in the setting of a nonfunctioning remnant; the authors recommend this occur within 6 months of the initial surgery.

POSTOPERATIVE SURVEILLANCE AND MANAGEMENT OF PERSISTENT OR RECURRENT DISEASE

Following parathyroidectomy, the overall risk of recurrence is estimated to be 40% to 60% at 10 years, and therefore, the importance of regular surveillance must be emphasized to patients.[9] Initially, the authors monitor calcium and PTH at 2 weeks, 6 months postoperatively, and then annually thereafter to monitor for persistent or recurrent disease. The diagnosis of persistent or recurrent disease is made biochemically. Persistent HPT is defined as hypercalcemia with inappropriately normal or elevated serum intact PTH within 6 months of surgery. If hypercalcemia occurs more than 6 months after parathyroidectomy, this is considered recurrent disease.

Management of recurrent disease is more complex than the index operative procedure. The risk of complication is higher in reoperative cervical exploration (12%–33%).[10,11] Surgeon experience with remedial surgery should be considered because high-volume parathyroid surgeons are known to have lower complication rates.[12] Preoperative imaging in reoperative surgery is an essential part of the preoperative planning. The authors perform ultrasound of the neck in addition to sestamibi scan and 4D CT in order to localize the pathogenic gland. If an autograft was previously performed in the forearm, this portion of the body should be included in the sestamibi study to evaluate for hyperplasia of transplanted gland. Bilateral upper-extremity PTH levels also may help determine if the autograft is the source of the excess hormone. If the operative procedure was performed at an outside institution, every effort should be made to obtain the operative and pathology reports and specimen to help confirm what was removed previously and where remnant tissue may be located. All patients undergo preoperative laryngoscopy before reoperative surgery to demonstrate vocal cord function. If function is abnormal, it warrants careful consideration of the timing and extent of the operation. In addition, in reoperative parathyroid surgery, the authors use intraoperative PTH assay to help plan their operative procedure. If preoperative imaging suggests an additional missed gland, they focus their attention to that location, and if the intraoperative PTH does not fall by 50% of the preincision value, the authors then will look to debulk their remnant. If debulking of the remnant gland does not result in a 50% ioPTH drop or if they encounter a significant amount of scarring and they think any future operative exploration would be ill advised, they will then consider removing the remainder of the remnant tissue and performing autotransplantation into the nondominant brachioradialis muscle. If this approach is to be used, cryopreservation of a portion of the remnant gland should be considered, if available, should the forearm autograft fail.

Enteropancreatic Neuroendocrine Tumors

The incidence of EP-NET in patients with MEN1 varies from 30% to 70% and is a major cause of premature death in MEN1 patients.[13,14] Many of these tumors secrete excessive amounts of hormone (gastrin, insulin, vasoactive intestinal polypeptide, glucagon).[3]

EP-NETs encountered in patients with MEN1 syndrome tend to present at an earlier age, are more frequently multiple, and have a higher rate of metastatic disease at presentation.[3] The multifocality of disease and occurrence of functional tumors concurrently with nonfunctional tumors make accurate diagnosis and management complex. It cannot be assumed by the surgeon that the tumor or tumors visualized on cross-sectional imaging correlate with the site of hormone excess, and thus, thoughtful consideration of the intraoperative localization and resection is essential. The main aim in treating MEN1-associated EP-NETs is to maintain the patient disease and symptom free for as long as possible while maintaining an acceptable quality of life.

SURGICAL MANAGEMENT

Although surgical resection is the mainstay of treatment of enteropancreatic tumors, the indication for and timing of operative intervention vary by hormone production, size, and location of the tumor. Whereas most agree that patients with MEN1 and non-gastrinoma functional EP-NETs should undergo surgery because of the high cure rate associated with surgical resection, this is not always the case with MEN1 patients with gastrinoma or nonfunctional PNETs. Therefore, this section focuses on the surgical management of the 2 most frequently occurring and often difficult-to-cure EP-NETs in MEN1 syndrome, gastrinoma and nonfunctioning PNETs.

Gastrinoma

Gastrinomas represent the most common functional EP-NET in MEN1 patients, causing symptoms and complications related to elevated gastric acid levels. Although the use of proton pump inhibitors has made complications from ulcer disease a rare cause of morbidity or death, these neoplasms have a propensity for malignant transformation, with up to 70% of patients having lymph node metastases at the time of operative intervention.[15–17] It has been demonstrated in multiple studies that most (85%–100%) of MEN1-associated gastrinomas are small and duodenal in origin.[16,18,19]

Currently, there is no clear consensus on the timing or extent of operative resection for gastrinoma in MEN1 patients. Recommendations on timing of the operation vary from at diagnosis, once the tumor size is $\geq$2 cm, or only after failed medical management. The most recent guidelines from the European Neuroendocrine Tumor Society and the North American Neuroendocrine Society recommend a conservative approach to patients with gastrinoma less than 2 cm due to increasing evidence suggesting that patients with small lesions that can be managed medically have an excellent prognosis.[20,21] The extent of operation also varies from routine Thompson procedure (distal pancreatectomy, enucleation of pancreatic head lesions, duodenotomy with excision of duodenal lesions, and peripancreatic lymphadenectomy), routine pancreaticoduodenectomy, total pancreatectomy, or some combination of the above listed procedures. The goal of surgery is to reduce the risk of distant metastatic disease with the lowest morbidity possible and to preserve endocrine and exocrine pancreatic function for as long as possible.

The operative strategy used at the authors' institution is depicted in **Fig. 1** and has previously been described by Dickson and colleagues.[16] In MEN1 patients with hypergastrinemia, operative exploration is performed when concomitant pancreatic neoplasms (usually nonfunctional) are ≥2 cm, when surveillance imaging demonstrates interval growth of smaller neoplasms, or when there is radiographic evidence of duodenal or regional lymph node disease. Duodenal evaluation and regional lymph node dissection (RLND) are performed in all patients undergoing abdominal exploration for hypergastrinemia. Duodenal evaluation includes intraoperative duodenotomy and digital palpation or duodenectomy in patients undergoing as part of a pancreaticoduodenectomy or total pancreatectomy. The limits of formal, anatomically based RLND are illustrated in **Fig. 2**. RLND begins with the Kocher maneuver extending to the left lateral border of the aorta with elevation of the duodenum, head, and uncinate process of the pancreas off the retroperitoneum. The periduodenal and peripancreatic lymph nodes posterior to the duodenum, and head, uncinate, and neck of pancreas and anterior to the aorta and vena cava are removed. The portal nodes from the right

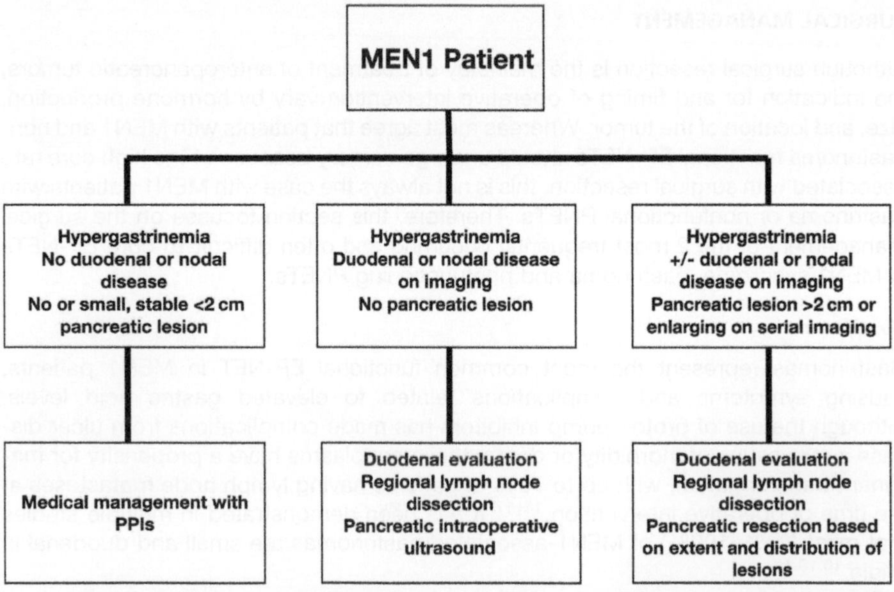

Fig. 1. Operative strategy for management of gastrinoma in the setting of known MEN1. PPIs, proton pump inhibitors. (*From* Dickson PV, Rich TA, Xing Y, et al. Achieving eugastrinemia in MEN1 patients: both duodenal inspection and formal lymph node dissection are important. Surgery 2011;150(6):1143–1152; with permission.)

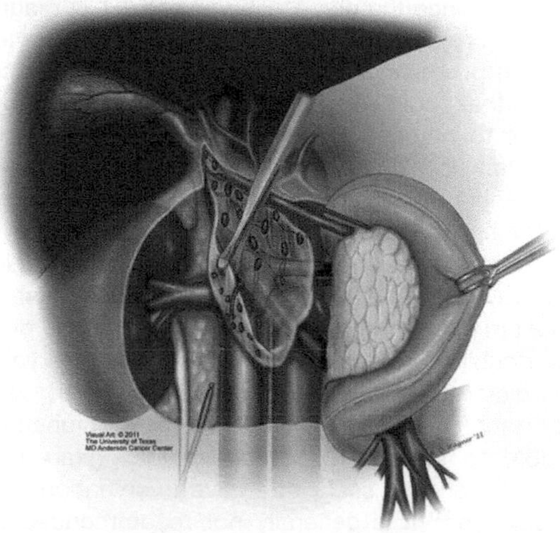

Fig. 2. Anatomic boundaries of formal regional lymphadenectomy performed routinely in patients with MEN1-associated hypergastrinemia. (*From* Dickson PV, Rich TA, Xing Y, et al. Achieving eugastrinemia in MEN1 patients: both duodenal inspection and formal lymph node dissection are important. Surgery 2011;150(6):1143–1152; with permission.)

lateral border and posterior aspect of the portal vein as well as hepatic artery lymph nodes are also excised. The extent of pancreatectomy is determined by the location of the lesions, their size, and the relationship of the lesion to the main pancreatic duct. If the operative indication is duodenal or regional lymph node disease and no pancreatic lesions are seen on preoperative cross-section imaging, intraoperative ultrasound and manual palpation of pancreas are performed to identify any occult lesions. This approach in the authors' institution seems to be associated with likelihood of both long-term eugastrinemia and locoregional control.[16]

POSTOPERATIVE SURVEILLANCE AND MANAGEMENT OF PERSISTENT OR RECURRENT DISEASE

The risk of persistent or recurrent gastrinoma after the index procedure is high (23%–100%), and management of recurrent disease is complex.[3,14,17,22] After initial resection, patients should be followed at least annually with biochemical markers and cross-sectional imaging. Reoperation is considered when a patient has persistent or recurrent hypergastrinemia and a lesion greater than 1 cm is visualized on cross-sectional imaging or endoscopic ultrasound. If the index operative procedure was performed at an outside institution, every effort should be made to obtain the operative and pathology reports to help confirm whether duodenal exploration and RLND were completed because these are often sites of missed disease and should be considered in the setting of recurrent/persistent disease. The extent of resection for recurrent disease is dictated by the location and extent of recurrence. Again, total pancreatectomy or pancreaticoduodenectomy should be avoided if possible because of the effect on patient quality of life.

Nonfunctioning Pancreatic Neuroendocrine Tumors

Nonfunctioning pancreatic tumors are not associated with clinical symptoms and therefore may result in delayed diagnosis without routine surveillance imaging in

MEN1 patients. However, once the non-functioning PNET is diagnosed, the goal of treatment is to reduce morbidity and mortality associated with metastatic or locally advanced disease while preserving endocrine and exocrine pancreas function and avoiding complications that occur with surgical resection. The risk of metastatic disease has been reported to increase with tumor size with studies demonstrating that 25% to 40% of patients with PNET greater than 4 cm develop hepatic metastases and 50% to 70% of patients with PNET greater than 2 to 3 cm in size have lymph node metastases at the time of exploration.[14,22,23]

As in gastrinomas, there is no clear consensus on the optimal timing or indication for surgical resection; however, most agree that surgical resection should be pursued in tumors greater than 2 cm or in tumors less than 2 cm that have demonstrated significant growth, that is, doubling in size over a 3- to 6-month interval. The extent of the surgical resection is dictated intraoperatively by the number, size, and location of the lesions. It is important for the surgeon to recall that nonfunctioning PNETs occur microscopically in 80% to 100% of patients with MEN1, are multiple, and occur throughout the pancreas, and as such, operative intervention is unlikely to render the patient free of disease.[20] It is generally not recommended to perform a total pancreatectomy at the time of the index operation, given the quality of life-changing effects.

In the authors' institution, operative intervention is considered when lesions are ≥2 cm in size or are enlarging on serial imaging. The extent of the resection is based on the distribution of the neoplasms with all attempts to avoid pancreaticoduodenectomy and total pancreatectomy. In patients with multiple lesions, smaller lesions less than 2 cm in the pancreatic head are enucleated provided this can be performed without disruption of the main pancreatic duct, and lesions in the pancreatic body and tail are resected with a formal distal pancreatectomy. Unlike in gastrinoma, there is no role for routine RLND in resection nonfunctioning PNET; therefore, RLND is only performed if nodal disease is present on imaging or palpated intraoperatively.

POSTOPERATIVE SURVEILLANCE AND MANAGEMENT OF PERSISTENT OR RECURRENT DISEASE

Similar to gastrinoma, the risk of persistent or recurrent nonfunctioning PNET after the index procedure is high, and management of recurrent disease is complex.[14,17,23] After initial resection, patients should be followed at least annually with cross-sectional imaging, with consideration of MRI to decrease radiation exposure. Reoperation is considered when a patient has a lesion ≥2 cm visualized on cross-sectional imaging or endoscopic ultrasound. The extent of resection for recurrent disease is dictated by the location and extent of recurrence. Again, total pancreatectomy or pancreaticoduodenectomy should be avoided if possible due to the effect on patient quality of life.

MULTIPLE ENDOCRINE NEOPLASIA TYPE 2

MEN2 is an autosomal-dominant disorder that occurs due to missense gain-of-function mutations in the *RET* proto-oncogene located on chromosome 10 (10q11.2). Specific *RET* mutations are associated with a particular phenotype and clinical course, with strong genotype-phenotype correlations.[24] More than 100 *RET* point mutations, duplications, insertions, deletions, and fusions have been identified in MEN2A kindreds, whereas fewer *RET* mutations (918 and 883) have been identified in MEN2B kindreds. The specific mutation often guides the clinical decision making and recommendations for management as well as assigns patients to risk groups.

Within MEN2, there are 2 commonly described syndromes, MEN type 2A (MEN2A) and MEN type 2B (MEN2B). These subtypes and the clinical features are depicted in **Table 2**.

This section focuses on the preoperative planning, goals of surgery, extent of surgery, intraoperative considerations, and management of recurrent disease for medullary thyroid carcinoma (MTC), pheochromocytoma, and primary HPT in the setting of known MEN2 syndrome.

Medullary Thyroid Carcinoma

MTC originates from the parafollicular C cells of the thyroid gland, which are derived from the neural crest.[1] MTC begins as C-cell hyperplasia that progresses to early medullary microcarcinoma and eventually will become grossly invasive macroscopic MTC if left untreated. Prevention or cure of MTC can only be achieved by surgery, and success is often determined by the timing and adequacy of the initial operation. Surgery for MTC in the setting of MEN2 should ideally be performed before malignant progression occurs. Given that all parafollicular C cells harbor the *RET* mutation in MEN2, the disease is often multicentric and bilateral and requires total thyroidectomy. Because C cells concentrate in the bilateral superior poles of the thyroid, removal of all thyroid tissue, including at the laryngeal insertion of the recurrent laryngeal nerve, is essential to prevent recurrence. The timing of early or prophylactic thyroidectomy is determined by the specific *RET* mutation and its associated age risk of developing MTC. **Table 3** depicts the American Thyroid Association (ATA) risk level based prophylactic thyroidectomy recommendations.

SURGICAL MANAGEMENT

The surgical management of the thyroid gland in MEN2 is ultimately determined by the timing of the operation in relation to disease progression/extent of disease. Preoperative planning for both prophylactic thyroidectomy and thyroidectomy in the setting of biopsy-proven MTC should include comprehensive thyroid, central neck, and lateral neck ultrasound to evaluate the thyroid gland and its draining lymph node basins as well as a preoperative serum calcitonin and carcinoembryonic antigen (CEA) and discussion in a multidisciplinary setting when available.[25,26] Preoperative ultrasound helps to determine the extent of locoregional disease to allow for appropriate surgical planning. Calcitonin levels help to assess the risk of distant metastatic disease. In addition, biochemical evaluation for pheochromocytoma and primary HPT should be performed in patients harboring *RET* mutations associated with these diseases. In children under the age of 5 years old, there is no indication to obtain plasma or urine metanephrines before prophylactic thyroidectomy, because pheochromocytoma

Table 2
Multiple endocrine neoplasia 2 variants and clinical features

MEN2 Syndrome	Clinical Features (% Penetrance)
MEN2A	MTC (>90%), pheochromocytoma (40%–60%), parathyroid hyperplasia (20%–30%), cutaneous lichen amyloidosis, Hirschsprung disease
MEN2B	MTC (>98%), pheochromocytoma (40%–60%), intestinal and mucosal neuromas (98%), Marfanoid habitus, inability to make tears, everted eye lids, ptosis, prominent corneal nerves

Table 3
American Thyroid Association risk level based prophylactic thyroidectomy recommendations

ATA Risk Level	Codon	Age of Prophylactic Procedure
A	768	Consider thyroidectomy before age 5
	790	May delay surgery if:
	791	• Normal annual serum calcitonin
	804	• Less aggressive family history
	891	• Family preference
B	609	
	611	
	618	
	620	
	630	
C	634	Thyroidectomy before 5 y of age

presents later in life.[25,26] However, in patients older than 11 to 16 years of age with known *RET* mutations associated with pheochromocytoma, biochemical evaluation with plasma metanephrines before thyroidectomy is warranted to avoid unanticipated intraoperative hemodynamic instability that can be associated with an undiagnosed and untreated pheochromocytoma.[25–29] Similarly, HPT associated with specific MEN2A mutations often presents later in life; however, obtaining a serum calcium and PTH level before operative intervention is warranted in MEN2A patients over the age of 10 years old.

The goals of surgical intervention are to perform a total thyroidectomy with particular attention to the superior poles of the gland given the location of parafollicular C cells, while preserving bilateral recurrent laryngeal nerves and normal parathyroid glands and removing metastatic regional lymph nodes by means of a compartment-oriented, en bloc lymphadenectomy.

Ultimately, the extent of thyroidectomy and lymph node dissection is determined by a combination of patient age, *RET* mutation, biopsy-proven evidence of locoregional disease, and/or presence of distant metastases.

Table 4 depicts the most commonly encountered clinical scenarios and the management strategy used at the authors' institution. The authors perform routine preoperative comprehensive neck ultrasound and obtain calcitonin and CEA levels on all patients undergoing thyroidectomy for known MEN2 syndromes to evaluate for locoregional and assess the risk of metastatic disease. In patients with preoperative calcitonin levels greater than 500 pg/mL or extensive locally aggressive disease in the neck, the authors will obtain a preoperative staging evaluation, which consists of CT neck and chest with intravenous contrast, and triple-phase CT of the abdomen and pelvis to evaluate for liver metastases. In patients without evidence of local disease, that is, in patients undergoing a prophylactic procedure, the authors perform a total thyroidectomy, usually without central neck dissection to avoid added risk of devascularizing the parathyroid glands. Parathyroid preservation is particularly important in the patient population undergoing prophylactic thyroidectomy, because many are children. In the pediatric population, frequent blood draws and calcium supplementation can be exceedingly challenging in the setting of postoperative hypocalcemia. Total thyroidectomy with level VI compartment dissection (central lymph node dissection) is the procedure of choice for patients with biopsy-proven MTC without evidence of lateral neck disease. Lateral compartmental dissection is performed in the setting of radiographic and/or biopsy-proven disease, and the authors' practice is

Table 4
Recommended surgical management of the thyroid in multiple endocrine neoplasia 2

Clinical Scenario	Recommended Surgical Intervention	Special Considerations
MEN2A or MEN2B with no evidence of MTC (no lymph node metastases, all thyroid nodules <5 mm, calcitonin <40 pg/mL)	Total thyroidectomy Level VI compartment if clinical lymph node metastases Lateral neck compartmental dissection of biopsy-positive compartments	If MEN2B patient presents at age >1-year-old prophylactic level VI, compartment dissection should be considered Preserve all parathyroid function
MEN2A or MEN2B with biopsy-proven MTC in thyroid no lymph node disease	Total thyroidectomy and level VI compartmental dissection	If calcitonin >500 pg/mL or patient has biopsy-proven lateral neck lymph node disease, the patient should be staged with CT neck and chest and dedicated triple phase CT or MRI of liver and bone scintigraphy before surgery Treat concomitant pheochromocytoma before MTC
MEN2A or MEN2B with biopsy-proven MTC in thyroid and in lateral neck compartment	Total thyroidectomy Level VI compartmental dissection Compartmental lateral lymph node dissection on the side or sides affected	
MEN2A or MEN2B with biopsy-proven MTC in thyroid and distant metastatic disease	Consider total thyroidectomy and level VI compartmental dissection with lateral compartmental dissection for biopsy-proven disease	Goal of surgery is locoregional disease control and prevention of central neck morbidity If extensive metastatic disease, resection of primary can be performed for palliative purposes if needed for airway compromise

not to perform lateral compartmental dissection based on calcitonin levels. Great care is taken to preserve parathyroid tissue in situ; however, if parathyroid glands are devascularized or removed during surgical intervention, autotransplantation is performed. In patients with MEN2B, the autograft is placed in the sternocleidomastoid muscle; however, in patients with MEN2A, particularly in MEN2A patients with strong family history of parathyroid hyperplasia or a *RET* mutation associated with parathyroid hyperplasia, the authors elect to place the autograft in the nondominant brachioradialis muscle for easier access should the patient develop HPT in the future.

POSTOPERATIVE SURVEILLANCE AND MANAGEMENT OF PERSISTENT OR RECURRENT DISEASE

Because of the risk of recurrent or persistent disease after thyroidectomy for MTC in MEN2, routine surveillance with history, physical examination, biochemical evaluation (calcitonin, CEA, thyrotropin, free T4), and ultrasound of the neck is required. The ATA and National Comprehensive Cancer Network recommend a basal calcitonin and CEA level at 3 months postoperatively.[26,30] If calcitonin and CEA are undetectable and normal, respectively, the patient can be followed with active surveillance, which includes serum calcitonin and CEA and ultrasound of central and lateral neck compartments every 6 months for a year and then annually thereafter. If the patient has a detectable basal calcitonin or elevated CEA level, imaging should be performed to evaluate for residual locoregional or distant disease with extent of imaging guided by calcitonin level. If the calcitonin level is greater than 150 pg/mL cross-sectional imaging of the chest and abdomen in addition to bone imaging, either scintigraphy or skeletal MRI, should be pursued to evaluate for distant disease. Functional imaging, most recently Gallium 68 DOTATATE, may be considered when cross-sectional imaging fails to reveal the source of elevated calcitonin. If imaging is unable to localize disease, the patient should then be followed every 6 months with CEA, calcitonin, and reimaging based on trend of the biochemical markers.[26,30]

The timing of remedial surgery for locally recurrent MTC in the setting of MEN2 is complex and nuanced. Although the goal is to render the patient free of disease without morbidity, this is often difficult to achieve in the setting of reoperation, and therefore, the risks and benefits of remedial surgery need to be considered. If the operative procedure was performed at an outside institution, every effort should be made to obtain the operative and pathology reports and specimen to help confirm the location of previous lymph node dissection and the potential locations of residual parathyroid tissue. All patients undergo preoperative laryngoscopy before reoperative surgery to demonstrate vocal cord function. If function is abnormal, it warrants careful consideration of the timing and extent of the operation. When determining the timing of reintervention, factors such as rate of tumor growth, rate of calcitonin and CEA doubling time, location of recurrent disease, and risk to vital structures as well as degree of patient concern/distress should be considered with earlier reintervention warranted in progressive disease encroaching on vital structures. Surgical resection of persistent or recurrent locoregional MTC should include compartmental dissection of biopsy-positive disease in level VI or lateral (levels II–V) compartments. Limited procedures that excise only the area of disease should be avoided unless the compartment was previously completely dissected.[26]

Pheochromocytoma

Pheochromocytomas are neuroendocrine tumors that arise from paraganglia cells derived from the neural crest. Adrenal-based pheochromocytomas arise in the sympathetic adrenal chromaffin cells. Almost all adrenal-based pheochromocytomas produce, store, metabolize, and secrete catecholamines and/or their metabolites.[31,32] The uncontrolled release of catecholamines by pheochromocytoma results in several physiologic and end-organ effects, such as tachycardia, tachyarrhythmia, relative hypovolemia secondary to vasoconstriction, hypertension, hyperglycemia, and stress-induced cardiomyopathy and therefore warrant early intervention once diagnosed.[32]

Pheochromocytomas occur in 40% to 60% of all MEN2 patients and have a unique biologic behavior in that they are frequently bilateral but rarely malignant.[33,34] Approximately 50% of patients who present with unilateral pheochromocytoma will develop a contralateral pheochromocytoma 10 years after resection.[34] However, the performance of empiric bilateral adrenalectomy in the absence of image-localized bilateral disease is ill advised given lifelong adrenal insufficiency, steroid dependence, and altered quality of life.[35]

SURGICAL MANAGEMENT

Adrenalectomy remains the treatment of choice for pheochromocytoma. Before operative intervention, multiple preoperative factors must be considered.

All hormonally productive pheochromocytomas require preoperative medical management with alpha-blockade. Although nonselective phenoxybenzamine is the alpha-antagonist most commonly described for preoperative blockade, several studies have demonstrated similar effectiveness with selective alpha-antagonists, such as doxazosin and terazosin or calcium channel antagonists.[36–39] Beta-blockade can be added after alpha-blockade if the patient remains hypertensive. Overall, the goals of preoperative blockade are to normalize blood pressure, heart rate, and volume status to prevent surgically induced catecholamine storm and its downstream effects on the cardiovascular system.

The approach to the adrenal gland (open, laparoscopic, robotic, retroperitoneoscopic) and the extent of adrenalectomy cortical-sparing versus total adrenalectomy depends on multiple factors, including location of the tumor, whether the patient has unilateral or bilateral tumors, patient body habitus, size of tumor, surgeon experience, and previous operative procedure. The goal of surgery for pheochromocytoma in MEN2 is to resect the tumor leaving behind intact functioning cortex to avoid lifelong steroid dependence, the risk of adrenal insufficiency and Addisonian crisis, and recurrent disease.

Cortical-sparing adrenalectomy can be performed successfully in MEN2 patients, allowing a low risk of chronic steroid hormone replacement and Addisonian crisis with low risk of recurrence.[40–42] Planning a successful cortical-sparing procedure requires cross-sectional imaging (triple-phase CT or MRI) with axial, coronal, and sagittal reconstruction aid in localization of the adrenal tumor or tumors, identification of the course of the adrenal vein, and facilitation of the planning of which portion of cortex can most successfully be spared.

If the tumor is unilateral with favorable anatomy for a cortical-sparing adrenalectomy, that is, the tumor is small and located in a caudad location, 20% to 30% of the adrenal cortex can be spared, and the tumor can be removed without full mobilization and disruption of the arterial vessels feeding the cortical portion of the adrenal gland. The authors' practice is to perform a cortical-sparing approach at the first operation for unilateral disease, using a retroperitoneoscopic approach if possible. The authors use a cortical-sparing approach at first operation to avoid the situation in which contralateral disease develops metachronously and cortex is not able to be preserved because of tumor size, location, or multiplicity.[41]

If a patient presents with bilateral disease, cortical-sparing adrenalectomy is first performed on the side most conducive to this approach to ensure remnant viability followed by contralateral total adrenalectomy. The authors do not routinely perform bilateral cortical-sparing adrenalectomy to decrease the risk of bilaterally recurrent disease.

POSTOPERATIVE SURVEILLANCE AND MANAGEMENT OF PERSISTENT OR RECURRENT DISEASE

Immediate and close postoperative surveillance is critical in patients who undergo bilateral adrenalectomy or unilateral adrenalectomy with a contralateral cortical-sparing adrenalectomy to detect and treat adrenal insufficiency. Management of the patient, often in conjunction with endocrinology colleagues, is essential preoperatively and postoperatively to provide patients with the appropriate counseling and education on management of adrenal insufficiency and its signs and symptoms. Patients at high risk for adrenal insufficiency must be given medical ID bands that document the necessity of glucocorticoid supplementation should they become ill or injured.

Biochemical confirmation of successful resection of pheochromocytoma should be performed postoperatively. Lifelong surveillance should be maintained with annual plasma metanephrines after resection because of risk of recurrence and/or novel contralateral disease. If plasma metanephrines are elevated, cross-sectional imaging should be obtained to localize the site of recurrent disease, and resection should be pursued with the same preoperative routine as described previously.

Primary Hyperparathyroidism

Primary HPT occurs in 20% to 30% of MEN2A patients. In comparison to sporadic or HPT associated with MEN1, the HPT associated with MEN2 is typically mild, presents in the third decade of life, and is rarely the first clinical manifestation of MEN2A.[43,44] Also, in contrast to MEN1, HPT in MEN2a does not routinely affect all 4 glands.

SURGICAL MANAGEMENT

The treatment of HPT in the setting of MEN2A is surgical resection. The indications for surgical intervention are the same as previous described in **Box 1**. Again, the goals of surgery are to achieve and maintain eucalcemia for the longest time possible, to avoid iatrogenic hypoparathyroidism and the associated life-altering hypocalcemia, to avoid operative complications, and to minimize the need for, but to facilitate the ease of, future surgery for recurrent disease.

The most common operative approach is resection of only affected glands, using intraoperative PTH assay.

Most frequently, HPT in MEN2 presents after thyroidectomy for MTC, and therefore, parathyroid surgery occurs in a reoperative setting. Preoperative localization studies should be obtained. As previously stated, it is the authors' practice to perform ultrasound of the neck in addition to sestamibi scan and 4D CT in order to localize the pathogenic gland. If an autograft was previously performed in the forearm, this portion of the body should be included in the sestamibi study to evaluate for hyperplasia of transplanted gland. Bilateral upper-extremity PTH levels also may help determine if the autograft is the source of the excess hormone. If the operative procedure was performed at an outside institution, every effort should be made to obtain the operative and pathology reports and specimen to help confirm previous removal of glands, if an autograft was performed and where remnant tissue may be located. All patients undergo preoperative laryngoscopy before reoperative surgery to demonstrate vocal cord function. If function is abnormal, it warrants careful consideration of the timing and extent of the operation.

If the abnormal gland or glands are localized, the authors prefer to perform a targeted parathyroidectomy with intraoperative PTH assay leaving unaffected glands in situ. If the intraoperative PTH drops by 50% after removal of the targeted gland or glands, the authors conclude the operation without further exploration. In a reoperative setting, consideration of immediate autografting or cryopreservation of parathyroid tissue must be made if there is concern for viability of remaining glands.

SUMMARY

MEN encompasses a group of rare hereditary disorders of the endocrine system, which are typically characterized by the occurrence of tumors involving 2 or more endocrine glands in the same patient. The overall goal in any surgery for tumors associated with MEN1 or MEN2 is to treat the disease while minimizing the complications and the physiologic effects and the impact on quality of life that occurs with the loss of hormones produced by the target organ. In addition, because of the known risk of recurrence of disease in all tumors associated with MEN1 and MEN2, routine surveillance and thoughtful consideration of the timing and extent of reoperative surgery are necessary.

REFERENCES

1. Brandi ML, Gagel RF, Angeli A, et al. Guidelines for diagnosis and therapy of MEN type 1 and type 2. J Clin Endocrinol Metab 2001;86(12):5658–71.
2. Thakker RV. Multiple endocrine neoplasia type 1 (MEN1). Best Pract Res Clin Endocrinol Metab 2010;24(3):355–70.
3. Thakker RV, Newey PJ, Walls GV, et al. Clinical practice guidelines for multiple endocrine neoplasia type 1 (MEN1). J Clin Endocrinol Metab 2012;97(9): 2990–3011.
4. Lambert LA, Shapiro SE, Lee JE, et al. Surgical treatment of hyperparathyroidism in patients with multiple endocrine neoplasia type 1. Arch Surg 2005;140(4): 374–82.
5. Giusti F, Tonelli F, Brandi ML. Primary hyperparathyroidism in multiple endocrine neoplasia type 1: when to perform surgery? Clinics (Sao Paulo) 2012;67(Suppl 1): 141–4.
6. Lourenco DM Jr, Coutinho FL, Toledo RA, et al. Biochemical, bone and renal patterns in hyperparathyroidism associated with multiple endocrine neoplasia type 1. Clinics (Sao Paulo) 2012;67(Suppl 1):99–108.
7. Nobecourt PF, Zagzag J, Asare EA, et al. Intraoperative decision-making and technical aspects of parathyroidectomy in young patients with MEN1 related hyperparathyroidism. Front Endocrinol (Lausanne) 2018;9:618.
8. Pieterman CR, van Hulsteijn LT, den Heijer M, et al. Primary hyperparathyroidism in MEN1 patients: a cohort study with longterm follow-up on preferred surgical procedure and the relation with genotype. Ann Surg 2012;255(6):1171–8.
9. Schneider DF, Mazeh H, Chen H, et al. Predictors of recurrence in primary hyperparathyroidism: an analysis of 1386 cases. Ann Surg 2014;259(3):563–8.
10. Karakas E, Muller HH, Schlosshauer T, et al. Reoperations for primary hyperparathyroidism–improvement of outcome over two decades. Langenbecks Arch Surg 2013;398(1):99–106.
11. Tonelli F, Marcucci T, Fratini G, et al. Is total parathyroidectomy the treatment of choice for hyperparathyroidism in multiple endocrine neoplasia type 1? Ann Surg 2007;246(6):1075–82.
12. Melfa G, Porello C, Cocorullo G, et al. Surgeon volume and hospital volume in endocrine neck surgery: how many procedures are needed for reaching a safety level and acceptable costs? A systematic narrative review. G Chir 2018; 39(1):5–11.
13. Doherty GM, Olson JA, Frisella MM, et al. Lethality of multiple endocrine neoplasia type I. World J Surg 1998;22(6):581–6 [discussion: 586–7].
14. Triponez F, Dosseh D, Goudet P, et al. Epidemiology data on 108 MEN 1 patients from the GTE with isolated nonfunctioning tumors of the pancreas. Ann Surg 2006;243(2):265–72.
15. Carty SE, Helm AK, Amico JA, et al. The variable penetrance and spectrum of manifestations of multiple endocrine neoplasia type 1. Surgery 1998;124(6): 1106–13 [discussion: 1113–4].
16. Dickson PV, Rich TA, Xing Y, et al. Achieving eugastrinemia in MEN1 patients: both duodenal inspection and formal lymph node dissection are important. Surgery 2011;150(6):1143–52.
17. Norton JA, Alexander HR, Fraker DL, et al. Comparison of surgical results in patients with advanced and limited disease with multiple endocrine neoplasia type 1 and Zollinger-Ellison syndrome. Ann Surg 2001;234(4):495–505 [discussion: 505–6].

18. Donow C, Pipeleers-Marichal M, Schroder S, et al. Surgical pathology of gastrinoma. Site, size, multicentricity, association with multiple endocrine neoplasia type 1, and malignancy. Cancer 1991;68(6):1329–34.
19. Thompson NW, Vinik AI, Eckhauser FE. Microgastrinomas of the duodenum. A cause of failed operations for the Zollinger-Ellison syndrome. Ann Surg 1989; 209(4):396–404.
20. Jensen RT, Norton JA. Treatment of pancreatic neuroendocrine tumors in multiple endocrine neoplasia type 1: some clarity but continued controversy. Pancreas 2017;46(5):589–94.
21. Kulke MH, Anthony LB, Bushnell DL, et al. NANETS treatment guidelines: well-differentiated neuroendocrine tumors of the stomach and pancreas. Pancreas 2010;39(6):735–52.
22. Norton JA. Surgical treatment and prognosis of gastrinoma. Best Pract Res Clin Gastroenterol 2005;19(5):799–805.
23. Norton JA, Fraker DL, Alexander HR, et al. Surgery to cure the Zollinger-Ellison syndrome. N Engl J Med 1999;341(9):635–44.
24. Raue F, Frank-Raue K. Update on multiple endocrine neoplasia type 2: focus on medullary thyroid carcinoma. J Endocr Soc 2018;2(8):933–43.
25. Kloos RT, Eng C, Evans DB, et al. Medullary thyroid cancer: management guidelines of the American Thyroid Association. Thyroid 2009;19(6):565–612.
26. Wells SA Jr, Asa SL, Dralle H, et al. Revised American Thyroid Association guidelines for the management of medullary thyroid carcinoma. Thyroid 2015;25(6): 567–610.
27. Machens A, Brauckhoff M, Holzhausen HJ, et al. Codon-specific development of pheochromocytomachromocytoma in multiple endocrine neoplasia type 2. J Clin Endocrinol Metab 2005;90(7):3999–4003.
28. Pacak K. Preoperative management of the pheochromocytomachromocytoma patient. J Clin Endocrinol Metab 2007;92(11):4069–79.
29. Skinner MA, DeBenedetti MK, Moley JF, et al. Medullary thyroid carcinoma in children with multiple endocrine neoplasia types 2A and 2B. J Pediatr Surg 1996; 31(1):177–81 [discussion: 181–2].
30. Haddad RI, Nasr C, Bischoff L, et al. NCCN guidelines insights: thyroid carcinoma, version 2.2018. J Natl Compr Canc Netw 2018;16(12):1429–40.
31. Chen H, Sippel RS, O'Dorisio MS, et al. The North American Neuroendocrine Tumor Society consensus guideline for the diagnosis and management of neuroendocrine tumors: pheochromocytomachromocytoma, paraganglioma, and medullary thyroid cancer. Pancreas 2010;39(6):775–83.
32. Kiernan CM, Solorzano CC. Pheochromocytomachromocytoma and paraganglioma: diagnosis, genetics, and treatment. Surg Oncol Clin N Am 2016;25(1): 119–38.
33. Bryant J, Farmer J, Kessler LJ, et al. Pheochromocytomachromocytoma: the expanding genetic differential diagnosis. J Natl Cancer Inst 2003;95(16):1196–204.
34. Lairmore TC, Ball DW, Baylin SB, et al. Management of pheochromocytomachromocytomas in patients with multiple endocrine neoplasia type 2 syndromes. Ann Surg 1993;217(6):595–601 [discussion: 601–3].
35. Telenius-Berg M, Ponder MA, Berg B, et al. Quality of life after bilateral adrenalectomy in MEN 2. Henry Ford Hosp Med J 1989;37(3–4):160–3.
36. Kiernan CM, Du L, Chen X, et al. Predictors of hemodynamic instability during surgery for pheochromocytomachromocytoma. Ann Surg Oncol 2014;21(12): 3865–71.

37. Prys-Roberts C, Farndon JR. Efficacy and safety of doxazosin for perioperative management of patients with pheochromocytomachromocytoma. World J Surg 2002;26(8):1037–42.
38. Siddiqi HK, Yang HY, Laird AM, et al. Utility of oral nicardipine and magnesium sulfate infusion during preparation and resection of pheochromocytomachromocytomas. Surgery 2012;152(6):1027–36.
39. Weingarten TN, Cata JP, O'Hara JF, et al. Comparison of two preoperative medical management strategies for laparoscopic resection of pheochromocytomachromocytoma. Urology 2010;76(2):508.e6-11.
40. Asari R, Scheuba C, Kaczirek K, et al. Estimated risk of pheochromocytomachromocytoma recurrence after adrenal-sparing surgery in patients with multiple endocrine neoplasia type 2A. Arch Surg 2006;141(12):1199–205 [discussion: 1205].
41. Grubbs EG, Rich TA, Ng C, et al. Long-term outcomes of surgical treatment for hereditary pheochromocytomachromocytoma. J Am Coll Surg 2013;216(2): 280–9.
42. Lee JE, Curley SA, Gagel RF, et al. Cortical-sparing adrenalectomy for patients with bilateral pheochromocytomachromocytoma. Surgery 1996;120(6):1064–70 [discussion: 1070–1].
43. Alevizaki M, Saltiki K. Primary hyperparathyroidism in MEN2 syndromes. Recent Results Cancer Res 2015;204:179–86.
44. Machens A, Dralle H. Advances in risk-oriented surgery for multiple endocrine neoplasia type 2. Endocr Relat Cancer 2018;25(2):T41–52.

The Importance of Family History in the Management of Endocrine Disease

Raymon H. Grogan, MD, MS*

KEYWORDS

- Familial genetic disorders • Familial endocrine surgery disorders • Family history
- Endocrine surgery workup • Endocrine patient workup • Familial endocrinopathies
- Family history questions • Endocrine disorder genetic testing

KEY POINTS

- There are more than 25 familial or genetic syndromes that affect the thyroid, parathyroid, adrenal, and endocrine pancreas.
- Family history is the gateway to the decision whether or not to pursue genetic testing; until genetic testing becomes routine for every patient, the family history remains vital.
- Knowing an endocrine patient has a familial syndrome can change the workup, operation, follow-up, and screening and diagnosis of additional family members.
- Multiple endocrine neoplasia syndromes are among the most well-characterized genetic disorders in humans, an excellent example of how detailed genotype–phenotype correlations can lead to improved care.

INTRODUCTION

The family history is an integral part of any complete history and physical examination done in a surgical clinic. However, the family history may hold more or less relevance to the care of a patient depending on the particular subspecialty. For example, when a surgeon sees a patient for an urgent or emergent operation such as an appendectomy, cholecystectomy, or incarcerated hernia repair, the family history has a minimal role in deciding when or how to operate on that patient. However, for other surgical specialties, family history becomes more significant, because it can provide insight into a patient's risk for developing certain cancers or even give a hint as to how aggressively a particular patient's cancer might behave. One of the surgical specialties that relies heavily on the family history is endocrine surgery. There are at least 25

Disclosures: The authors have nothing to disclose.
Baylor St. Luke's Medical Center, Michael E. DeBakey Department of Surgery, Baylor College of Medicine, 7200 Cambridge Street, 7th floor, Houston, Texas 77030, USA
* Corresponding author.
E-mail address: rgrogan@bcm.edu

Surg Clin N Am 99 (2019) 711–720
https://doi.org/10.1016/j.suc.2019.04.016 surgical.theclinics.com

distinct familial syndromes that affect the endocrine organs and may lead to an operation at some point in that patient's life. Thyroid disorders, hyperparathyroidism, adrenal tumors, and pancreatic neuroendocrine tumors all have the possibility to be linked to some form of heritable disorder. Importantly, once known to be present, these familial syndromes can dictate the type and extent of operation, the amount of follow-up, and the amount of screening necessary for an individual patient or an entire family. It is not a stretch to say that, without a thorough and accurate family history, for many endocrine surgery disorders, a patient has not been completely worked up or cared for appropriately.

As technology and our understanding of genetics and genomics evolves, the family history continues to play an ever more important role in caring for patients. We are now at a time when whole genome or exome sequencing is a possibility, but not a routine clinical reality. There may come a time when whole genome sequencing is a standard part of a patient's workup, no different than a complete blood count or Chem-7 panel, but until that time, the gateway to genetic testing remains a thorough family history and an astute interpretation of the findings. A family history that is found to be suspicious is what currently triggers possible further genetic workup. And as genetic testing becomes more advanced, the ability to take clinical action using that information will continue to develop. There is likely no better example of the use of genetic testing for clinical decision making than in the case of multiple endocrine neoplasia (MEN) 2. Today it is possible for genetic testing for MEN2 to lead to a prophylactic thyroidectomy in a young child, and is almost completely dependent on the particular type of mutation found in the family. There are very few genetic syndromes so well-characterized in any other specialty in medicine. And endocrine surgery is full of examples like this. In this article, we explore the endocrine disorders that can be associated with familial syndromes. Interestingly, some of these genetic disorders affect multiple endocrine organs. To do this, we first examine the individual syndromes that affect multiple endocrine organs. Then we will also look specifically at each of the endocrine systems that are routinely encountered by endocrine surgeons, namely, the thyroid, parathyroid, adrenal, and endocrine pancreas to describe any familial syndromes that only affect 1 organ at a time.

THE GENOTYPE–PHENOTYPE CORRELATION

In the absence of genetic testing, the family history is used to help family members understand their risk of disease and develop a screening protocol for family members. In essence, when a physician asks a patient for their family history, what they are really asking is whether or not a particular genetic phenotype exists within a family. Keeping this concept in mind will help to better inform the manner in which the family history is obtained. A person's phenotype is the set of observable physical properties of an individual. The phenotype is partially determined by the genotype, but can be altered by the environment. In the setting of familial syndromes the phenotype is used to describe the types of organs affected by a disorder, whether any particular tumor is benign or malignant, and how aggressive a cancer might act. This phenotype is typically what one is truly asking about when is collecting the family history. The family history paints a picture of the phenotype, which should then alert the physician to further questioning regarding the family history or lead to genetic testing if available and clinically warranted. A genotype–phenotype correlation is when a particular genetic mutation can be linked to developing a particular familial or heritable phenotype. In some cases, the genotype–phenotype correlation is very strong and can predict tumor behavior with great accuracy. A good example of this is the genotype–phenotype correlation in MEN2A and MEN2B. In this example, specific point mutations in the MEN gene are used to predict with great accuracy how aggressive a cancer might be in a family and can even be used to consider prophylactic thyroidectomy in children. In other cases, the genotype–phenotype correlation is less well-understood. An example of this is von Hippel-Lindau (VHL) syndrome in which there is significant overlap in the genotype–phenotype correlation between families and within individuals, regardless of the particular mutation, making the specific genetic change less useful for prognostication. Regardless of accuracy, the majority of the familial endocrine disorders have a specific gene or loci that has been linked to a particular broad phenotype. One exception to this rule is familial nonmedullary thyroid cancer, which has no single specific genetic loci associated with the development of this syndrome. The only way to conduct a thorough family history in these patients is to understand what to look for in the family history and to know what questions to ask (see **Box 3**). To this end, we briefly describe the majority of familial endocrine disorders with their major defining criteria.

SYNDROMES THAT AFFECT MULTIPLE ENDOCRINE ORGANS

Multiple Endocrine Neoplasia Syndromes

The MEN syndromes are a group of disorders that affect multiple endocrine organs with both benign and malignant tumors.[1–5] The diagnosis is typically made when at least 2 specific endocrine organs are affected. Other nonendocrine organs can also be affected in the MEN syndromes. The MEN syndromes are some of the most well-defined and broadly studied genetic syndromes in humans. These syndromes are best described according to the phenotype they are associated with.

Multiple endocrine neoplasia type 1

MEN1 is an autosomal-dominant syndrome with a prevalence of 1 in 30,000 people. The syndrome is caused by a mutation in the *MEN1* gene. Mutations in this gene lead to alterations tin the function of the MENIN protein. The classic triad of the syndrome is characterized by tumors of the pituitary, parathyroid, and islet cells of the pancreas. In addition, MEN1 is also associated with benign nonfunctional adrenal cortical tumors, carcinoid tumors, facial angiofibromas, collagenomas, lipomas, leiomyomas, meningiomas, and ependymomas. These tumors can cause a wide variety of clinical syndromes related to excess hormone production from these organs. Possible hormone excess includes prolactin (lactation), growth hormone (excess growth of jaw and other tissue), adrenocorticotrophic hormone (hypercortisolism/Cushing's), gastrin (stomach and duodenal ulcers), glucagon (diabetes and skin rash), vasoactive intestinal peptide (diarrhea), and parathyroid hormone (hyperparathyroidism/kidney stones/osteoporosis).

Multiple endocrine neoplasia type 2

There are 3 subtypes of MEN2, namely, MEN2A, MEN2B, and familial medullary thyroid cancer. All 3 subtypes are autosomal-dominant syndromes with a prevalence of 1 in 30,000 people. The syndrome is caused by a mutation in the *RET* gene. MEN2A is responsible for approximately 75% of all MEN2 cases, MEN2B is responsible for approximately 5% of cases, and familial medullary thyroid cancer is responsible for the remaining 20% of cases of MEN2. Patients with either any of the 3 subtypes almost universally will develop medullary thyroid cancer at some point in their lifespan.

Multiple endocrine neoplasia type 2A

Nearly 100% of patients with MEN2A will develop medullary thyroid cancer, 50% will develop pheochromocytomas, and 10% will develop primary hyperparathyroidism.

The clinical diagnosis of MEN2A is suspected when at least 2 of the tumors in the syndrome are found either in the same individual or in first-degree relatives in a family.

Multiple endocrine neoplasia type 2B

Nearly 100% of patients with MEN2B will develop medullary thyroid cancer; 50% will develop pheochromocytomas; 95% will have mucosal neuromas of the lips, tongue, or gastrointestinal tract; and 95% will have joint or spine problems. In addition, there can be a subtle change in facial appearance in up to 75% of individuals associated with swollen lips and thickened eye lids.

Familial medullary thyroid cancer

Nearly 100% of patients with familial medullary thyroid cancer develop medullary thyroid cancer. There are no other known components of this particular MEN2 syndrome.

Von Hippel-Lindau syndrome

VHL syndrome is an autosomal-dominant syndrome with a prevalence of 1 in 36,000 people. The syndrome is caused by several different types of mutations in the *VHL* gene. The VHL syndrome affects multiple organs and can manifest with central nervous system hemangioblastomas, retinal hemangioblastomas, endolymphatic sac tumors, benign asymptomatic lung lesions, pancreatic cysts and cancers, pheochromocytomas, paragangliomas, benign asymptomatic liver lesions, renal cysts, renal cell carcinoma, and cystadenomas of the gonads (both male and female). Clinical signs and symptoms of VHL include headaches, retinal detachment, blindness, hearing loss, tinnitus, pancreatic cysts or neuroendocrine tumors, renal cell carcinoma, pheochromocytoma, and cysts of the broad ligament or epididymis.

Carney complex

Carney complex is an autosomal-dominant syndrome with a very rare prevalence. There have only been a few hundred cases reported worldwide. The syndrome is caused by mutations of the *PRKAR1A* gene, which leads to problems with the protein kinase A protein. Clinical signs and symptoms include spotty skin pigmentation, benign myxomas, atrial myxomas, breast ductal adenomas, acromegaly, Sertoli cell tumors, papillary thyroid cancer, schwannomas, blue nevi, and osteochondromyxomas. Hormone excess can include excess cortisol, prolactin, or insulin-like growth factor-1. The presence of café-au-lait spots or blue nevi in conjunction with a myxoma is highly suspicious for the syndrome.

Li-Fraumeni syndrome

Li-Fraumeni syndrome is an autosomal-dominant syndrome initially thought to be rare. However, new diagnostic criteria have changed its prevalence such that it is thought that it is as frequent as 1 in 5000 to 1 in 20,000 individuals. The syndrome is caused by mutations of the *TP53* gene or the *CHEK2* gene, which leads to problems with the P53 and CHK2 proteins. Both of these proteins are tumor suppressors; thus, alterations of their activity can lead to multiple benign tumors and cancers. The most common cancers found in Li-Fraumeni syndrome include osteosarcoma, soft tissue sarcoma, leukemia, breast cancer, brain cancer, and adrenal cortical carcinoma. In addition, less commonly found cancers have been reported, including stomach, colon, pancreas, esophagus, lung, and gonadal cancers. New diagnostic criteria called the Chompret Criteria can help in the diagnosis of Li-Fraumeni syndrome. In this system, there are 3 criterion and any person or family that meets any 1 of these 3 criteria should undergo genetic testing. Criterion 1 is any of the noted tumors in someone under the age of 46 along with any first-degree relative with any of these cancers before age 56 (with the exception of breast cancer if the index case also has breast cancer). Criterion 2 is a person with at least 2 of the Li-Fraumeni syndrome cancers with one of them being diagnosed before age 46. Criterion 3 is anyone diagnosed with adrenal cortical carcinoma or a choroid plexus tumor, regardless of family history.

Familial adenomatous polyposis coli

Familial adenomatous polyposis coli (FAP) is an autosomal-dominant syndrome with a prevalence of 1 in 7000 to 1 in 22,000 people worldwide. The syndrome is caused by mutations in the *APC* gene or a mutation in the *MUTYH* gene. There are 4 subtypes of FAP that include classic FAP, attenuated FAP, Gardner syndrome, and Turcot syndrome. All the syndromes are associated with multiple colorectal polyps that increase a person's risk for colon cancer. Classic FAP is diagnosed when a person has more than 100 colorectal polyps. Attenuated FAP is associated with an individual who has between 20 and 100 colorectal polyps. Gardner syndrome is multiple colorectal polyps along with epidermoid cysts, fibromas, desmoid tumors, and osteomas. Turcot syndrome is associated with multiple colon polyps and brain cancer, either glioblastoma or medulloblastoma. In addition to the noted tumors, patients are at risk for small bowel tumors, pancreas cancer, hepatoblastoma, stomach cancer, bile duct cancer, adrenal cortical carcinoma, and papillary thyroid cancer. There is a very specific subtype of papillary thyroid cancer known as the cribriform-morullar variant of papillary thyroid cancer. When this type of thyroid cancer is found, it is highly suspicious of FAP syndrome.

Tuberous sclerosis

Tuberous sclerosis is a rare, autosomal-dominant syndrome with a prevalence estimated to be 1 in 1 million individuals. The syndrome has been linked to mutations in the *TSC1* or *TSC2* genes. Some major features of the syndrome are angiofibromas, skin lesions, brain tumors, renal angiomyolipomas, hemangioblastomas, pancreatic cysts, pancreatic neuroendocrine tumors, and pheochromocytomas.

McCune-Albright syndrome

McCune-Albright syndrome is not associated with a particular inheritance pattern; rather, it is a result of genetic mosaicism resulting from a random mutation of the *GNAS* gene early in development. It has a prevalence between 1 in 1000 and 1 in 1 million people. The severity of the disorder depends on how many copies of the mutated gene an individual has. Even though it is not a familial syndrome, it is included here because it has a syndromic presentation that can be confused for a familial syndrome. It is characterized by fibrous bony lesions that can lead to bone deformity and asymmetry, café-au-lait spots, early puberty, hyperthyroidism, multinodular goiter, pituitary adenoma and excess growth hormone, and adrenal cortical adenomas causing Cushing's syndrome. Gastrointestinal polyps are also sometimes found.

Thyroid

Pendred syndrome

Pendred syndrome is an autosomal-recessive syndrome with an unknown prevalence caused by a mutation in the *SLC26A4* gene, which codes for the pendrin protein. The syndrome is characterized by congenital or early onset hearing loss and goiter. It is thought to account for 7% to 8% of all cases of congenital hearing loss.

Werner syndrome

Werner syndrome is an autosomal-recessive syndrome with a prevalence of 1 in 200,000 people worldwide. However, founder populations have been noted in Japan and Sardinia, Italy, where the estimated prevalence is closer to 1 in 30,000 individuals in those populations. It is caused by mutations in the *WRN* gene, which codes for the Werner protein. The syndrome is associated with premature aging such as developing gray hair, wrinkles, and hair loss in the 20s, followed by development of cataracts, skin ulcers cataracts, or osteoporosis in the 30s. In addition, individuals with Werner's syndrome are at increased risk for cancers, including papillary thyroid cancer, melanoma, soft tissue sarcoma, and osteosarcoma.

Familial nonmedullary papillary thyroid cancer

Familial nonmedullary papillary thyroid cancer seems to be an autosomal-dominant syndrome that accounts for approximately 5% of all cases of papillary thyroid cancer.[6] Several genetic loci have been linked to familial nonmedullary papillary thyroid cancer; however, most of these loci have been found in single families. There is no one dominant genetic loci that has been found to date that can be used to screen for familial nonmedullary papillary thyroid cancer. It is characterized by multiple members of a single family being diagnosed with papillary or in some cases follicular thyroid cancer. The diagnosis is a clinical diagnosis based on family history, and is made when at least 3 first-degree relatives are found to have nonmedullary thyroid cancer in the same family. These cancers are often found to be more aggressive than sporadic papillary thyroid cancer. Genetic anticipation has been noted in some families, with the earliest known age of a diagnosis of papillary thyroid cancer associated with familial nonmedullary papillary thyroid cancer being 8 years of age. In addition to thyroid cancer, many family members also have multinodular goiter.

Cowden's syndrome

Cowden's syndrome is an autosomal-dominant syndrome with a prevalence of 1 in 200,000 people worldwide. The syndrome is caused by mutations in the *PTEN* gene. Cowden's syndrome is characterized by a high risk of tumors of the breast, thyroid, endometrium, colorectal, kidney, and skin. In addition to these tumors, benign conditions including skin tags, papillomas, and macrocephaly can be found in individuals with the syndrome. The 2 most common cancers in Cowden's syndrome are breast cancer (50%–85%) and thyroid cancer (30%–40%). Thyroid cancer is typically follicular thyroid cancer, however papillary thyroid cancer can also be associated with the syndrome. The occurrence of breast and thyroid cancer in a single individual is suspicious for Cowden's syndrome. Likewise, a strong family history of breast and thyroid cancer in multiple first-degree relatives is also suspicious for the syndrome. Finally, anyone with thyroid cancer and a large head circumference should raise concern for the possibility of Cowden's syndrome.

Parathyroid

Hyperparathyroidism jaw-tumor syndrome

Hyperparathyroidism jaw-tumor syndrome is an autosomal-dominant syndrome with an unknown prevalence caused by a mutation in the *HRPT2* gene, which codes for the parafibromin protein. There have been approximately 200 cases reported in the worldwide literature. The syndrome is characterized by hyperparathyroidism, jaw tumors, and an increased risk of parathyroid carcinoma. Most commonly, a single parathyroid adenoma is found; however, multigland disease is also frequent. There is an increased risk for parathyroid carcinoma; approximately 15% of these patients develop this rare cancer. Only 25% to 50% present with the benign fibroma of the jaw that is also characteristic of the syndrome. In addition, uterine tumors and kidney tumors are found in this syndrome.

Benign familial hypocalciuric hypercalcemia

Benign familial hypocalciuric hypercalcemia is an autosomal-dominant syndrome with an estimated prevalence of 1 in 78,000.[7] The true prevalence is unknown because many of the symptoms are subclinical and may never be diagnosed. The syndrome is caused by a mutation in the *CASR* gene, which causes a loss of function of the calcium-sensing receptor protein. The syndrome is associated with mildly elevated calcium along with hypocalciuria, hypophosphatemia, and hypermagnesemia. Parathyroid hormone levels are usually at the upper limits of normal or mildly elevated, and the parathyroid glands may be mildly enlarged. Parathyroidectomy will not cure the syndrome and has no role in its management.

Familial isolated hyperparathyroidism

Familial isolated hyperparathyroidism is an autosomal-dominant syndrome with an unknown prevalence that can be caused by mutations in *MEN1*, *HRPT2*, or *CASR* genes. There are also families with a family history of isolated hyperparathyroidism in which a particular mutation has not been identified. As the name implies, it is associated with isolated hyperparathyroidism without any other known clinical sequelae in multiple family members.

Adrenal

Familial hyperaldosteronism

Familial hyperaldosteronism is an autosomal-dominant syndrome with an unknown prevalence that is thought to account for fewer than 1 in 10 cases of hyperaldosteronism. There are 3 types that are associated with differing onset and severity of hypertension. In type I the hypertension is mild to severe and occurs in early childhood. It is associated with a fusion of the *CYP11B1* and *CYP11B2* genes. In type II, the hypertension occurs in middle adulthood and the genetic cause is unknown. In type III, there is severe hypertension that starts in childhood and often results in end-organ damage to the heart and kidneys. The adrenal glands in type III are enlarged up to 6 times normal. Type III is associated with mutations in the *KCNJ5* gene, which encodes for a potassium transporter protein.

Hereditary paraganglioma–pheochromocytoma syndromes

Hereditary paraganglioma–pheochromocytoma syndromes are a group of autosomal-dominant syndromes with an estimated prevalence of 1 in 1 million people. Mutations in the *SDHB*, *SDHC*, *SDHD*, and *SDHAF2* genes that code for different subunits of the succinate dehydrogenase protein have been associated with the syndrome. Mutations in several other genes have also recently been associated with the syndrome. The syndrome is associated with the development of paragangliomas of both the sympathetic and parasympathetic ganglia. Pheochromocytomas are a particular type of sympathetic paraganglioma that occurs in the adrenal glands. Parasympathetic paragangliomas typically arise in the head and neck region and often do not produce excess hormone. There is an increased risk for developing malignant tumors relative to sporadic paragangliomas.

Neurofibromatosis type 1 (von Recklinghausen's disease)

Neurofibromatosis type 1 (von Recklinghausen's disease) is an autosomal-dominant syndrome with a prevalence of 1 in 3000 people. The syndrome is caused by a mutation in the *NF1* gene. Mutations in this gene lead to alterations tin the function of the Neurofibromin protein that cause neurocutaneous manifestations. The classic patients develop café-au-lait spots and neurofibromas. In addition, they can develop brain tumors, pheochromocytomas, muscle tumors, and spinal cord tumors. These patients are also at risk for developing gastrointestinal stromal tumors and neuroendocrine tumors of the intestines. Neurofibromatosis type 2 is caused by mutations in the *NF2* gene, and can appear similar to type 1 in that patients develop café-au-lait spots and neurofibromas. However, type 2 patients do not typically develop pheochromocytomas.

Beckwith-Wiedemann syndrome

Beckwith-Wiedemann syndrome is inherited in an autosomal-dominant pattern. The syndrome is caused by imprinting of the short arm of chromosome 11 (11p15.5). Imprinting causes 1 copy of the gene/chromosomal region to be deactivated. The most common cause of gene deactivation in Beckwith-Wiedemann syndrome is abnormal DNA methylation patterns. In addition, it can be caused by paternal inheritance of both copies of the gene or genetic mutations. Beckwith-Wiedemann syndrome has a prevalence of 1 in 13,700 people worldwide. Beckwith-Wiedemann syndrome is characterized by macrosomia, abdominal wall defects, childhood tumors, newborn hypoglycemia, cleft palate, port wine stain, and pits or creasing of the ear. Childhood tumors include Wilms tumor, hepatoblastoma, neuroblastoma, and rhabdomyosarcoma. In addition, these patients are at increased risk for adrenal cortical carcinoma. Approximately 20% of all patients with Beckwith-Wiedemann syndrome develop adrenal cortical carcinoma.

Lynch syndrome or hereditary nonpolyposis coli

Lynch syndrome or hereditary nonpolyposis coli is a very common, autosomal-dominant syndrome with a prevalence estimated to be as high as 1 in 300 individuals. The syndrome has been linked to mutations in at least 5 different DNA mismatch repair genes including *MLH1*, *MSH2*, *MSH6*, *PMS2*, and *EPCAM*. Patients have an increased lifetime risk of developing colorectal cancer, endometrial cancer, and ovarian cancer.

Box 1
Key family history questions for thyroid patients

For papillary thyroid cancer

Has anyone else in the family been diagnosed with thyroid cancer?

If so, are they first-degree relatives?

Is there a history of goiter?

Is there a history of early aging in the family, that is, excessive skin wrinkling and gray hair in their 20s?

Is there a history of osteosarcoma?

Is there a history of endometrial cancer?

Is there a history of kidney cancer?

Is there a history of breast cancer?

Is there a history of enlarged head circumference?

For medullary thyroid cancer

Is there a history of pheochromocytoma?

Is there a history of hyperparathyroidism?

For benign goiter

Is there a history of hearing loss at birth?

Box 2 Key family history questions for parathyroid patients
Is there a history of pituitary tumors?
Is there a history of pancreatic neuroendocrine tumors?
Is there a history of pheochromocytoma?
Is there a history of jaw tumors?
Is there a history of uterine cancer?
Is there a history of kidney cancer?
Is there a history of hyperparathyroidism in the family?

It is thought that 3% of all cases of adrenal cortical carcinoma are associated with Lynch syndrome. This is similar to the prevalence of Lynch syndrome in both colorectal and endometrial cancer.

Congenital adrenal hyperplasia

Congenital adrenal hyperplasia is a group of rare autosomal-recessive syndromes associated with mutations in several different genes that encode proteins that are part of the pathway that produces hormones in the adrenal gland. It has a prevalence of approximately 1 in 15,000 individuals. These mutations cause relative adrenal hormone deficiencies, which leads to the overproduction of other hormone precursors to compensate for the missing hormone. The resulting hormone overproduction leads to adrenal hyperplasia as well as other downstream consequences, depending on which hormone is deficient.

SUMMARY

The family history is an important part of the history and physical for any patient; however, its relevance and impact vary by specialty. Endocrine surgery is a subspecialty in which the family history has a vital role. A thorough family history of an patient undergoing endocrine surgery can change the diagnosis, change the operation, reveal new diagnosis, and dictate screening and surveillance for the future. With the use of electronic medical records, asking a thorough family history is made easier as a standard set of questions can be templated into the note (**Boxes 1–3**). It is of utmost importance that this portion of the history and physical examination not be overlooked.

Box 3 Key family history questions for adrenal patients
Is there a history of hypertension at a young age, or difficult to control hypertension in middle age?
Is there a history of neurofibromas or café-au-lait spots?
Is there a history of early childhood tumors?
Is there a history of cleft palate or abdominal wall defects?
Is there a history of colorectal cancer?
Is there a history of ovarian cancer?
Is there a history of endometrial cancer?

REFERENCES

1. National Institute of Health. NIH genetics home reference. Available at: https://ghr.nlm.nih.gov/. Accessed February 1, 2019.
2. Rare Diseases Clinical Research Network. Available at: https://www.rarediseasesnetwork.org. Accessed February 1, 2019.
3. American Society of Clinical Oncology. Cancer.net. Available at: https://www.cancer.net/cancer-types. Accessed February 1, 2019.
4. Clark OH, Duh Q-Y, Kebebew E, et al, editors. Textbook of endocrine surgery. 3rd edition. London: Jaypee; 2016. https://doi.org/10.5005/jp/books/12798.
5. Angelos P, Grogan RH, editors. Difficult decisions in endocrine surgery. 1st edition. New York: Springer International Publishing; 2018. https://doi.org/10.1007/978-3-319-92860-9.
6. Nixon IJ, Suarez C, Simo R, et al. The impact of family history on non-medullary thyroid cancer. Eur J Surg Oncol 2016;42(10):1455–63.
7. Lee JY, Shoback DM. Familial hypocalciuric hypercalcemia and related disorders. Best Pract Res Clin Endocrinol Metab 2018;32(5):609–19.

Evaluation of an Adrenal Incidentaloma

Dylan S. Jason, MD, Sarah C. Oltmann, MD*

KEYWORDS

• Adrenal incidentaloma • Adrenal mass • Adrenal neoplasm • Adrenal work up

KEY POINTS

- Adrenal incidentalomas are, by definition, adrenal masses found incidentally on imaging.
- A standardized algorithm to approach the workup of patients with adrenal incidentaloma will ensure proper diagnosis and treatment.
- It is critical not to miss a functional or malignant adrenal mass.
- Those patients not requiring surgical resection need an appropriate follow-up plan based on the initial assessment, be that subsequent imaging and/or biochemical evaluation, or no further evaluation.

INTRODUCTION

Use of cross-sectional imaging has continued to increase over the past few decades, often resulting in the detection of previously unrecognized adrenal masses. Cross-sectional imaging of both the chest and abdomen will include the region of the adrenal glands. Occasionally, thoracic and lumbar spine imaging also may capture them. The term "adrenal incidentaloma" was coined to describe these findings.[1] With a reported incidence of up to 10%,[2,3] with higher incidences noted with advancing age, it is possible that a high-volume center would detect multiple adrenal incidentalomas per day.

Although many of these incidentalomas are benign and inert (up to 80%), a small percentage will cause hormonal overproduction (cortisol, aldosterone, or catecholamine/metanephrine) or may represent a malignancy (primary adrenal tumor or metastatic from another source). Hormonal overproduction can have significant morbidity associated with it, and in some cases may result in mortality. Adrenocortical carcinoma (ACC) is an extremely rare and aggressive cancer arising from the adrenal gland. Surgery, when ACC is caught early, is the only chance for cure.

Disclosure Statement: The authors have nothing to disclose.
Department of Surgery, The University of Texas Southwestern Medical Center, 5323 Harry Hines Boulevard, E6.104B, Dallas, TX 75390, USA
* Corresponding author.
E-mail address: sarah.oltmann@utsouthwestern.edu

Surg Clin N Am 99 (2019) 721–729
https://doi.org/10.1016/j.suc.2019.04.009 surgical.theclinics.com
0039-6109/19/

Once an adrenal mass is detected, it is important that patients are appropriately screened for hormonal activity. This evaluation may be performed by primary care, or referred on to subspecialists depending on the local expertise and the resources available. Given the potential for a high volume of these lesions, even an expedient, cost-effective, efficient, and accurate workup may cause strain on the health care system. A complete patient history and review of systems can help guide the extent of hormonal workup required. Furthermore, testing often requires specific instructions to the patient about medications to avoid, and timing on how to ensure the screening results provide credible data. A methodical, consistent approach to patient evaluation for adrenal incidentalomas may facilitate timely identification of pathology, while ensuring benign lesions are simply observed. Each medical system should consider creating a dedicated work flow for the workup and referral that fits within their structure.

NORMAL ADRENAL ANATOMY AND PATHOPHYSIOLOGY

The adrenal glands are found within the retroperitoneum, atop the kidneys. Arterial blood flow is obtained through multiple, small, un-named arterioles, and venous outflow is through a single adrenal vein. On the right side, this is a small, short branch directly off the inferior vena cava, and on the left side, the adrenal vein branches off of the phrenic vein, close to its insertion into the left renal vein. The adrenal gland consists of a cortex and a medulla.

The cortex is composed of 3 layers: the zona glomerulosa, the zona fasciculate, and the zona reticularis. The zona glomerulosa is the site of mineralocorticoid production, specifically aldosterone. Aldosterone production is normally stimulated through the renin-angiotensin system, and acts on the distal tubules and collecting ducts of the nephrons resulting in the active reabsorption of sodium, and the excretion of potassium. Blood volume and blood pressure are indirectly impacted as a result. The zona fasciculate is the site of glucocorticoid production, with cortisol serving as the main glucocorticoid. Cortisol influences both the metabolic and immunologic activities of the body. Finally, the zona reticularis is the site of androgen production, dehydroepiandrosterone (DHEA), and DHEA sulfate (DHEA-S), precursors to testosterone.

The medulla is derived from embryonic neural crest cells, which produce and release catecholamines and metanephrines, as well as to a lesser extent, dopamine. The adrenal medulla is the location of phenylethanolamine N-methyltransferase (PNMT), the enzyme needed to convert catecholamines to metanephrines.

CLINICAL PRESENTATION AND EXAMINATION

When evaluating adrenal masses, the focus should be on determining the functional status of the tumor, if it is malignant, and are there any associated symptoms reported by the patient. Although most of these masses will be nonfunctional, approximately 80% in some series,[4] there is a real risk of functional adenoma (5%), pheochromocytoma (5%), ACC (<4%), and metastatic lesions (<2%).[5]

History and physical should be completed and focused on excluding or including a functional tumor (**Table 1**). During the review of systems, physicians should inquire about the following: headaches, flushing, palpitations/arrhythmias, tremor, anxiety, easy bruising or bleeding, insomnia, fatigue, weakness, muscle cramping, poor wound healing, sudden changes in weight, hair loss, and easy tearing of skin/thinning of skin. Besides symptoms that may be associated with hormonal production, questions should be asked regarding potential mass effect in the abdomen: abdominal/flank or back pain, early satiety, nausea, or vomiting. Additional personal history to

Table 1
Signs and symptoms of adrenal tumor by type

Tumor Type	Symptoms	Signs
Cortisol producing	Muscle weakness, easy bruising/ bleeding, poor wound healing, decrease libido, psychiatric disturbances, insomnia, flushing, palpitations	Moon facies, buffalo hump, hirsutism, abdominal striae, central obesity with peripheral wasting, thinning of skin, hypertension, hyperglycemia
Aldosteronoma	Muscle cramping, muscle weakness, fatigue, headache, polydipsia, polyuria	Refractory hypertension, hypokalemia
Pheochromocytoma	Episodic headache, sweating, palpitations, pallor, anxiety, sense of impending doom, flushing/hot flashes	Hypertension, tachycardia, cardiac arrhythmias, acute myocardial infarction, congestive heart failure, tremor
Adrenocortical carcinoma (ACC)	Large: mass effect Productive: Cushing's syndrome, virilization	Large: none, may be able to palpate Productive: related to the hormone produced
Secondary metastasis to the adrenal gland	Generally none related to the adrenal tumor	Findings consistent with primary tumor source, adrenal insufficiency if adrenal tissue compromised
Nonfunctional mass	Small: none Large: vague abdominal complaints/mass effect/pain	Small: none Large: none, may be able to palpate

clarify includes any history of hypertension, hypertensive crisis, cardiovascular disease, previous myocardial infarction or cerebrovascular accident, pathologic fractures, or recent onset of hyperglycemia/diabetes mellitus. Inquiry into age-appropriate cancer screening should be done, as well as elucidating any particular personal risk factors for malignancy. A direct inquiry of a family history of adrenal masses or early sudden death from presumed stroke or heart attack should be performed.

A complete physical examination follows. Attention is paid to heart rate and blood pressure, looking for tachycardia and/or hypertension. Additional physical findings to note: moon facies, buffalo hump, increased supraclavicular fat pads, striae, central obesity with peripheral wasting, cardiac arrhythmias, tremor, ecchymosis of extensor surfaces of upper extremities, thinning of skin or hair, and/or agitation. Based on patient age, mass characteristics, and other risk factors, consideration should be given to a complete breast examination to rule out masses, a skin examination to evaluate for melanoma, stool guaiac, and/or colonoscopy for colorectal screening, and a chest radiograph to look for pulmonary masses.

BIOCHEMICAL EVALUATION

Diagnostic procedures for adrenal incidentalomas start with laboratory evaluation to assess for hormone excess. The focused laboratory assessment includes studies to evaluate for cortisol excess, pheochromocytoma, and in those patients with hypertension, primary hyperaldosteronism (**Table 2**).[6]

To assess for cortisol excess, a low-dose dexamethasone suppression test is a reliable starting point. In the evening (before 2300), 1 mg of dexamethasone is taken

Table 2
Screening evaluation for adrenal incidentaloma based on clinical concerns

Clinical Diagnosis	Laboratory Test
Cortisol producing	• Low-dose dexamethasone suppression test • 24-h urine free cortisol
Pheochromocytoma	• Serum fractionated metanephrines • 24-h urine fractionated metanephrines and fractionated catecholamines
Primary hyperaldosteronism	• Plasma aldosterone concentration • Plasma renin activity
Adrenocortical carcinoma	• Low-dose dexamethasone suppression test • Serum dehydroepiandrosterone sulfate

with a fasting blood sample collected at 0800 the next morning. Those patients who do not at all appear to suppress (cortisol levels >5.0 μg/dL or >138 nmol/L), and have low adrenocorticotropic hormone levels, there is clear evidence of Cushing's syndrome. However, some patients will appear to not completely suppress (cortisol levels ranging from 1.9 to 5 μg/dL or 51–138 nmol/L), which is concerning for subclinical Cushing's syndrome. These patients benefit from further investigation with either a 24-hour urine free cortisol measurement, or midnight salivary cortisol measurements. If there is any question about the patient's compliance with taking the dexamethasone appropriately, serum dexamethasone levels also can be drawn. If a 24-hour urine measurement is performed, it is important to remember to control for possible user error by also obtaining a 24-hour urine creatinine measurement. Those patients found to have excess cortisol production should also then be screened for hypertension, type 2 diabetes, and osteopenia/osteoporosis. Treatment directed at these additional conditions should be initiated as appropriate.

If during evaluation a patient is noted to be hypertensive, the patient should be screened for primary hyperaldosteronism. This involves the measurement of plasma aldosterone and plasma renin. Potassium levels also can be checked; however, not all patients with primary hyperaldosteronism will have hypokalemia. Once aldosterone and renin levels have been drawn, the plasma aldosterone concentration (PAC) to plasma renin activity (PRA) ratio must be determined.[7] In patients with primary hyperaldosteronism, the PRA is usually low (<1 ng/mL per hour) and the PAC is elevated (>15 ng/dL). An elevated PAC, a low PRA, and a PAC-PRA ratio that is >20 is consistent with the diagnosis of primary hyperaldosteronism.

All patients should be screened for pheochromocytoma. Plasma-fractionated metanephrines, or 24-hour urine fractionated metanephrines and catecholamines should be measured. Although plasma measurements may be more convenient for the patient, it is important to note the good sensitivity (96%–100%) but poor specificity (85%–90%).[8,9] If plasma-fractionated metanephrines are elevated, a 24-hour urine collection should be used as a confirmatory test due to its much greater specificity. Levels greater than twofold over the normal reference range are considered diagnostic for pheochromocytoma.

For patients with imaging worrisome for ACC, or reported signs and symptoms of hirsutism or virilization, additional testing should be performed. Evaluation of sex steroid hormone levels is appropriate in this setting. DHEA-S is the most common; however, androstenedione, testosterone, 17-OH-progesterone, and 17-B-estradiol also can be measured.

IMAGING CHARACTERISTICS

Computed tomography (CT) is the most common imaging modality that reveals an incidentaloma. It is important for the clinician to understand the reason for the initial imaging and the method used to evaluate the images (**Table 3**).

On noncontrasted CT images, Hounsfield unit (HU) measurements can provide helpful information to stratify the mass. If an adrenal mass has a smooth border and measures less than 10 HU (indicating a high fat density) it is very likely to be a benign adenoma.[10] Masses measuring greater than 20 HU are more concerning, and require further evaluation to rule out adrenal cortical carcinoma, pheochromocytoma, or a secondary metastasis to the adrenal gland.

Those nodules with indeterminate or concerning features on noncontrast imaging benefit from a dedicated adrenal protocol CT scan to further delineate characteristics. Adrenal protocoling generally involves thin cuts (2–3 mm) through the adrenal glands, with 4 phases of image capture: noncontrast, early arterial, venous, and delayed washout. A nodule with a rapid washout (>50% at 10 minutes after contrast administration) is consistent with adenoma, whereas delayed washout (<50% at 10 minutes after contrast administration) is concerning for adrenal carcinoma, pheochromocytoma, or metastases.[11]

Although CT is the most commonly used adrenal imaging, MRI is also used. On MRI, benign adenomas will have isointensity with the liver on both T1-weighted and

Table 3
Radiographic characteristics

Tumor Type	Computed Tomography	MRI
Benign adenoma	Unilateral homogeneous mass <4 cm, smooth contour, clear margination Low (<10 HU) unenhanced attenuation Rapid contrast washout (>50% at 10 min)	Isointensity with liver on both T1 and T2. Lipid shift evident.
Pheochromocytoma	Highly vascular Increased attenuation (>20 HU) on unenhanced CT Delayed washout (<50% at 10 min) Hemorrhagic and cystic changes Variable sizes and laterality (possible bilateral)	High signal intensity on T2.
Adrenocortical carcinoma	Large (>4 cm), heterogeneous with central low attenuation due to tumor necrosis, irregular shape, calcifications, unilateral Delayed washout (<50% at 10 min) Evidence of local invasion	Hypointense to the liver on T1. Moderate to high signal intensity on T2. Evidence of local invasion.
Adrenal metastases	Irregular, heterogeneous, possibly bilateral High attenuation (>20 HU) on unenhanced CT Delayed washout (<50% at 10 min)	Isointense to the liver on T1. Moderate to high signal intensity on T2.
Others	Adrenal cysts Myelolipomas Adrenal hemorrhage	Characteristic appearance.

T2-weighted images; they will also display chemical shift that is consistent with lipid on out of phase images. Pheochromocytomas will display high intensity on T2 series, and may also display cystic and hemorrhagic changes. ACC will be hypointense to the liver on T1 and have moderate to high intensity on T2 images. MRI is very useful in delineating the extent of local invasion of ACC.[12]

The maximum diameter of the mass is predictive of malignancy, with 90% of ACCs being larger than 4 cm in diameter at time of diagnosis.[13] As ACC also tends to extend into the adrenal vein as a tumor thrombus, it is critical to evaluate for vascular involvement or extension. Irregular shape and heterogeneous-appearing masses are concerning for adrenal metastases. Tumor necrosis and calcifications also should raise concern for carcinoma.

ADRENAL BIOPSY

The role of adrenal biopsy is controversial at baseline. A fine-needle aspiration biopsy may be considered in a multidisciplinary fashion if all the following are true: the mass is proven to be hormonally inactive, the mass is indeterminate on imaging, and the management of the patient would be altered by the histology results. This is generally in the setting of a known primary malignancy elsewhere with a newly discovered adrenal mass.[14] Risks of adrenal biopsy include hematoma (adrenal, renal, liver), pancreatitis, abdominal pain, pneumothorax, hematuria, abscess formation, and seeding of tumor cells along the needle track.[15] If ACC is suspected, the mass should not be biopsied.

TREATMENT

For functional unilateral adrenal masses that do not have radiological features concerning for malignancy, patients should be referred for laparoscopic adrenalectomy. Appropriate medical perioperative management is imperative to ensure patient safety. Masses highly suspicious for ACC should be referred for open adrenalectomy. Other unilateral adrenal masses with indeterminate findings on imaging or size >4 cm should be offered surgical intervention. Surgical approach for these may be laparoscopic or open, depending on the individual patient factors.

Unilateral adrenal myelolipomas are diagnosed based on imaging characteristics alone due to the presence of large amounts of fat in the adrenal mass.[16] These masses do not generally require surgical intervention; however, surgery can be considered if the myelolipoma is causing symptoms of mass effect, or rapid growth is noted.

Laparoscopic adrenalectomy is the gold standard for most adrenal masses. Laparoscopic adrenalectomy has been shown to have the least postoperative pain, shorter length of stay, and decreased blood loss, as well as faster recovery time.[17] Patients should ideally be referred to a high-volume adrenal surgeon (>4 adrenalectomies a year) for optimal clinical outcomes.[18,19] Patients with known or suspected ACC should be considered for open adrenalectomy due to the high risk of local recurrence and peritoneal carcinomatosis.[20]

FOLLOW-UP

A fair number of adrenal incidentalomas will be small, benign-appearing, and nonfunctional lesions, so there needs to be an appropriate plan for follow-up if surgical intervention is not planned (**Table 4**). These lesions can be followed with repeat imaging at 6 to 12 months to reevaluate for interval size increase or development of suspicious features.[21] Further imaging intervals (6, 12, or 24 months) and the type of imaging

Table 4
Society guidelines regarding adrenal incidentaloma follow-up

Society	Imaging Follow-up	Biochemical Follow-up
American Association of Clinical Endocrinologists (AACE), American Association of Endocrine Surgeons (AAES)[23]	Mass <4 cm, no concerning features = repeat imaging at 3 and 6 mo then annually for 1–2 y.	Annually for up to 5 y.
American College of Radiology (ARC)[22]	Benign mass (myelolipoma, cyst, hemorrhage) = no additional workup or follow-up imaging. 1–2 cm in size but no diagnostic benign features = repeat imaging at 12 mo. 2–4 cm in size but no diagnostic benign features = repeat imaging in 6–12 mo depending on clinical context.	Per AACE/AAES recommendations.
ESE (European Society of Endocrinology)[6]	No repeat imaging on masses <4 cm in size with clear benign features. Indeterminate mass on imaging = repeat imaging at 6–12 mo. Resection if >20% increase in size or development of concerning features. Repeat images at 6–12 mo if size increase is <20%.	No repeat hormonal workup if initial workup was normal unless development of clinically apparent endocrine activity or worsening of comorbidities.

should be guided by the individual case and the physician's clinical judgment. Interval enlargement of more than 1 cm warrants consideration of resection. Repeat biochemical workup also should be repeated at 12 months and then at further intervals depending on the clinical situation.

SUMMARY

The adrenal incidentaloma is becoming more common in part because of more widely used cross-sectional imaging such as CT and MRI. Using a combination of imaging findings, a thorough history and physical examination, and biochemical workup, a definitive diagnosis for incidentalomas can be reached. Due to the increasing number of these masses being detected, it is important that each center have an approach to the workup that takes into account the resources available. The clinicians caring for these patients must be well versed in the differential, workup, treatment, and follow-up.

ACKNOWLEDGMENTS

Dedman Family Scholar in Clinical Care - Support for SCO.

REFERENCES

1. Zeiger MA, Thompson GB, Duh QY, et al, American Association of Clinical Endocrinologists, American Association of Endocrine Surgeons. American Association of Clinical Endocrinologists and American Association of Endocrine Surgeons

Medical Guidelines for the management of adrenal incidentalomas: executive summary of recommendations. Endocr Pract 2009;15(5):450–3.
2. Kloos RT, Gross MD, Francis IR, et al. Incidentally discovered adrenal masses. Endocr Rev 1995;16(4):460–84.
3. Gajraj H, Young AE. Adrenal incidentaloma. Br J Surg 1993;80(4):422–6.
4. Young WF Jr. Management approaches to adrenal incidentalomas. A view from Rochester, Minnesota. Endocrinol Metab Clin North Am 2000;29(1):159–85, x.
5. Grumbach MM, Biller BM, Braunstein GD, et al. Management of the clinically inapparent adrenal mass ("incidentaloma"). Ann Intern Med 2003;138(5):424–9.
6. Fassnacht M, Arlt W, Bancos I, et al. Management of adrenal incidentalomas: European Society of Endocrinology clinical practice guideline in collaboration with the European Network for the Study of Adrenal Tumors. Eur J Endocrinol 2016; 175(2):G1–34.
7. Funder JW, Carey RM, Mantero F, et al. The management of primary aldosteronism: case detection, diagnosis, and treatment: an Endocrine Society clinical practice guideline. J Clin Endocrinol Metab 2016;101(5):1889–916.
8. Sawka AM, Jaeschke R, Singh RJ, et al. A comparison of biochemical tests for pheochromocytoma: measurement of fractionated plasma metanephrines compared with the combination of 24-hour urinary metanephrines and catecholamines. J Clin Endocrinol Metab 2003;88(2):553–8.
9. Lenders JW, Pacak K, Walther MM, et al. Biochemical diagnosis of pheochromocytoma: which test is best? JAMA 2002;287(11):1427–34.
10. Hamrahian AH, Ioachimescu AG, Remer EM, et al. Clinical utility of noncontrast computed tomography attenuation value (Hounsfield units) to differentiate adrenal adenomas/hyperplasias from nonadenomas: Cleveland Clinic experience. J Clin Endocrinol Metab 2005;90(2):871–7.
11. Szolar DH, Korobkin M, Reittner P, et al. Adrenocortical carcinomas and adrenal pheochromocytomas: mass and enhancement loss evaluation at delayed contrast-enhanced CT. Radiology 2005;234(2):479–85.
12. Israel GM, Korobkin M, Wang C, et al. Comparison of unenhanced CT and chemical shift MRI in evaluating lipid-rich adrenal adenomas. AJR Am J Roentgenol 2004;183(1):215–9.
13. Herrera MF, Grant CS, van Heerden JA, et al. Incidentally discovered adrenal tumors: an institutional perspective. Surgery 1991;110(6):1014–21.
14. Jhala NC, Jhala D, Eloubeidi MA, et al. Endoscopic ultrasound-guided fine-needle aspiration biopsy of the adrenal glands: analysis of 24 patients. Cancer 2004; 102(5):308–14.
15. Arellano RS, Harisinghani MG, Gervais DA, et al. Image-guided percutaneous biopsy of the adrenal gland: review of indications, technique, and complications. Curr Probl Diagn Radiol 2003;32(1):3–10.
16. Craig WD, Fanburg-Smith JC, Henry LR, et al. Fat-containing lesions of the retroperitoneum: radiologic-pathologic correlation. Radiographics 2009;29(1):261–90.
17. Thompson GB, Grant CS, van Heerden JA, et al. Laparoscopic versus open posterior adrenalectomy: a case-control study of 100 patients. Surgery 1997;122(6): 1132–6.
18. Lindeman B, Hashimoto DA, Bababekov YJ, et al. Fifteen years of adrenalectomies: impact of specialty training and operative volume. Surgery 2018; 163(1):150–6.
19. Park HS, Roman SA, Sosa JA. Outcomes from 3144 adrenalectomies in the United States: which matters more, surgeon volume or specialty? Arch Surg 2009;144(11):1060–7.

20. Gonzalez RJ, Shapiro S, Sarlis N, et al. Laparoscopic resection of adrenal cortical carcinoma: a cautionary note. Surgery 2005;138(6):1078–85 [discussion: 1085–6].
21. Terzolo M, Stigliano A, Chiodini I, et al. AME position statement on adrenal incidentaloma. Eur J Endocrinol 2011;164(6):851–70.
22. Mayo-Smith WW, Song JH, Boland GL, et al. Management of incidental adrenal masses: a white paper of the ACR incidental findings committee. J Am Coll Radiol 2017;14(8):1038–44.
23. Zeiger MA, Thompson GB, Duh QY, et al, American Association of Clinical Endocrinologists, American Association of Endocrine Surgeons. The American Association of Clinical Endocrinologists and American Association of Endocrine Surgeons medical guidelines for the management of adrenal incidentalomas. Endocr Pract 2009;15(Suppl 1):1–20.

Evaluation and Management of Primary Hyperaldosteronism

Frances T. Lee, MD[a], Dina Elaraj, MD[b,*]

KEYWORDS

- Hyperaldosteronism • Primary hyperaldosteronism • Adrenal hyperplasia
- Aldosterone excess • Adenoma

KEY POINTS

- Primary hyperaldosteronism is an important and increasingly prevalent cause of hypertension that is characterized by unregulated aldosterone excess.
- More than 90% of primary hyperaldosteronism cases are attributable to either idiopathic adrenal hyperplasia or aldosterone-producing adenomas.
- The approach to the diagnosis of primary hyperaldosteronism should be step-wise, starting with screening of at-risk populations, confirmatory testing for positively screened patients, and subtype classification in order to direct surgical or medical management.
- Based on current guidelines, subtype classification of primary hyperaldosteronism should be determined with both imaging and adrenal vein sampling (AVS), reserving deferment of AVS for a selective subset of patients.

INTRODUCTION

In 1953 an American endocrinologist by the name of Jerome W. Conn[1] described a young female patient who presented with a syndrome of intermittent muscle spasms, weakness, and paralysis lasting 7 years. He noted that her medical work-up was significant for hypertension, hypokalemia, and alkalosis. Under the hypothesis that the patient's symptoms were caused by hypersecretion of a salt-retaining corticoid, Dr Conn conducted urine assays, which detected exceedingly high levels of aldosterone, further supporting his working diagnosis. The patient was ultimately referred for surgical exploration of her adrenal glands and was found to have a unilateral adrenal tumor. It was noted that on removal of the tumor the patient's symptoms subsided and her

Disclosures: The authors have nothing to disclose.
[a] Department of General Surgery, Northwestern University Feinberg School of Medicine, 675 North Saint Clair Street, Suite 3-150, Chicago, IL 60611, USA; [b] Section of Endocrine Surgery, Northwestern University Feinberg School of Medicine, 676 North Saint Clair Street, Suite 650, Chicago, IL 60611, USA
* Corresponding author.
E-mail address: delaraj@nm.org

Surg Clin N Am 99 (2019) 731–745
https://doi.org/10.1016/j.suc.2019.04.010
surgical.theclinics.com

metabolic abnormalities had normalized, a phenomenon that helped characterize a new clinical entity termed Conn syndrome. Although this disease is more commonly known today as primary hyperaldosteronism, it remains a prevalent but curable form of hypertension among the general population. This article reviews the evaluation and management of primary hyperaldosteronism.

EPIDEMIOLOGY

The reported prevalence of primary hyperaldosteronism varies among published studies and depends on (1) the criteria and thresholds used to define and confirm cases, and (2) the denominator population (ie, all patients vs hypertensives only) of patients selected.[2,3] Nonetheless, studies have reported the prevalence of primary hyperaldosteronism as less than 10% in all hypertensive patients, and closer to 20% in those resistant to 3 or more antihypertensive agents.[2,4,5] Similarly, conflicting reports on prevalence rates among the 2 most common causes of primary hyperaldosteronism, namely aldosterone-producing adenoma (APA) and idiopathic bilateral adrenal hyperplasia (IHA), are present in the literature and vary according to the selectivity of screening.[6] When selective screening for primary hyperaldosteronism is performed using the aldosterone/renin ratio (ARR), the prevalence for APA exceeds IHA (60% vs 35%, respectively).[7,8] However, when nonselective (broader) screening is applied in the primary care setting, the inverse prevalence pattern is noted in that IHA exceeds APA (65% vs 30%, respectively) and is associated with milder clinical and biochemical manifestations of primary hyperaldosteronism.[9,10] Moreover, although APA and IHA make up most of the sporadic cases of primary hyperaldosteronism, about 5% of cases are familial.[11]

Although primary hyperaldosteronism can affect patients at any age, studies have shown that the mean age at diagnosis is around 50 years, which implicates some degree of late recognition of the disease.[12] It can take up to 10 years for some hypertensive patients to be referred for evaluation of primary hyperaldosteronism, a delay that can have significant impact on their outcomes.[13] Primary hyperaldosteronism affects both men and women with equal prevalence, although APA specifically has been shown to have a higher prevalence in women.[14]

ANATOMY AND PATHOPHYSIOLOGY

The adrenal glands are retroperitoneal organs that produce and secrete various hormones. Each gland can be functionally organized as 2 anatomic components: the adrenal cortex and the adrenal medulla. Although the medulla is primarily the site of catecholamine production, the cortex is where cholesterol-based adrenal steroids (mineralocorticoids, glucocorticoids, and sex hormones) are synthesized. From outermost to innermost, the zona glomerulosa, zona fasiculata, and zona reticularis are the layers that make up the adrenal cortex and synthesize aldosterone, cortisol, and androgens/estrogens, respectively.

Primary hyperaldosteronism is caused by independent and unregulated production of aldosterone by the adrenal cortex. Normal production of aldosterone is regulated by the renin-angiotensin-aldosterone (RAA) axis, in which the kidney, in response to a decrease in renal perfusion, produces renin as an upstream mediator in the mechanisms of volume expansion. Through a series of steps, renin allows the synthesis of angiotensin II from angiotensinogen produced by the liver. Subsequently, angiotensin II increases effective circulating volume indirectly by acting on the adrenal cortex to produce aldosterone, which subsequently acts back on the kidney to reabsorb salt and water.

In primary hyperaldosteronism, the excess aldosterone is autonomously produced most commonly by a primary adrenal tumor (APA) or adrenal gland hyperplasia (IHA) and it is not regulated by the RAA system. Although the cause of either APA or IHA is not entirely understood, basic science research has elucidated various somatic mutations in aldosterone-regulating genes (ie, *KCNJ5*, *CACNA1D*, *ATP1A1*, *ATP2B3*, *CTNNB1*) that can be present in either subtype of primary hyperaldosteronism.[15] These genetic mutations affect the cells in the zona glomerulosa by promoting increased expression of CYP11B2, the gene that codes for aldosterone synthase, an important enzyme in the biosynthesis of aldosterone. Mutations in the potassium channel–encoding gene, *KCNJ5*, are the most common and occur in nearly half of APA cases.[16] Different mutations can be harbored by different nodules within the same adrenal gland in cases of multinodular adrenals with APA.[17] Although the pathophysiology of IHA has been less understood than that of APA, a recent study that evaluated adrenal gland specimens from a unique cohort of patients with IHA suggests that the formation of adrenal-producing cell clusters with associated mutations, specifically in the *CACNAID* gene, may precede the development of IHA.[18,19]

Rarer causes of primary hyperaldosteronism and a brief overview of secondary hyperaldosteronism are detailed in **Table 1**. Regardless of the primary or secondary causes of hyperaldosteronism, high levels of serum aldosterone become homeostatic over time and can cause resistant hypertension (along with its associated complications) and electrolyte abnormalities, which can manifest in a variety of symptoms. Studies have shown an increased risk of cardiovascular complications (stroke, coronary artery disease, atrial fibrillation, and heart failure) in patients with primary hyperaldosteronism compared with counterparts with essential hypertension.[20,21] Thus, treatment of hyperaldosteronism is critical for reducing the cardiovascular morbidity and mortality in afflicted patients.[22]

CLINICAL PRESENTATION AND FINDINGS

Patients who are referred for evaluation of primary hyperaldosteronism typically have long-standing, moderate to severe hypertension that is increasingly refractory to multiple blood pressure medications. On initial evaluation they are often asymptomatic, but when symptoms are present they are generally nonspecific and can be attributed to hypokalemia and excess serum aldosterone. These symptoms include musculoskeletal spasms, weakness, fatigue, headache, polyuria, and polydipsia. Although hypokalemia (serum K <3.5 mmol/L) can result from the direct effect of aldosterone on the distal nephron to augment potassium excretion, it only occurs in less than 40%

Table 1
Causes of hyperaldosteronism

Primary Hyperaldosteronism		Secondary Hyperaldosteronism
Most Common Causes	**Rare Causes**	**Causes**

• Adrenal adenoma (APA)
• Adrenal hyperplasia; bilateral, also termed IHA
• Adrenal hyperplasia; unilateral
	• Ectopic aldosterone-secreting tumors
	• Adrenocortical adenocarcinoma
	• Familial hyperaldosteronism
	  ○ Type 1 (glucocorticoid-remediable aldosteronism)
	  ○ Type 2
	  ○ Type 3
		• Renal artery stenosis
		• Congestive heart failure
		• Cirrhosis with ascites
		• Nephrotic syndrome

of patients with primary hyperaldosteronism and is even less frequent in cases caused by adrenal hyperplasia.[23] Thus, hypokalemia is neither a sensitive nor specific marker for disease.[24,25] Nevertheless, hypokalemia when present can be accompanied by other metabolic derangements, such as alkalosis, mild hypernatremia, and hypomagnesemia.[26,27]

SCREENING AND CASE DETECTION FOR AT-RISK PATIENTS

Because of the increasing prevalence of primary hyperaldosteronism and its known impact on cardiovascular morbidity, early case detection is of paramount importance. At-risk populations that should be screened for primary hyperaldosteronism are outlined in **Box 1**. Screening, or biochemical testing, should be initiated by measuring the ratio of the plasma aldosterone concentration (PAC) to plasma renin activity (PRA) or to direct renin concentration (DRC; less commonly used). This ratio of PAC/PRA, commonly referred to as the ARR, is a sensitive marker that detects and integrates the pathophysiologic deviations in primary hyperaldosteronism: increased plasma aldosterone in conjunction with suppressed renin levels. Thus, the ARR is a computational screening tool that is superior to measuring isolated serum aldosterone, DRC, or potassium levels. Nonetheless, determining a patient's ARR requires conscientious preparation to avoid inaccurate results (ie, false-positives or false-negatives) that can be caused by certain medications and conditions.[28,29] Medications that can affect ARR testing are often common antihypertensives, all of which cannot be discontinued before testing. One approach to testing is to withdraw medications that markedly affect the ARR for at least 4 weeks (mineralocorticoid receptor antagonists, amiloride, triamterene, potassium-wasting diuretics) and then interpret the ARR in the context of the patient's remaining antihypertensive medications. If the results of the ARR are not diagnostic, additional medications (β-blockers, central alpha antagonists, angiotensin-converting enzyme inhibitors, angiotensin receptor blockers, renin inhibitors, dihydropyridine calcium channel antagonists) should be held for 2 weeks. These medications can be substituted safely in the interim with α-blockers (prazosin, doxazosin, terazosin), nondihydropyridine calcium channel

Box 1
Patient populations with increased prevalence of hyperaldosteronism

Case detection for primary hyperaldosteronism: at-risk populations for screening

General patients

- Sustained blood pressure greater than 150/100 mm Hg on 3 measurements obtained on different days

Hypertensives (with hypertension defined as blood pressure >140/90 mm Hg)

- Uncontrolled blood pressure more than 140/90 mm Hg that is resistant to 3 conventional antihypertensive drugs
- Controlled blood pressure less than 140/90 mm Hg on 4 or more antihypertensive drugs
- Hypertension and spontaneous or diuretic-induced hypokalemia
- Hypertension and adrenal incidentaloma
- Hypertension and sleep apnea
- Hypertension and a family history of early-onset hypertension or cardiovascular accident younger than 40 years of age
- Hypertension with first-degree relative diagnosed with primary aldosteronism

Adapted from Funder JW, Carey RM, Mantero F, et al. The management of primary aldosteronism: case detection, diagnosis, and treatment: an Endocrine Society clinical practice guideline. J Clin Endocrinol Metab 2016;101(5):1889–916; with permission.

blockers (slow-release verapamil), or vasodilators (hydralazine, moxonidine), which have minimal to no effects on renin or aldosterone levels. In addition, certain conditions, such as electrolyte abnormalities, renal disease, age, gender, phases of the menstrual cycle, and pregnancy, should be optimized or considered when interpreting results. More details on optimizing ARR testing conditions can be found in **Table 2**.

When determining the cutoff for a positive ARR to detect primary hyperaldosteronism, it must be kept in mind that different thresholds affect the sensitivity or specificity of the screening test. When using PAC (ng/dL)/PRA (ng/mL) for ARR (as opposed to using PAC/DRC, which may be inaccurate under certain conditions[30]), the cutoff values can range from 20 to 40, with 30 being the most commonly adopted threshold. In some cases, false-positive ARRs can result if both the PAC and PRA are low; this is seen in a subset of patients with essential hypertension that have suppressed renin levels in addition to low plasma aldosterone.[31,32] Thus in cases of low-renin hypertensives, which can compromise up to 30% of hypertensive patients, some investigators advocate combining a positive ARR test with a minimum PAC of greater than 15 ng/mL to increase the positive predictive value for cases of true primary hyperaldosteronism.[33]

DIAGNOSIS AND CONFIRMATORY TESTING FOR PRIMARY HYPERALDOSTERONISM

On adequate interpretation of a positive ARR screening test, clinicians should establish or exclude the diagnosis of primary hyperaldosteronism with one of several available confirmatory tests. The purpose of confirmatory testing is to assess whether or not aldosterone secretion is suppressible, because it would be insuppressible in true primary hyperaldosteronism. However, according to the most recent published Endocrine Society guidelines, one clinical scenario that may be exempt from confirmatory testing involves the following criteria: spontaneous hypokalemia with plasma renin at less than detection levels and a PAC of greater than 20 ng/dL.[34] For all other cases, confirmatory testing is recommended as the next step after a positive ARR screen in order to limit unnecessary, invasive supplemental procedures (explained later in relation to diagnostic procedures) in cases of false-positives.

At present, there are 4 confirmatory tests approved for the diagnosis of primary hyperaldosteronism: oral sodium loading, saline infusion test (SIT), fludrocortisone

Table 2
Preconditions that influence the accuracy of screening for primary hyperaldosteronism

Optimal Test Conditions for Accurate Determination of ARR					
Time of Day	Patient Activity	Patient Position	Patient Medications	Patient Metabolism	Patient Diet
Morning	Has been out of bed for at least 2 h	Seated for at least 5 min	All interfering BP medications discontinued for at least 2 wk Any initiated MR antagonists stopped for at least 4 wk if possible	Potassium repleted to $[K^+]$ of 4.0 if initially hypokalemic	Overnight fasting Unrestricted sodium intake

Abbreviations: BP, blood pressure; MR, mineralocorticoid receptor.

Data from Tiu SC, Choi CH, Shek CC, et al. The use of aldosterone-renin ratio as a diagnostic test for primary hyperaldosteronism and its test characteristics under different conditions of blood sampling. J Clin Endocrinol Metab 2005;90(1):72–8; and Tomaschitz A, Pilz S. Aldosterone to renin ratio–a reliable screening tool for primary aldosteronism? Horm Metab Res 2010;42(6):382–91.

suppression test (FST), and captopril challenge.[35] Although there is no 1 optimal test or gold standard, each test can offer specific advantages or disadvantages that allow a patient-centered decision. As done for ARR screening, the cessation of interfering medications and optimization of confounding conditions (ie, plasma potassium, time of day, posture, dietary salt) should continue during confirmatory testing. Of note, there is 1 other test, which is most commonly performed in Japan and is known as the furosemide upright test; however, it has not been approved by the Endocrine Society guidelines to use in the diagnosis of primary hyperaldosteronism.

There is ongoing evaluation on 2 modified confirmatory tests that may enhance the sensitivity for primary hyperaldosteronism: the dexamethasone-enhanced fludrocortisone suppression test (FDST) and the seated SIT (SSIT). The FDST is a modified form of the FST in which dexamethasone is given on the last day of the test to eliminate any potential stimulatory effect of endogenous, stress-induced adrenocorticotropic hormone (ACTH) on aldosterone secretion.[36] The SSIT is a modified form of the SIT, in which the patient receives a saline infusion in a seated, upright position (for at least 30 minutes) rather than in a recumbent position.[37] Based on the notion that aldosterone levels can be posture dependent (higher in upright positions), preliminary studies that used this modified confirmatory test have reported favorable results with improved sensitivity for diagnosing primary hyperaldosteronism. Nonetheless, further studies will be needed to validate any benefits from the modifications described earlier.

SUBTYPE CLASSIFICATION OF PRIMARY HYPERALDOSTERONISM

Thus far this article has outlined the initial steps in diagnosing primary hyperaldosteronism: screening followed by confirmatory testing. Once the diagnosis is confirmed, the next step in the evaluation is to distinguish between the different subtypes of primary hyperaldosteronism (IHA or APA), because each may be treated differently. Subtype classification of primary hyperaldosteronism can be determined largely by (1) adrenal imaging, and (2) adrenal vein sampling (AVS).

Adrenal Imaging

High-resolution computed tomography (CT) is a useful, noninvasive tool in the initial approach for subtyping primary hyperaldosteronism. Specifically, an adrenal-based CT protocol in which thin (<3.0 mm) image slices are obtained has the best sensitivity (~80%–85%) and specificity (~70%–75%) for identifying an APA; there is no added benefit from MRI.[38,39] CT findings can be interpreted as one of the following possibilities: (1) normal-appearing adrenal glands; (2) unilateral, adrenal macroadenoma (>1 cm); (3) bilateral adenomas of either macrocharacteristics or microcharacteristics; (4) minimal, unilateral adrenal limb thickening. Although some characteristics of a unilateral adrenal mass (>1 cm) on CT may support the subtype of APA (**Table 3**), there is significant overlap in quantitative CT analyses between APA and IHA, making it especially difficult to distinguish either subtype in cases of small, inconspicuous APAs or nodular hyperplasia.[40] In addition, unilateral adrenal adenomas detected on CT may be nonfunctional but are radiographically indistinguishable from APAs, posing a risk for inappropriate management.

Surgical management of primary hyperaldosteronism with adrenalectomy requires ascertainment of APA rather than IHA, which is difficult to achieve with CT studies alone. This difficulty is especially troublesome for unilateral micro-APAs (<1 cm) that are either undetected by CT or misinterpreted as IHA and may subsequently exclude patients from appropriate surgery.[41] In contrast, CT can also produce false-positives and can incorrectly direct adrenalectomy in patients with IHA whose disease process

Table 3
Comparison of computed tomography and adrenal vein sampling in subtype classification of primary hyperaldosteronism

	CT	AVS
APA Characteristics	• Unilateral, hypodense adrenal mass • ≤10 HU on noncontrast CT • Early wash-in and washout of contrast on adrenal protocol CT • Absolute percentage washout of ≥60% and relative percentage washout of ≥40% on adrenal protocol CT with delayed enhancement[66]	• LI of ≥2.0–4.0 in affected adrenal gland (depending on whether ACTH infusion is not/is used) with verified SI
IHA Characteristics	• Larger size in adrenal glands compared with those of patients with APA[67] • Mean width of adrenal limb ≥3–5 mm • Hyperplasia can be nodular or diffuse • Quantitative measures of CT densitometry and washout similar to adenoma[40]	• LI of <2.0–4.0 among bilateral adrenal glands (depending on whether ACTH infusion is not/is used)
Advantages	• Widely available among institutions • Inexpensive • Noninvasive • Provides structural information	• Best sensitivity and specificity for APA (gold standard) • Provides functional information
Disadvantages	• Limited sensitivity for microadenomas (<1 cm) • Poor specificity for nonfunctional adenomas • Discordance in findings with AVS results in up to 50% of patients[59]	• Lack of centers that perform AVS • Lack of standardization of the procedure (sequential vs simultaneous cannulation of adrenal veins; administration of ACTH) • Lack of standardization in cutoff values for SI and LI • Invasive with associated risks • Costly • Increased radiation exposure relative to CT • Requires thorough patient preparation and discontinuation of interfering medications • Technically demanding and time consuming
Complications	Related to IV contrast: • Allergic reactions, anaphylaxis • Nephropathy	Risks (<1%)[54] • Venous injury • Hemorrhage • Infection • Hematoma • Contrast-induced nephropathy • Contrast allergic reaction • Venous thrombosis • Adrenal insufficiency • Hypertensive crisis

(continued on next page)

Table 3
(*continued*)

	CT	AVS
Potential Contraindications or Deferment	Contraindications for CT: • Reported allergy to IV contrast • Renal disease	Deferment for AVS[46]: • Patients <35–40 y old with marked primary hyperaldosteronism and unilateral adenoma on CT • Nonsurgical candidates because of unacceptable surgical risks or patient preference for medical management • Patients with adrenal masses highly suspicious for malignancy • Contrast-related concerns

Abbreviations: AVS, adrenal vein sampling; HU, Hounsfield units; IV, intravenous; LI, lateralization index; SI, selectivity index.

is misclassified as unilateral microadenomas.[42,43] Moreover, CT does not provide any information on the functionality of detected, unilateral masses and, because the prevalence of nonfunctioning adrenal masses increases with age, it is important to discern a true APA from any resembling counterpart in older patients.

Adrenal Vein Sampling

To address CT limitations and increase the accuracy of subtypification and localization of an APA, AVS has been advocated.[44] AVS is an invasive procedure in which catheterization of the patient's bilateral adrenal veins is achieved by venography to provide functional information from each gland.[45] Similar to screening and confirmatory testing, AVS requires thorough preprocedural preparation. During AVS, plasma levels of aldosterone and cortisol are either sequentially or simultaneously acquired from bilateral adrenal veins and a peripheral vein. Successful cannulation of the adrenal veins is defined by an adrenal/peripheral vein cortisol ratio of at least 2.0 (or $\geq$3.0 if performed with cosyntropin administration), which is termed the selectivity index. Lateralization of 1 adrenal gland that is likely to harbor an APA is manifested by a lateralization index of at least 2.0 (or $\geq$4.0 if performed with cosyntropin administration), in which the aldosterone/cortisol ratio of the affected gland is least 2-fold to 4-fold higher than that of the contralateral normal gland. Administration of cosyntropin (ACTH) during AVS is practiced by many centers under the theory that hormonal variation of cortisol and aldosterone is controlled when ACTH stimulates their secretion by the adrenal gland, subsequently improving selectivity in catheterization.[46] Despite this potential benefit, cosyntropin use with AVS remains controversial, because there are no standard guidelines for its use and confounding results have also been shown with suboptimal dosing that may cause incorrect lateralization.[47–50] Although it can be a technically challenging procedure, most notable in catheterization of the right adrenal vein (because of its shorter and more posterosuperior course), AVS can have a technical success rate of greater than 95% in experienced centers.[51] Thus, because of its high sensitivity (95%) and specificity (100%) when successfully performed, it is currently considered the gold standard in lateralization of distinguishing APA from IHA.[52,53]

Because of the lack of availability[54] and standardization among centers as well as many other disadvantages of AVS (see **Table 3**), there is growing effort to find alternative measures and more specific predictors of APA that are not detailed in this article.

Ongoing investigations are focused on the utility and efficacy of such modalities (ie, nuclear imaging, PET-CT imaging, steroid profiling) in lateralization of APA.[55] At present, there are a few clinical scenarios in which AVS may be deferred in lateralization of an APA. These scenarios include young patients (<35–40 years old) who show a unilateral adenoma (>1.0 cm) on CT with a normal contralateral adrenal gland in the setting of marked primary hyperaldosteronism and may be taken directly to surgery.[56,57] Similarly, an ARR greater than 50 and preserved glomerular filtration rate ($\geq$100 mL/min/1.73 m^2) are other markers that have been shown to improve diagnostic accuracy of unilateral APA when present with a CT-detected adenoma associated with hypokalemia and hyperaldosteronism.[12,58] Although this selective use of AVS is advocated by several groups, note that CT findings have been shown to be discordant with AVS lateralization in up to 50% of patients and have been associated with inferior postsurgical outcomes compared with patients who have undergone AVS.[59,60] Thus, despite rare exceptions, the use of CT alone to diagnose an APA is unreliable because of various limitations described earlier, and most surgical candidates should undergo AVS when possible.[61–63]

CLINICAL OUTCOMES

Outcomes of Adrenalectomy for Unilateral Primary Hyperaldosteronism

Theoretically, adrenalectomy for unilateral primary hyperaldosteronism should cure the aldosterone excess, resulting in the cure of hypokalemia, if present, and the improvement, if not cure, of hypertension. However, outcomes of patients undergoing adrenalectomy for unilateral primary hyperaldosteronism vary widely throughout the literature, which is thought to be caused, at least in part, by the lack of standardized criteria to report outcomes.

In 2017 an international panel of experts, the Primary Aldosteronism Surgery Outcome group, published a study reporting the consensus reached in defining clinical and biochemical outcomes for patients undergoing total unilateral adrenalectomy for unilateral primary hyperaldosteronism as defined by adrenal venous sampling (**Table 4**).[13] In their published cohort analysis of 705 patients from 12 international centers, 94% achieved complete biochemical success but only 37% achieved complete clinical success. Partial clinical success, defined as correction of hypokalemia, if present preoperatively, and improvement in blood pressure control, was achieved in an additional 47% of patients for a total of 84% of patients who experienced some degree of clinical improvement. Only 2% of patients experienced absent biochemical and 16% of patients experienced absent clinical success.

Note that clinical outcomes are not only dependent on biochemical outcome but also on other factors, predominantly related to the duration of aldosterone-induced hypertension and preexisting detrimental effects on the cardiovascular and renal systems. Younger patients and female patients were more likely to have complete or partial clinical success after surgery, likely related to the shorter duration of hypertension and the vasoprotective role of estrogens in premenopausal women. Patients with higher body mass indices were found to have an increased likelihood of absent clinical or biochemical success, hypothesized to be related to higher aldosterone levels in patients with obesity.[64]

Outcomes of Mineralocorticoid Receptor Antagonist Treatment of Bilateral Primary Hyperaldosteronism

Multiple studies have examined outcomes of patients with primary hyperaldosteronism treated mineralocorticoid receptor antagonist (MRA) therapy. Note that although

Table 4
Definitions of complete, partial, and absent clinical and biochemical success of unilateral total adrenalectomy for unilateral primary hyperaldosteronism as defined by the Primary Aldosteronism Surgery Outcome group

	Clinical	Biochemical
Complete Success (Remission)	Normal BP off antihypertensive medications	1. Correction of hypoK(if present preoperatively) And 2. Normalization of ARR Or 3. Suppressed aldosterone during confirmatory testing if increased ARR postoperatively
Partial Success (Improvement)	Stable BP on less antihypertensive medication or lower BP on the same amount or reduced antihypertensive medications	1. Correction of hypoK (if present preoperatively) and increased ARR postoperatively And 2. ≥50% decrease in baseline aldosterone level Or 3. Abnormal but improved postoperative aldosterone during confirmatory testing
Absent Success (Persistence)	Unchanged or increased BP on the same amount or increased antihypertensive medications	1. Persistent hypoK (if present preoperatively) Or 2. Persistent increased ARR postoperatively And 3. Failure to suppress aldosterone secretion during confirmatory testing

Confirmatory testing refers to saline infusion test, oral sodium loading test, fludrocortisone suppression test, or captopril challenge test.
Abbreviation: HypoK, hypokalemia.

the dose of an MRA is usually titrated to normokalemia, there is no way of knowing whether all of the mineralocorticoid receptors are being blocked. Furthermore, patients treated with MRA therapy may be undertreated in order to avoid hyperkalemia.

A large cohort study examined outcomes of patients with primary hyperaldosteronism treated with MRA therapy (n = 602) compared with age-matched controls with essential hypertension (n = 41,853) over a 15-year period.[20] The investigators found a 1.9-fold increase in cardiovascular events (myocardial infarction, coronary revascularization, hospital admission for congestive heart failure or stroke) and a 1.3-fold increase in mortality in patients with primary hyperaldosteronism treated with MRA therapy compared with the control group. Of note, 344 of the patients with hyperaldosteronism in this study (57%) had undergone AVS for subtype classification with 54 patients lateralizing (ie, found to have an APA). Outcomes of these patients were not analyzed separately. However, the investigators also conducted an exploratory analysis of outcomes in patients with primary hyperaldosteronism treated with MRA therapy versus adrenalectomy (n = 309) and found that patients treated surgically had a significantly lower risk of composite cardiovascular events (hazard ratio,

0.58; 95% confidence interval, 0.35–0.97) compared with the cohort of patients with essential hypertension.

The effect of adrenalectomy versus MRA therapy on left ventricular (LV) hypertrophy has been studied by multiple investigators and was analyzed as a meta-analysis of 4 prospective cohort studies including 355 patients by a group of Italian researchers in 2015.[65] The prevalence of LV hypertrophy was similar in patients treated with adrenalectomy (n = 178) or MRA therapy (n = 177) (56% vs 52%, respectively). At an average duration of follow-up of 4 years, the meta-analysis showed that both surgical and medical treatment decreased LV mass but that there was no difference in LV mass change between the two groups ($-12.5\% \pm 5.1\%$ vs $-7.1\% \pm 4.8\%$, respectively). The conclusion of the study was that, because no difference was seen with respect to LV hypertrophy in patients with primary aldosteronism (PA) treated surgically or medically, the recommendation for adrenalectomy in patients with PA who are surgical candidates should be reconsidered. However, one of the major limitations of this conclusion is that patients were not randomized and all patients who underwent surgery had an APA, and most patients (172 out of 177 patients) treated with MRA therapy had IHA.

SUMMARY

Primary hyperaldosteronism is a prevalent cause of hypertension that is caused by autonomous aldosterone secretion, with most cases caused by either 1 (APA) or both (IHA) adrenal glands. The initial screening test involves measuring the ARR and interpreting the results in the context of the patient's antihypertensive medication regimen. Some drugs may need to be discontinued before testing. A positive screening ARR should be followed by confirmatory testing in most cases. Once primary hyperaldosteronism has been diagnosed, a CT scan of the abdomen should be done followed by subtype classification with AVS, unless the CT scan shows a large adrenal mass for which adrenalectomy would be indicated a priori. Patients who lateralize on AVS are probably best treated with adrenalectomy, whereas those who are diagnosed with IHA should be treated with an MRA. Most patients who undergo adrenalectomy for primary hyperaldosteronism derive some clinical and biochemical benefit from surgery. Patients treated with MRA therapy may have similar outcomes with respect to LV hypertrophy compared with patients who have undergone adrenalectomy but have worse cardiovascular outcomes compared with matched patients with essential hypertension.

REFERENCES

1. Conn JW. Presidential address. I. Painting background. II. Primary aldosteronism, a new clinical syndrome. J Lab Clin Med 1955;45(1):3–17.
2. Funder JW. Primary aldosteronism: the next five years. Horm Metab Res 2017; 49(12):977–83.
3. Hannemann A, Wallaschofski H. Prevalence of primary aldosteronism in patient's cohorts and in population-based studies–a review of the current literature. Horm Metab Res 2012;44(3):157–62.
4. Douma S, Petidis K, Doumas M, et al. Prevalence of primary hyperaldosteronism in resistant hypertension: a retrospective observational study. Lancet 2008; 371(9628):1921–6.
5. Young WF Jr. Diagnosis and treatment of primary aldosteronism: practical clinical perspectives. J Intern Med 2019;285(2):126–48.

6. Plouin PF, Amar L, Chatellier G. Trends in the prevalence of primary aldosteronism, aldosterone-producing adenomas, and surgically correctable aldosterone-dependent hypertension. Nephrol Dial Transplant 2004;19(4):774–7.
7. Omura M, Saito J, Yamaguchi K, et al. Prospective study on the prevalence of secondary hypertension among hypertensive patients visiting a general outpatient clinic in Japan. Hypertens Res 2004;27(3):193–202.
8. Mulatero P, Stowasser M, Loh KC, et al. Increased diagnosis of primary aldosteronism, including surgically correctable forms, in centers from five continents. J Clin Endocrinol Metab 2004;89(3):1045–50.
9. Monticone S, Burrello J, Tizzani D, et al. Prevalence and clinical manifestations of primary aldosteronism encountered in primary care practice. J Am Coll Cardiol 2017;69(14):1811–20.
10. Fogari R, Preti P, Zoppi A, et al. Prevalence of primary aldosteronism among unselected hypertensive patients: a prospective study based on the use of an aldosterone/renin ratio above 25 as a screening test. Hypertens Res 2007;30(2):111–7.
11. Mulatero P, Tizzani D, Viola A, et al. Prevalence and characteristics of familial hyperaldosteronism: the PATOGEN study (Primary Aldosteronism in TOrinoGENetic forms). Hypertension 2011;58(5):797–803.
12. Blumenfeld JD, Sealey JE, Schlussel Y, et al. Diagnosis and treatment of primary hyperaldosteronism. Ann Intern Med 1994;121(11):877–85.
13. Williams TA, Lenders JWM, Mulatero P, et al. Outcomes after adrenalectomy for unilateral primary aldosteronism: an international consensus on outcome measures and analysis of remission rates in an international cohort. Lancet Diabetes Endocrinol 2017;5(9):689–99.
14. Ferriss JB, Beevers DG, Brown JJ, et al. Clinical, biochemical and pathological features of low-renin ("primary") hyperaldosteronism. Am Heart J 1978;95(3):375–88.
15. Fernandes-Rosa FL, Williams TA, Riester A, et al. Genetic spectrum and clinical correlates of somatic mutations in aldosterone-producing adenoma. Hypertension 2014;64(2):354–61.
16. Scholl UI, Healy JM, Thiel A, et al. Novel somatic mutations in primary hyperaldosteronism are related to the clinical, radiological and pathological phenotype. Clin Endocrinol 2015;83(6):779–89.
17. Fernandes-Rosa FL, Giscos-Douriez I, Amar L, et al. Different somatic mutations in multinodular adrenals with aldosterone-producing adenoma. Hypertension 2015;66(5):1014–22.
18. Omata K, Satoh F, Morimoto R, et al. Cellular and genetic causes of idiopathic hyperaldosteronism. Hypertension 2018;72(4):874–80.
19. Zennaro MC, Fernandes-Rosa F, Boulkroun S, et al. Bilateral idiopathic adrenal hyperplasia: genetics and beyond. Horm Metab Res 2015;47(13):947–52.
20. Hundemer GL, Curhan GC, Yozamp N, et al. Cardiometabolic outcomes and mortality in medically treated primary aldosteronism: a retrospective cohort study. Lancet Diabetes Endocrinol 2018;6(1):51–9.
21. Monticone S, D'Ascenzo F, Moretti C, et al. Cardiovascular events and target organ damage in primary aldosteronism compared with essential hypertension: a systematic review and meta-analysis. Lancet Diabetes Endocrinol 2018;6(1):41–50.
22. Prejbisz A, Warchol-Celinska E, Lenders JW, et al. Cardiovascular risk in primary hyperaldosteronism. Horm Metab Res 2015;47(13):973–80.

23. Magill SB, Raff H, Shaker JL, et al. Comparison of adrenal vein sampling and computed tomography in the differentiation of primary aldosteronism. J Clin Endocrinol Metab 2001;86(3):1066–71.
24. Rossi GP, Bernini G, Caliumi C, et al. A prospective study of the prevalence of primary aldosteronism in 1,125 hypertensive patients. J Am Coll Cardiol 2006; 48(11):2293–300.
25. Gyamlani G, Headley CM, Naseer A, et al. Primary aldosteronism: diagnosis and management. Am J Med Sci 2016;352(4):391–8.
26. Gregoire JR. Adjustment of the osmostat in primary aldosteronism. Mayo Clin Proc 1994;69(11):1108–10.
27. Agus ZS. Mechanisms and causes of hypomagnesemia. Curr Opin Nephrol Hypertens 2016;25(4):301–7.
28. Tiu SC, Choi CH, Shek CC, et al. The use of aldosterone-renin ratio as a diagnostic test for primary hyperaldosteronism and its test characteristics under different conditions of blood sampling. J Clin Endocrinol Metab 2005;90(1):72–8.
29. Tomaschitz A, Pilz S. Aldosterone to renin ratio–a reliable screening tool for primary aldosteronism? Horm Metab Res 2010;42(6):382–91.
30. Stowasser M, Ahmed A, Guo Z, et al. Can screening and confirmatory testing in the management of patients with primary aldosteronism be improved? Horm Metab Res 2017;49(12):915–21.
31. Gordon RD, Laragh JH, Funder JW. Low renin hypertensive states: perspectives, unsolved problems, future research. Trends Endocrinol Metab 2005;16(3): 108–13.
32. Sealey JE, Gordon RD, Mantero F. Plasma renin and aldosterone measurements in low renin hypertensive states. Trends Endocrinol Metab 2005;16(3):86–91.
33. Sahay M, Sahay RK. Low renin hypertension. Indian J Endocrinol Metab 2012; 16(5):728–39.
34. Funder JW, Carey RM, Mantero F, et al. The management of primary aldosteronism: case detection, diagnosis, and treatment: an Endocrine Society clinical practice guideline. J Clin Endocrinol Metab 2016;101(5):1889–916.
35. Mulatero P, Monticone S, Bertello C, et al. Confirmatory tests in the diagnosis of primary aldosteronism. Horm Metab Res 2010;42(6):406–10.
36. Gouli A, Kaltsas G, Tzonou A, et al. High prevalence of autonomous aldosterone secretion among patients with essential hypertension. Eur J Clin Invest 2011; 41(11):1227–36.
37. Ahmed AH, Cowley D, Wolley M, et al. Seated saline suppression testing for the diagnosis of primary aldosteronism: a preliminary study. J Clin Endocrinol Metab 2014;99(8):2745–53.
38. Mulatero P, Bertello C, Rossato D, et al. Roles of clinical criteria, computed tomography scan, and adrenal vein sampling in differential diagnosis of primary aldosteronism subtypes. J Clin Endocrinol Metab 2008;93(4):1366–71.
39. Lingam RK, Sohaib SA, Rockall AG, et al. Diagnostic performance of CT versus MR in detecting aldosterone-producing adenoma in primary hyperaldosteronism (Conn's syndrome). Eur Radiol 2004;14(10):1787–92.
40. Park SY, Park BK, Park JJ, et al. Differentiation of Adrenal Hyperplasia From Adenoma by Use of CT Densitometry and Percentage Washout. AJR Am J Roentgenol 2016;206(1):106–12.
41. Omura M, Sasano H, Fujiwara T, et al. Unique cases of unilateral hyperaldosteronemia due to multiple adrenocortical micronodules, which can only be detected by selective adrenal venous sampling. Metabolism 2002;51(3):350–5.

42. Young WF, Stanson AW, Thompson GB, et al. Role for adrenal venous sampling in primary aldosteronism. Surgery 2004;136(6):1227–35.
43. Kempers MJ, Lenders JW, van Outheusden L, et al. Systematic review: diagnostic procedures to differentiate unilateral from bilateral adrenal abnormality in primary aldosteronism. Ann Intern Med 2009;151(5):329–37.
44. England RW, Geer EB, Deipolyi AR. Role of venous sampling in the diagnosis of endocrine disorders. J Clin Med 2018;7(5) [pii:E114].
45. Kahn SL, Angle JF. Adrenal vein sampling. Tech Vasc Interv Radiol 2010;13(2): 110–25.
46. Rossi GP, Auchus RJ, Brown M, et al. An expert consensus statement on use of adrenal vein sampling for the subtyping of primary aldosteronism. Hypertension 2014;63(1):151–60.
47. Rossi GP, Pitter G, Bernante P, et al. Adrenal vein sampling for primary aldosteronism: the assessment of selectivity and lateralization of aldosterone excess baseline and after adrenocorticotropic hormone (ACTH) stimulation. J Hypertens 2008;26(5):989–97.
48. Seccia TM, Miotto D, De Toni R, et al. Adrenocorticotropic hormone stimulation during adrenal vein sampling for identifying surgically curable subtypes of primary aldosteronism: comparison of 3 different protocols. Hypertension 2009; 53(5):761–6.
49. Rossi GP, Ganzaroli C, Miotto D, et al. Dynamic testing with high-dose adrenocorticotrophic hormone does not improve lateralization of aldosterone oversecretion in primary aldosteronism patients. J Hypertens 2006;24(2):371–9.
50. Rossitto G, Maiolino G, Lenzini L, et al. Subtyping of primary aldosteronism with adrenal vein sampling: Hormone- and side-specific effects of cosyntropin and metoclopramide. Surgery 2018;163(4):789–95.
51. Daunt N. Adrenal vein sampling: how to make it quick, easy, and successful. Radiographics 2005;25(Suppl 1):S143–58.
52. Carr CE, Cope C, Cohen DL, et al. Comparison of sequential versus simultaneous methods of adrenal venous sampling. J Vasc Interv Radiol 2004;15(11):1245–50.
53. Nwariaku FE, Miller BS, Auchus R, et al. Primary hyperaldosteronism: effect of adrenal vein sampling on surgical outcome. Arch Surg 2006;141(5):497–502 [discussion: 502–3].
54. Rossi GP, Barisa M, Allolio B, et al. The Adrenal Vein Sampling International Study (AVIS) for identifying the major subtypes of primary aldosteronism. J Clin Endocrinol Metab 2012;97(5):1606–14.
55. Lenders JWM, Eisenhofer G, Reincke M. Subtyping of patients with primary aldosteronism: an update. Horm Metab Res 2017;49(12):922–8.
56. Minami I, Yoshimoto T, Hirono Y, et al. Diagnostic accuracy of adrenal venous sampling in comparison with other parameters in primary aldosteronism. Endocr J 2008;55(5):839–46.
57. Zarnegar R, Bloom AI, Lee J, et al. Is adrenal venous sampling necessary in all patients with hyperaldosteronism before adrenalectomy? J Vasc Interv Radiol 2008;19(1):66–71.
58. Kupers EM, Amar L, Raynaud A, et al. A clinical prediction score to diagnose unilateral primary aldosteronism. J Clin Endocrinol Metab 2012;97(10):3530–7.
59. Dekkers T, Prejbisz A, Kool LJS, et al. Adrenal vein sampling versus CT scan to determine treatment in primary aldosteronism: an outcome-based randomised diagnostic trial. Lancet Diabetes Endocrinol 2016;4(9):739–46.

60. Williams TA, Burrello J, Sechi LA, et al. Computed tomography and adrenal venous sampling in the diagnosis of unilateral primary aldosteronism. Hypertension 2018;72(3):641–9.
61. McAlister FA, Lewanczuk RZ. Primary hyperaldosteronism and adrenal incidentaloma: an argument for physiologic testing before adrenalectomy. Can J Surg 1998;41(4):299–305.
62. Harper R, Ferrett CG, McKnight JA, et al. Accuracy of CT scanning and adrenal vein sampling in the pre-operative localization of aldosterone-secreting adrenal adenomas. QJM 1999;92(11):643–50.
63. Wachtel H, Zaheer S, Shah PK, et al. Role of adrenal vein sampling in primary aldosteronism: Impact of imaging, localization, and age. J Surg Oncol 2016; 113(5):532–7.
64. Rossi GP, Belfiore A, Bernini G, et al. Body mass index predicts plasma aldosterone concentrations in overweight-obese primary hypertensive patients. J Clin Endocrinol Metab 2008;93(7):2566–71.
65. Marzano L, Colussi G, Sechi LA, et al. Adrenalectomy is comparable with medical treatment for reduction of left ventricular mass in primary aldosteronism: meta-analysis of long-term studies. Am J Hypertens 2015;28(3):312–8.
66. Park JJ, Park BK, Kim CK. Adrenal imaging for adenoma characterization: imaging features, diagnostic accuracies and differential diagnoses. Br J Radiol 2016; 89(1062):20151018.
67. Lingam RK, Sohaib SA, Vlahos I, et al. CT of primary hyperaldosteronism (Conn's syndrome): the value of measuring the adrenal gland. AJR Am J Roentgenol 2003;181(3):843–9.

When to Intervene for Subclinical Cushing's Syndrome

Lily B. Hsieh, MD[a], Erin Mackinney, MD[b],
Tracy S. Wang, MD, MPH[c,*]

KEYWORDS

- Subclinical Cushing's syndrome • Adrenal incidentaloma
- Minimally invasive adrenalectomy • Subclinical hypercortisolism
- Subclinical glucocorticoid hypersecretion

KEY POINTS

- Patients with adrenal incidentalomas should undergo a biochemical evaluation.
- The diagnosis of subclinical Cushing's syndrome (SCS) may be difficult, given ongoing controversy regarding criteria for diagnosis. These can be guided by recommendations from various endocrine societies.
- SCS has been associated with significant morbidity, including hypertension, diabetes, hyperlipidemia, osteoporosis, and cardiovascular disease.
- A multidisciplinary approach between the endocrinologist and the endocrine surgeon should be used for management of SCS.
- Once SCS is diagnosed, adrenalectomy is recommended for SCS patients who are appropriate surgical candidates, with comorbidities than can be attributed to excess cortisol, especially with young age and/or worsening comorbidities despite optimal medical treatment.

INTRODUCTION

Adrenal incidentalomas are adrenal masses found on imaging performed for other reasons than evaluation of the adrenal gland. Autopsy studies show the presence of adrenal masses ranging from 1% to 8.7%. In radiologic studies, the frequency of adrenal incidentalomas is around 4% in those in middle age (30–50 years) and can be as high as 10% in the elderly, peaking around the fifth and seventh decade.[1] With the

Disclosure Statement: The authors have nothing to disclose.
[a] Division of Surgical Oncology, Medical College of Wisconsin, 8701 Watertown Plank Road, Milwaukee, WI 53226, USA; [b] Department of General Surgery, Southern Illinois University School of Medicine, PO Box 19638, Springfield, IL 62794-9638, USA; [c] Section of Endocrine Surgery, Medical College of Wisconsin, Division of Surgical Oncology, 8701 Watertown Plank Road, Milwaukee, WI 53226, USA
* Corresponding author.
E-mail address: tswang@mcw.edu

Surg Clin N Am 99 (2019) 747–758
https://doi.org/10.1016/j.suc.2019.04.011 surgical.theclinics.com

increasing number of adrenal incidentalomas identified and patients undergoing biochemical evaluation, an increasing number of patients are diagnosed with subclinical Cushing's syndrome (SCS).[2] Although the prevalence of SCS in the overall population is estimated to be between 0.2% to 2%, the frequency of SCS in adrenal incidentalomas is estimated to be approximately 20%.[3–5]

The optimal management of patients with SCS is unclear and remains a topic of controversy. Significant comorbidities are associated with SCS, and studies have demonstrated improvement in associated comorbidities after adrenalectomy.[2,6] Guidelines for the evaluation of adrenal incidentalomas, written by multiple national and international endocrine societies, have sought to clarify the criteria for the diagnosis as well as optimal treatment of SCS. This article reviews the biochemical evaluation of adrenal nodules, criteria for the diagnosis of SCS, and the role for adrenalectomy in the treatment of SCS, including postoperative outcomes.

DEFINITION

SCS has multiple synonyms: pre-clinical Cushing, subclinical autonomous glucocorticoid hypersecretion, subclinical hypercortisolism, and dysregulated hypercortisolism.[1] It has been suggested that it be considered a distinct entity from Cushing's syndrome because several studies have not shown progression to overt Cushing's syndrome.[2,7–9] There is general consensus regarding the main 3 components of SCS from the guidelines of the National Institutes of Health (NIH) state-of-the-science statement, the Endocrine Society (ES), the French Society of Endocrinology (FSE), American Association of Clinical Endocrinologists (AACE)/American Association of Endocrine Surgeons (AAES), the Italian Association of Clinical Endocrinologists (AME), the European Society of Endocrinology (ESE), and the Japan Endocrine Society (JES)[1,2,10–15]:

1. The presence of an adrenal incidentaloma or adrenal mass/lesion.
2. Cortisol excess based on biochemical evaluation.The criteria and the testing used vary depending on the various guidelines and will be elucidated in the Diagnosis section.
3. No classic clinical manifestations of overt Cushing's syndrome (ie, dorsocervical fat pad, moon facies, abdominal striae, proximal myopathy, easy bruising).

DIAGNOSIS

Biochemical Evaluation

Because patients with SCS do not have the overt clinical signs of Cushing's syndrome, as described above, the diagnosis begins with biochemical testing for cortisol excess once the presence of adrenal incidentaloma is confirmed. Cortisol secretion runs along a continuum from adrenal insufficiency to excessive secretion to the point of altering phenotype (Cushing's syndrome), and arbitrary cutoffs that are too stringent can hinder disease detection, whereas too lenient cutoffs can lead to overdiagnosis and possibly overtreatment.

Assessment of Excess Cortisol Secretion

Recommendations across guidelines are variable, but there is consensus that the 1-mg (low-dose) overnight dexamethasone suppression test (DST) is recommended as the initial screening test.[1–7] In patients with adrenocorticotropic hormone (ACTH)-dependent cortisol secretion, dexamethasone suppresses the hypothalamic-pituitary-adrenal (HPA) axis, which results in suppression of cortisol secretion. Patients with cortisol-secreting adenomas will not show suppression of cortisol secretion after oral dexamethasone. However, the threshold for what constitutes a positive test for diagnosing SCS varies between guidelines (**Table 1**). It is generally agreed on that a plasma cortisol level after a 1-mg DST of less than 1.8 μg/dL excludes autonomous cortisol secretion.[1,2,10–12,14] The AACE/AAES, JES, NIH, ESE, and AME recommend a result greater than 5 μg/dL after 1-mg DST, which has a specificity of 100%, but a sensitivity of only 58%, in diagnosing SCS.[1,2,10,12,13] Two societies, the ES and FSE, recommend a lower cutoff of greater than 1.8 μg/dL as a positive test result for SCS, which has a higher sensitivity (75%–100%) and a lower specificity (72%–82%), with the understanding that there will be a higher false positive rate.[11,14] The lower threshold is based on studies showing increased morbidity and mortality associated with excess cortisol secretion, using a cutoff of greater than 1.8 μg/dL after DST.[8,9] However, most guidelines consider cortisol levels between 1.8 μg/dL and 5 μg/dL indeterminate and suggest other tests to evaluate excess cortisol secretion (see **Table 1**).[1,2,10,12] Even with cortisol levels greater than 5 μg/dL meeting criteria for the diagnosis of SCS, the NIH, AACE/AAES, AME, and ESE still recommend further testing to evaluate for excess cortisol and ACTH-independent secretion.[1,2,10,13] **Table 1** elucidates the tests recommended by the various guidelines.

Other tests recommended to show excess cortisol secretion are late-night salivary cortisol (LNSC) and urinary free cortisol (UFC). LNSC testing has been established as a diagnostic test for Cushing's syndrome.[11,16,17] It is less cumbersome to perform than midnight serum cortisol to evaluate for the loss in the diurnal variation of cortisol secretion in patients with SCS; patients can obtain the samples at home with simple instructions. A meta-analysis of 7 studies involving more than 300 patients with Cushing's syndrome demonstrated a sensitivity of 92% and specificity of 96% of LNSC testing in diagnosing Cushing's syndrome.[17] Patients with hypercortisolism lose the diurnal variation of cortisol secretion seen in normal individuals and have elevated cortisol levels at the time of the usual midnight nadir. However, these results may not be reliable in an individual with an abnormal sleeping pattern, such as a nightshift worker. Also, some studies have shown that patients with SCS may not have disruption of the normal diurnal variation of cortisol secretion and have normal LNSC.[1,18,19] However, LNSC in conjunction with the 1-mg DST has been shown to have a higher sensitivity and specificity (88.9% and 85.2%) than LNSC alone (31.3% and 83.3%).[20]

UFC measures cortisol excretion over 24 hours to encompass a complete circadian rhythm. Both urinary and salivary assays are reflective of unbound serum cortisol.[6] A UFC 4 times the normal value is considered diagnostic of Cushing's syndrome, but factors such as chronic anxiety, depression, and obesity can contribute to as much as a 3-fold increase in UFC.[13] High fluid intake also affects UFC, increasing the cortisol excreted in urine.[21] The prevalence of UFC elevation in people with adrenal incidentalomas has been reported from 5% to 20%.[4,6,22] As with LNSC, a normal UFC does not exclude SCS.[23]

Testing for Adrenocorticotropic Hormone–independent Secretion

Plasma ACTH levels are used in evaluation of hypercortisolism to determine the source of cortisol secretion. In the setting of a cortisol-secreting adrenal mass, hypercortisolism is considered to be ACTH independent when serum ACTH levels are suppressed to less than 10 pg/mL.[6] However, ACTH levels are not always suppressed in the setting of SCS.[6] The lack of ACTH suppression has been attributed to inconsistencies in detecting low levels of ACTH in commercially available assays from antibody interference[24]; in cases of mild cortisol excess, there might not be ACTH suppression because some patients with SCS do not experience postadrenalectomy insufficiency requiring glucocorticoid replacement.[25,26] A lack of ACTH response (<30 pg/mL) during corticotropin-

Table 1
Testing recommended for diagnosing subclinical Cushing's syndrome

	Screening Test	Confirmatory Tests (CT)						
	1 mg DST	2-d Low-Dose DST	Midnight Serum Cortisol	Midnight Salivary Cortisol	ACTH	UFC	DHEAS	Adrenal Scintigraphy
NIH[1]	<1.8 μg/dL excludes, between 1.8 μg/dL and 5 μg/dL indeterminate, >5 μg/dL confirms	NM	NM	NN	NM	NM	NM	NM
AACE/AAES[3]	>5 μg/dL confirms	+	NM	NM	+	NM	+	NM
ES[2]	Between 1.8 μg/dL and 5 μg/dL	+	NM	+	+	+	+	NM
AME[5]	<1.8 μg/dL excludes, between 1.8 μg/dL and 5 μg/dL indeterminate, >5 μg/dL confirms	+	+	DNR	+	+	DNR	NM
JSE[4]	>1.8 μg/dL + CT	NM	+	+	+	+	DNR	NM
ESE /ENSAT[7]	<1.8 μg/dL is normal, between 1.8 μg/dL and 5 μg/dL possible autonomous cortisol secretion, >5 μg/dL confirms	NM	NM	+	+	+	NM	NM
JES[6]	≥1.8 μg/dL + 2 CT ≥3 μg/dL + 1 CT >5 μg/dL confirms	NM	+	+	+	NM	+	+

Abbreviations: +, endorsement of the diagnostic test for SCS; CT, computed tomography; DNR, do not recommend; NM, no mention.

releasing hormone stimulation test can be used in patients with borderline ACTH to distinguish ACTH-dependent from ACTH-independent cortisol secretion.[6,13]

Because there is no screening test with 100% sensitivity for SCS, multiple tests that target different aspects of the HPA axis are used in conjunction to confirm a diagnosis of SCS. Guidelines for evaluation of adrenal incidentalomas for SCS vary in their recommendations for confirmatory testing (as seen in **Table 1**), but all do recommend multiple tests to increase sensitivity and specificity in diagnosing SCS.

Clinical Evaluation

As discussed above, excess endogenous cortisol secretion may be either ACTH dependent or ACTH independent (autonomous cortisol production by the adrenal gland). Prolonged exposure of tissue to inappropriately high levels of cortisol results in signs and symptoms typical of Cushing's syndrome (easy bruising, facial plethora, proximal myopathy, striae).[11] Often, patients will also have other nonspecific signs caused by cortisol excess, such as hypertension, obesity, diabetes, and depression.[11] Indications for treating Cushing's syndrome is quite clear with the increased morbidity and mortality associated with Cushing's syndrome.[27,28] The ES Clinical Practice Guideline recommends testing for Cushing's syndrome (once exogenous causes have been ruled out) for patients with unusual features for age (eg, osteoporosis, hypertension), multiple features highly suggestive of Cushing's syndrome, adrenal incidentalomas, and in children, with decreasing height percentile and increasing weight.[11] Studies have shown that SCS is not an early form of Cushing's syndrome; it rarely progresses to full-blown Cushing's syndrome.[29–34]

Once an adrenal incidentaloma is identified and biochemical testing is suggestive of SCS, clinical evaluation is similar for evaluation of associated comorbidities of Cushing's syndrome, but not the typical physical manifestations, such as facial plethora, proximal myopathy, or striae. As seen with Cushing's syndrome, hypercortisolism can lead to cardiovascular and metabolic comorbidities and osteoporosis.[16] Most SCS-associated comorbidities overlap with those of metabolic syndrome: obesity, diabetes, hypertension, dyslipidemia, and cannot be directly attributed to cortisol excess, although they can be exacerbated by hypercortisolism.[11] Hypertension, glucose intolerance/type 2 diabetes mellitus, obesity, dyslipidemia, and osteoporosis have been associated with adrenal incidentalomas with SCS.[7,31,35–41] An increased rate of osteoporotic fractures has been shown in patients with SCS.[41–44] Cardiovascular disease is another comorbidity associated with SCS.[8,44,45] Finally, 2 long-term follow-up studies have suggested a higher mortality in SCS attributed to cardiovascular comorbidity compared with nonsecreting adrenal adenomas.[9,46]

The ESE and the European Network for the Study of Adrenal Tumors (ENSAT) has renamed SCS to autonomous cortisol secretion to reflect that SCS is not a pre-Cushing's syndrome and should be considered a separate entity.[2] In the setting of autonomous cortisol secretion, ESE/ENSAT recommends screening for hypertension, type 2 diabetes, and asymptomatic vertebral fractures and offering appropriate treatment of those conditions.[2] Patients with SCS/autonomous cortisol secretion should be evaluated for cortisol excess-related comorbidities to assess potential benefits of adrenalectomy.

INDICATIONS FOR SURGERY

Because progression of SCS to overt Cushing's syndrome is rare, surgical consideration must be based on associated comorbidities, and size of adrenal mass, as well as its appearance on imaging.[29–34] Two options for treatment of SCS are surveillance and medical management of excess cortisol-associated comorbidities, if any, or adrenalectomy. There are no large, randomized controlled trials to determine which option is best. Most studies that have assessed outcomes after adrenalectomy for SCS in the setting of adrenal incidentalomas are retrospective in nature with small cohorts.[6]

Before 2012, 4 studies, 3 retrospective cohort studies and 1 randomized controlled trial, have directly compared outcomes of comorbidities associated with SCS (hypertension, diabetes, and dyslipidemia) after adrenalectomy versus medical management of comorbidities (**Table 2**); in general, these studies were small (n = 20–45) and had follow-up ranging from 7 months to 7.7 years.[47–50] These studies reported improvement in diabetes, hypertension, and dyslipidemia in some of the SCS patients after adrenalectomy, and no improvement in the SCS patients who were medically managed.[48–51] Some patients in the medically managed group also showed worsening of the cardiovascular risk factors during the follow-up period.[48–51] In 2017, Petramala and colleagues[51] published a retrospective study with a relatively large cohort of 70 patients with SCS, with 26 patients undergoing laparoscopic unilateral adrenalectomy, and 44 patients were managed conservatively. Only patients undergoing surgery had statistically significant improvement in hypertension, obesity, and diabetes compared with the nonsurgical group, where those previously mentioned comorbidities all worsened.[51]

In a meta-analysis of 26 studies of patients with SCS (n = 584), adrenalectomy resulted in an overall improvement of cardiovascular risk factors: hypertension, diabetes, obesity, and dyslipidemia. However, when compared with the medically managed SCS patients, SCS patients undergoing adrenalectomy showed improvement only in hypertension and diabetes.[52] Another systematic review of outcomes after adrenalectomy for SCS patients (n = 139) evaluated 6 retrospective studies and 1 prospective, randomized trial.[53] These studies evaluated the outcomes of surgery on hypertension, glucose metabolism, lipid metabolism, obesity, and osteoporosis. Hypertension, glucose metabolism, lipid metabolism, and obesity were improved after adrenalectomy.[53]

In addition to improvement of cardiovascular risk factors in SCS patients after adrenalectomy, improvements in bone mineral density (BMD) have also been shown after adrenalectomy.[41] Salcuni and colleagues[54] showed improvement in BMD in patients with SCS after adrenalectomy. SCS patients in the surgery group (n = 32) had lower baseline BMD compared with the nonsurgical SCS group, but they showed improvement of BMD at lumbar spine during the follow-up period, reducing the risk of vertebral body fractures.

The ESE/ENSAT guidelines do not recommend adrenalectomy for all patients with autonomous cortisol secretion from adrenal lesions because of the lack of high-quality studies showing the benefits of adrenalectomy in SCS patients.[2] Although retrospective studies with small cohorts suggest improvement of comorbidities after adrenalectomy for SCS, currently, it is not possible to predict who will benefit from surgery. Each patient should be evaluated individually and should take into consideration the presence of cortisol excess–associated comorbidities, end organ damage, and age of patient.[2] The AACE and AAES recommend adrenalectomy in SCS patients with worsening hypertension, abnormal glucose tolerance, dyslipidemia, and osteoporosis because there is a lack of studies showing the long-term benefits of adrenalectomy in SCS patients.[11] If surgery is considered, cortisol secretion independent of ACTH must be proven to ensure cortisol excess is from the adrenal lesion.

For surgical candidates with a diagnosis of SCS, surgery is recommended for those with treatment-resistant or worsening comorbidities associated with cortisol excess: hypertension, obesity, diabetes, dyslipidemia, and a decrease in BMD.[1,12,13] **Fig. 1**

Table 2
Outcomes of subclinical Cushing's syndrome–associated comorbidities after adrenalectomy and medical management of comorbidities

				Improvement in Comorbidities											
				Weight			Blood Pressure			Impaired Glucose Regulation			Dyslipidemia		
Study (Type)	Total (N)	Adrenalectomy Group (AG)	Medical Management Group (MM)	AG N (%)	MM N (%)	*P* Value	AG N (%)	MM N (%)	*P* Value	AG N (%)	MM N (%)	*P* Value	AG N (%)	MM N (%)	*P* Value
Petramala et al,[51] 2017 (retrospective)	70	26	44	8 (29)	0	*P*<.05	7 (26)	0	*P*<.05	4 (15)	0	NS	2 (7)	0	NS
Toniato et al,[47] 2009 (randomized prospective)	45	23	22	12 (50)	0	NC	15 (67)	0	NC	14 (63)	0	NC	9 (38)	0	NC
Tsuiki et al,[48] 2008 (retrospective)	20	8	12	0	0	NC	7 (83)	0	NC	22 (2)	0	NC	5 (67)	0	NC
Iacobone et al,[49] 2012 (retrospective)	35	20	15	8 (40)	0	*P*<.05	11 (53)	0	*P*<.05	10 (50)	0	*P*<.05	4 (20)	0	NS
Chiodini et al,[50] 2010 (retrospective)	41	25	16	8 (32)	2 (12.5)	*P*<.05	14 (56)	0	*P*<.05	12 (48)	0	*P*<.05	NR	NR	NA

Abbreviations: NA, not applicable; NC, not calculated; NR, not reported; NS, not significant.

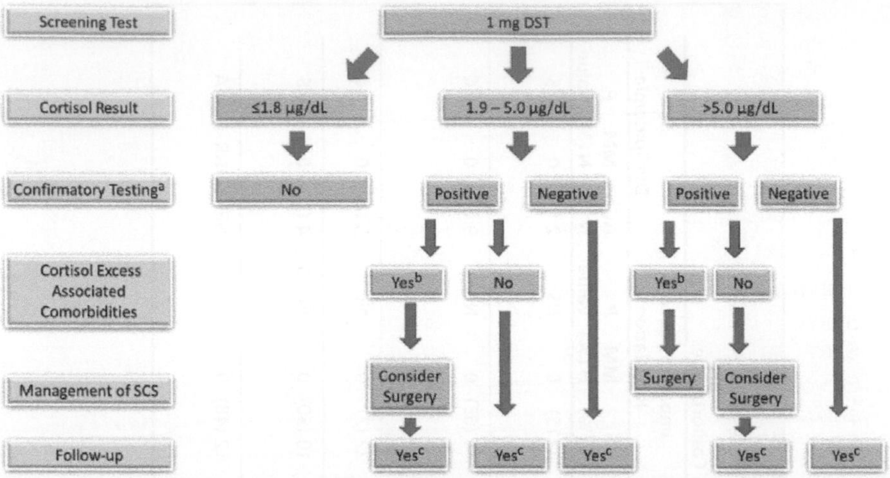

Fig. 1. Evaluation of patients for SCS with adrenal incidentaloma and no clinical signs of Cushing's syndrome. [a] ACTH, LNSC, UFC. Two-day low-dose DST (see **Table 1**). [b] Hypertension, type 2 diabetes, dyslipidemia, osteoporosis. [c] If the patient does not undergo adrenalectomy, reassess for cortisol excess and associated comorbidities during follow-up and reconsider surgery if cortisol excess or comorbidities worsen. Consider surgery if adrenal nodule increases in size. (*Adapted from* Fassnacht, M., et al., Management of adrenal incidentalomas: European Society of Endocrinology Clinical Practice Guideline in collaboration with the European Network for the Study of Adrenal Tumors. Eur J Endocrinol, 2016. 175(2): p. G1-G34, with permission.)

outlines a step-by-step approach for the diagnosis and management of SCS. Laparoscopic adrenalectomy is the preferred approach given the low morbidity and even lower perioperative mortality.[55]

SUMMARY

SCS is a clinical entity associated with significant comorbidities contrary to what the name "subclinical" might suggest. Diagnosing SCS is challenging, particularly with the wide range of recommendations across guidelines, and also a variety of confirmatory testing. There is no gold-standard testing for SCS. The lack of consensus regarding the diagnostic criteria for SCS can make interpretation of laboratory results challenging because there may be underdiagnosis or overdiagnosis of SCS patients. Because studies have shown improvement in SCS-associated comorbidities in only some SCS patients after adrenalectomy, it may be difficult to determine who may benefit from surgery versus who may benefit from medical management. A multidisciplinary approach with the endocrinologist and endocrine surgeon should be taken to manage SCS patients. With low morbidity and mortality associated with minimally invasive adrenalectomy, surgery should be considered in appropriate surgical candidates with SCS and associated comorbidities, such as hypertension, obesity, diabetes, and osteoporosis, which are refractory to medical management.

REFERENCES

1. Terzolo M, Stigliano A, Chiodini I, et al. AME position statement on adrenal incidentaloma. Eur J Endocrinol 2011;164(6):851–70.

2. Fassnacht M, Arlt W, Bancos I, et al. Management of adrenal incidentalomas: European Society of Endocrinology Clinical Practice Guideline in collaboration with the European Network for the Study of Adrenal Tumors. Eur J Endocrinol 2016; 175(2):G1–34.
3. Reincke M. Subclinical Cushing's syndrome. Endocrinol Metab Clin North Am 2000;29(1):43–56.
4. Chiodini I. Clinical review: diagnosis and treatment of subclinical hypercortisolism. J Clin Endocrinol Metab 2011;96(5):1223–36.
5. Terzolo M, Pia A, Reimondo G. Subclinical Cushing's syndrome: definition and management. Clin Endocrinol (Oxf) 2012;76(1):12–8.
6. Starker LF, Kunstman JW, Carling T. Subclinical Cushing syndrome: a review. Surg Clin North Am 2014;94(3):657–68.
7. Giordano R, Marinazzo E, Berardelli R, et al. Long-term morphological, hormonal, and clinical follow-up in a single unit on 118 patients with adrenal incidentalomas. Eur J Endocrinol 2010;162:779–85.
8. Morelli V, Reimondo G, Giordano R, et al. Long-term follow-up in adrenal incidentalomas: an Italian multicenter study. J Clin Endocrinol Metab 2014;99(3):827–34.
9. Di Dalmazi G, Vicennati V, Garelli S, et al. Cardiovascular events and mortality in patients with adrenal incidentalomas that are either non-secreting or associated with intermediate phenotype or subclinical Cushing's syndrome: a 15-year retrospective study. Lancet Diabetes Endocrinol 2014;2(5):396–405.
10. NIH state-of-the-science statement on management of the clinically inapparent adrenal mass ("incidentaloma"). NIH Consens State Sci Statements 2002;19(2): 1–25.
11. Nieman LK, Biller BM, Findling JW, et al. The diagnosis of Cushing's syndrome: an Endocrine Society Clinical Practice Guideline. J Clin Endocrinol Metab 2008;93(5):1526–40.
12. Yanase T, Oki Y, Katabami T, et al. New diagnostic criteria of adrenal subclinical Cushing's syndrome: opinion from the Japan Endocrine Society. Endocr J 2018; 65(4):383–93.
13. Zeiger MA, Thompson GB, Duh QY, et al, American Association of Clinical Endocrinologists; American Association of Endocrine Surgeons. American Association of Clinical Endocrinologists and American Association of Endocrine Surgeons medical guidelines for the management of adrenal incidentalomas: executive summary of recommendations. Endocr Pract 2009;15(5):450–3.
14. Tabarin A, Bardet S, Bertherat J, et al. Exploration and management of adrenal incidentalomas. French Society of Endocrinology Consensus. Ann Endocrinol (Paris) 2008;69(6):487–500.
15. Fassnacht M, Dekkers OM, Else T, et al. European Society of Endocrinology Clinical Practice Guidelines on the management of adrenocortical carcinoma in adults, in collaboration with the European Network for the Study of Adrenal Tumors. Eur J Endocrinol 2018;179(4):G1–46.
16. Carroll TB, Findling JW. The diagnosis of Cushing's syndrome. Rev Endocr Metab Disord 2010;11(2):147–53.
17. Carroll T, Raff H, Findling JW. Late-night salivary cortisol for the diagnosis of Cushing syndrome: a meta-analysis. Endocr Pract 2009;15(4):335–42.
18. Masserini B, Morelli V, Bergamaschi S, et al. The limited role of midnight salivary cortisol levels in the diagnosis of subclinical hypercortisolism in patients with adrenal incidentaloma. Eur J Endocrinol 2009;160(1):87–92.

19. Nunes ML, Vattaut S, Corcuff JB, et al. Late-night salivary cortisol for diagnosis of overt and subclinical Cushing's syndrome in hospitalized and ambulatory patients. J Clin Endocrinol Metab 2009;94(2):456–62.
20. Palmieri S, Morelli V, Polledri E, et al. The role of salivary cortisol measured by liquid chromatography-tandem mass spectrometry in the diagnosis of subclinical hypercortisolism. Eur J Endocrinol 2013;168(3):289–96.
21. Mericq MV, Cutler GB Jr. High fluid intake increases urine free cortisol excretion in normal subjects. J Clin Endocrinol Metab 1998;83(2):682–4.
22. Valli N, Catargi B, Ronci N, et al. Biochemical screening for subclinical cortisol-secreting adenomas amongst adrenal incidentalomas. Eur J Endocrinol 2001;144(4):401–8.
23. Kidambi S, Raff H, Findling JW. Limitations of nocturnal salivary cortisol and urine free cortisol in the diagnosis of mild Cushing's syndrome. Eur J Endocrinol 2007;157(6):725–31.
24. Yener S, Demir L, Demirpence M, et al. Interference in ACTH immunoassay negatively impacts the management of subclinical hypercortisolism. Endocrine 2017;56(2):308–16.
25. Kim HK, Yoon JH, Jeong YA, et al. The recovery of hypothalamic-pituitary-adrenal axis is rapid in subclinical cushing syndrome. Endocrinol Metab (Seoul) 2016;31(4):592–7.
26. Khawandanah D, ElAsmar N, Arafah BM. Alterations in hypothalamic-pituitary-adrenal function immediately after resection of adrenal adenomas in patients with Cushing's syndrome and others with incidentalomas and subclinical hypercortisolism. Endocrine 2019;63(1):140–8.
27. Plotz CM, Knowlton AI, Ragan C. The natural history of Cushing's syndrome. Am J Med 1952;13(5):597–614.
28. Etxabe J, Vazquez JA. Morbidity and mortality in Cushing's disease: an epidemiological approach. Clin Endocrinol (Oxf) 1994;40(4):479–84.
29. Barzon L, Scaroni C, Sonino N, et al. Risk factors and long-term follow-up of adrenal incidentalomas. J Clin Endocrinol Metab 1999;84:520–6.
30. Barzon L, Sonino N, Fallo F, et al. Prevalence and natural history of adrenal incidentalomas. Eur J Endocrinol 2003;149:273–85.
31. Terzolo M, Bovio S, Reimondo G, et al. Subclinical Cushing's syndrome in adrenal incidentalomas. Endocrinol Metab Clin North Am 2005;34:423–39.
32. Nieman LK. Update on subclinical Cushing's syndrome. Curr Opin Endocrinol Diabetes Obes 2015;22(3):180–4.
33. Bernini GP, Moretti A, Oriandini C, et al. Long-term morphological and hormonal follow-up in a single unit on 115 patients with adrenal incidentalomas. Br J Cancer 2005;92(6):1104–9.
34. Libè R, Dall'Asta C, Barbetta L, et al. Long-term follow-up study of patients with adrenal incidentalomas. Eur J Endocrinol 2002;147(4):489–94.
35. Terzolo M, Bovio S, Pia A, et al. Midnight serum cortisol as a marker of increased cardiovascular risk in patients with a clinically inapparent adrenal adenoma. Eur J Endocrinol 2005;153:307–15.
36. Tauchmanovà L, Rossi R, Biondi B, et al. Patients with subclinical Cushing's syndrome due to adrenal adenoma have increased cardiovascular risk. J Clin Endocrinol Metab 2002;87:4872–8.
37. Emral R, Uysal AR, Asik M, et al. Prevalence of subclinical Cushing's syndrome in 70 patients with adrenal incidentaloma: clinical, biochemical and surgical outcomes. Endocr J 2003;50(4):399–408.

38. Chiodini I, Albani A, Ambrogio AG, et al. Six controversial issues on subclinical Cushing's syndrome. Endocrine 2017;56(2):262–6.
39. Di Dalmazi G, Vicennati V, Rinaldi E, et al. Progressively increased patterns of subclinical cortisol hypersecretion in adrenal incidentalomas differently predict major metabolic and cardiovascular outcomes: a large cross-sectional study. Eur J Endocrinol 2012;166:669–77.
40. Fernandez-Real J, Engel WR, Simó R, et al. Study of glucose tolerance in consecutive patients harbouring incidental adrenal tumours. Study Group of Incidental Adrenal Adenoma. Clin Endocrinol (Oxf) 1998;49:53–61.
41. Chiodini I, Vainicher CE, Morelli V, et al. MECHANISMS IN ENDOCRINOLOGY: endogenous subclinical hypercortisolism and bone: a clinical review. Eur J Endocrinol 2016;175(6):R265–82.
42. Chiodini I, Torlontano M, Carnevale V, et al. Bone loss rate in adrenal incidentalomas: a longitudinal study. J Clin Endocrinol Metab 2001;86(11): 5337–41.
43. Morelli V, Eller-Vainicher C, Salcuni AS, et al. Risk of new vertebral fractures in patients with adrenal incidentaloma with and without subclinical hypercortisolism: a multicenter longitudinal study. J Bone Miner Res 2011;26(8):1816–21.
44. Di Dalmazi G, Pasquali R, Beuschlein F, et al. Subclinical hypercortisolism: a state, a syndrome, or a disease? Eur J Endocrinol 2015;173(4):M61–71.
45. Di Dalmazi G, Pasquali R. Adrenal adenomas, subclinical hypercortisolism, and cardiovascular outcomes. Curr Opin Endocrinol Diabetes Obes 2015;22(3): 163–8.
46. Debono M, Bradburn M, Bull M, et al. Cortisol as a marker for increased mortality in patients with incidental adrenocortical adenomas. J Clin Endocrinol Metab 2014;99(12):4462–70.
47. Toniato A, Merante-Boschin I, Opocher G, et al. Surgical versus conservative management for subclinical Cushing syndrome in adrenal incidentalomas: a prospective randomized study. Ann Surg 2009;249(3):388–91.
48. Tsuiki M, Tanabe A, Takagi S, et al. Cardiovascular risks and their long-term clinical outcome in patients with subclinical Cushing's syndrome. Endocr J 2008; 55(4):737–45.
49. Iacobone M, Citton M, Viel G, et al. Adrenalectomy may improve cardiovascular and metabolic impairment and ameliorate quality of life in patients with adrenal incidentalomas and subclinical Cushing's syndrome. Surgery 2012; 152(6):991–7.
50. Chiodini I, Morelli V, Salcuni AS, et al. Beneficial metabolic effects of prompt surgical treatment in patients with an adrenal incidentaloma causing biochemical hypercortisolism. J Clin Endocrinol Metab 2010;95(6):2736–45.
51. Petramala L, Cavallaro G, Galassi M, et al. Clinical benefits of unilateral adrenalectomy in patients with subclinical hypercortisolism due to adrenal incidentaloma: results from a single center. High Blood Press Cardiovasc Prev 2017; 24(1):69–75.
52. Bancos I, Alahdab F, Crowley RK, et al. THERAPY OF ENDOCRINE DISEASE: improvement of cardiovascular risk factors after adrenalectomy in patients with adrenal tumors and subclinical Cushing's syndrome: a systematic review and meta-analysis. Eur J Endocrinol 2016;175(6):R283–95.
53. Iacobone M, Citton M, Scarpa M, et al. Systematic review of surgical treatment of subclinical Cushing's syndrome. Br J Surg 2015;102(4):318–30.

54. Salcuni AS, Morelli V, Eller Vainicher C, et al. Adrenalectomy reduces the risk of vertebral fractures in patients with monolateral adrenal incidentalomas and subclinical hypercortisolism. Eur J Endocrinol 2016;174(3):261–9.
55. Gupta PK, Natarajan B, Pallati PK, et al. Outcomes after laparoscopic adrenalectomy. Surg Endosc 2011;25(3):784–94.

Adrenocortical Cancer Treatment

Samuel E. Long, MD*, Barbra S. Miller, MD

KEYWORDS

• Adrenal cancer • Adrenocortical carcinoma • Adrenalectomy • Mitotane • Cancer • Cortisol • Surgery

KEY POINTS

- Adrenocortical carcinoma is a rare cancer with poor prognosis.
- Evaluation of adrenal masses requires both assessment of imaging characteristics and investigation for evidence of adrenal hormone excess.
- Fine-needle aspiration of adrenal tumors is rarely indicated during evaluation of adrenal masses.
- Surgery is the primary treatment modality for management of early stage adrenocortical carcinoma.
- Mitotane and cisplatin-based chemotherapy are considered first-line treatment for metastatic adrenocortical carcinoma.

INTRODUCTION

Considered a rare malignancy with an incidence of 1 to 2 per million in the population, adrenocortical carcinoma (ACC) has historically been associated with poor outcomes; however, knowledge about ACC has increased significantly over the past 2 decades leading to advances in care.[1–3] Surgery remains the primary modality to achieve cure in patients with early stage disease. In those with advanced disease, mitotane, chemotherapy, and other surgical and nonsurgical interventional therapies are now used in various combinations. This has allowed for improved survival in a greater number of patients compared with historical controls. The following material focuses on the evaluation and management of patients with ACC.

PREOPERATIVE EVALUATION

The initial evaluation of any patient with suspected ACC begins with a thorough history and physical examination, assessing for any clinical evidence of adrenal

The authors have no disclosures to report.
Division of Endocrine Surgery, Department of Surgery, University of Michigan, 2920H Taubman Center, 1500 E. Medical Center Drive, Ann Arbor, MI 48109, USA
* Corresponding author.
E-mail address: selong@med.umich.edu

Surg Clin N Am 99 (2019) 759–771
https://doi.org/10.1016/j.suc.2019.04.012

hormone excess.[2–4] New onset hypertension, edema, weight gain, changes in secondary sexual characteristics, and features consistent with Cushing's syndrome may be associated with ACC. Patients should be questioned about a history of other previous malignancy or new symptoms that suggest an undiagnosed malignancy of nonadrenal origin as a suspicious adrenal mass may represent metastatic disease. Melanoma, breast cancer, renal cell cancer, and lymphoma are most commonly associated with involvement of the adrenal glands, but other malignancies have been described.[3,4]

More than half of patients with ACC will have biochemical evidence of adrenal hormone excess, most commonly cortisol and androgens (**Fig. 1**).[5] Excess aldosterone production alone is rarely seen in patients with ACC.[5,6] Benign aldosteronomas are generally small, ranging from 1 to 2 cm on average. Therefore, a larger aldosterone-producing tumor not meeting imaging criteria for being benign could be malignant. Malignant aldosterone-producing tumors are significantly smaller on average than other ACCs.[6,7] A comprehensive biochemical evaluation is carried out in systematic fashion (**Table 1**), investigating for end-products of steroid synthesis as well as intermediaries, both of which may be used as tumor markers going forward to assess for evidence of tumor recurrence or disease progression.[2,3,8] It is imperative to rule out pheochromocytoma by biochemical analysis before considering any operative intervention.[2,9,10]

IMAGING

Computed tomography (CT) is the most common modality used to evaluate adrenal masses; however, unless done using an adrenal protocol, it is unlikely the mass will be fully evaluated.[2,11] MRI[12] and/or PET-CT[13,14] also have a role in the evaluation of adrenal abnormalities, especially in heterogeneous tumors where percent washout on CT should not be calculated or when imaging may be discordant from clinical suspicion. ACC is typically ^{18}F-fluorodeoxyglucose (FDG) avid, although tumor necrosis is

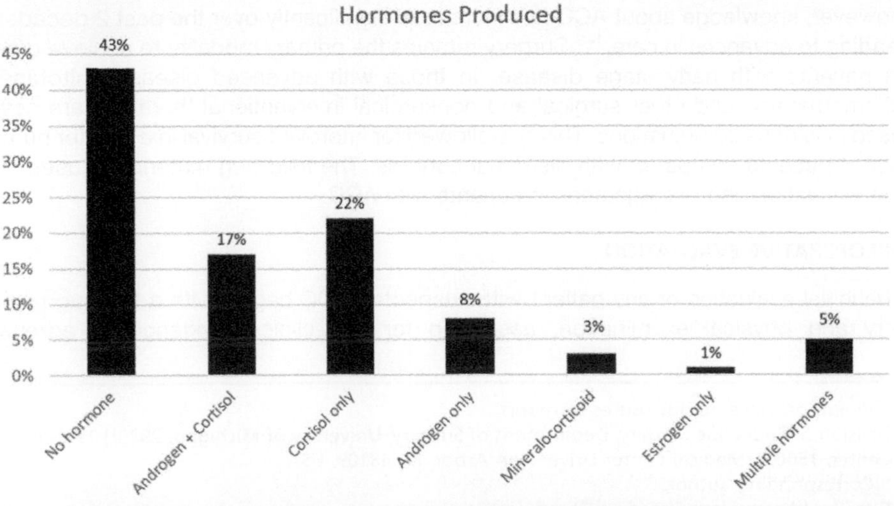

Fig. 1. Types of hormone secretion associated with adrenocortical carcinoma. (*Data from* Else, T, Williams A, Sabolch A, et.al. Adjuvant Therapies and Patient and Tumor Characteristics Associated With Survival of Adult Patients With Adrenocortical Carcinoma. J Clin Endocrinol Metab. 2014; 99(2):455-61.)

Table 1 Biochemical evaluation of adrenocortical carcinoma	
Initial Biochemical Evaluation of ACC	
Mineralocorticoids	Metabolic panel, aldosterone, renin
Glucocorticoids	ACTH, 24-h urine study for cortisol OR 1 mg DST
Androgens	DHEA-S, testosterone (women only), 17-beta-estradiol (men and postmenopausal women), 17-OH progesterone, 11-deoxycortisol, androstenedione
Catecholamines	Plasma and/or 24-h urine metanephrine and normetanephrines

Abbreviation: DST, dexamethasone suppression test.

common and may result in non-^{18}F-FDG avid areas of tumor.[13,14] **Table 2** lists the characteristics and criteria that may assist in differentiating benign from indeterminate adrenal masses.[15] Imaging should also be used to guide the surgical approach, identify the potential need for en-bloc resection of any adjacent structures, and identify any concerning lymph nodes or other potential sites of metastatic disease. In patients with suspected ACC, imaging should include the chest to evaluate for metastatic disease.[2,3,8,15]

In the past, the decision to intervene on an adrenal mass was often based on size. Tumor size greater than 4 to 6 cm was historically used as a cut-off to proceed with surgery given the increased rate of malignancy with larger tumors.[16] This has since been superseded by imaging characteristics (ie, washout patterns, lipid content, heterogeneity, etc.) which have more prognostic value than size alone.[2,3,8,15] A purely nonfunctional tumor with benign imaging characteristics does not necessarily need to be resected. If an incidental adrenal mass is noted but appears benign, short-term interval follow-up with repeat imaging at 6–12 months is now recommended.[17] If a benign-appearing tumor continues to reveal evidence of growth or causes compressive symptoms of adjacent structures, then it should be resected.

BIOPSY

Fine-needle aspiration has a limited role in the evaluation of adrenal masses.[18–20] Seeding of the needle tract has been reported when ACCs have been biopsied. The few instances in which biopsy may be indicated include the following: (1) when metastatic disease from another primary tumor is suspected; (2) if a patient has unresectable disease and tissue confirmation is required before beginning

Table 2
Imaging characteristics of benign and indeterminate adrenal tumors

	Size	CT	MRI	PET CT
Benign	<4 cm if other benign internal characteristics	<10 Hounsfield units, > 50% washout	>50% chemical shift	Tumor SUV <3.4 Tumor: Liver SUV ratio <1.45[14]
Indeterminate	>4–6 cm if other indeterminate characteristics[a]	>10 Hounsfield units, <50% washout	<50% chemical shift	Tumor SUV >3.4 Tumor: Liver SUV ratio >1.45[14]

[a] Indeterminate characteristics: Heterogeneous internal attenuation, calcification, necrosis, irregular borders, local invasion, intravascular tumor thrombus, adjacent lymphadenopathy.

chemotherapy; (3) the patient is a poor operative candidate with significant comorbidities. Other less common indications for biopsy include a suspected adrenal lymphoma or infectious causes such as tuberculosis or histoplasmosis, all of which usually present with bilateral abnormalities.[18] Fine-needle aspiration should never be performed until pheochromocytoma has been ruled out as hypertensive crisis may result.[10]

PREOPERATIVE CONSIDERATIONS

Patients should undergo standard evaluation for fitness for surgery. Patients with evidence of hormone excess, especially those producing cortisol, are at increased risk for complications and difficulty recovering from surgery.[2,8,15] There are several medications that can be used preoperatively to control the effects of hormone excess.[3,8] In patients with hypercortisolism, inhibitors of cortisol production (ketoconazole, mitotane, metyrapone, etomidate) as well as glucocorticoid receptor antagonists (mifepristone) can be used.[21] It is critical to remember that cortisol levels cannot be used to guide therapy when using glucocorticoid receptor antagonists and that dexamethasone should be used instead of hydrocortisone for treatment of Addisonian crisis when patients are taking mifepristone. For mineralocorticoid excess, either spironolactone or eplerenone can be used to control hypertension or hypokalemia in Conn syndrome and some cases of severe cortisol excess.[3,8] Additional medications for management of adrenal hormone excess are outlined in **Table 3**.

SURGICAL RESECTION

Minimally invasive adrenalectomy, whether performed by laparoscopic, retroperitoneoscopic, or robotically assisted approaches, has become the standard for resection of benign tumors of appropriate size.[2,15] Open resection is preferred for adrenal masses known or strongly suspected to be ACC.[2,22] For those with indeterminate tumors not meeting imaging criteria for being benign, controversy with regard to the operative approach remains.[23–27] Disease recurrence in some studies has been shown to occur earlier and more often in patients treated for ACC by minimally invasive approaches due to a higher rate of intraoperative tumor spill and positive margins in some studies.[23,25,27] Overall survival was also found to be shorter in Stage 1 and Stage 2 patients who underwent laparoscopic resection.[27]

Table 3
Medications used to decrease excess production of excess adrenal hormones in patients with adrenocortical carcinoma

Type of Hormone Excess	Primary Medication	Alternative Medications
Cortisol	Ketoconazole, mitotane, metyrapone, mifepristone [a]	Etomidate[b]
Aldosterone	Spironolactone	Eplerenone, amiloride
Testosterone	Spironolactone	Abiraterone[c], Ketoconazole[c]
Estrogen	Tamoxifen	Raloxifene, anastrozole, letrozole, exemestane

[a] Selection of medication depends on degree of hormone excess.
[b] Patients should be monitored in an intensive care unit setting.
[c] Off-label use.

RIGHT OPEN ADRENALECTOMY

Open adrenalectomy[28] is typically performed through a wide right subcostal incision that extends across to the left side (with or without extension to the xiphoid process). Other approaches, including a midline incision or Makuuchi incision[29] can be performed. A thoracoabdominal incision is rarely required. Systematic exploration of the abdomen is pursued, looking for evidence of metastatic disease. Ultrasound of the liver can be performed, looking for metastases that may not be visualized on preoperative imaging. With a right ACC, the vena cava is also inspected for either obvious invasion or intracaval tumor thrombus. A self-retaining tractor such as a Thompson or Omni retractor is then placed. This allows retraction of the ribs and for full mobilization of the liver to provide access to the inferior vena cava, right adrenal gland, and kidney. It is advantageous to release the left coronary and triangular ligaments as well to allow for full rotation of the liver. If tumor is found to be invading the posterior aspect of the liver, a thin rim of liver can be resected along with the specimen as part of the anterior margin. In general, the posterior peritoneal lining should be kept on the anterior surface of the tumor as part of the anterior margin. Dissection then occurs inferiorly over the superior half of the kidney, taking the posterior peritoneal lining and any fat over the superior half of the kidney to provide a sufficient inferior margin. This is continued to the plane between the adrenal gland and kidney. If there is any question of local invasion into the kidney parenchyma or renal hilar vessels, partial nephrectomy or total nephrectomy should be performed to ensure an R0 resection. The surgeon should refrain from trying to create a plane that does not exist, as this can result in tumor rupture, dissemination, and early recurrence. In some cases, the kidney may be able to be spared if the renal hilar vasculature is not involved and the renal capsule can be included as part of the inferior margin. The operation continues, taking all retroperitoneal fat surrounding the tumor to the abdominal side wall as part of the lateral and posterior margins, with dissection exposing and sometimes including part of the posterior musculature if necessary. The dissection is carried superiorly to the level of the diaphragm. If tumor seems to involve the diaphragm, a portion of the diaphragm can be excised and closed primarily or with mesh. Lastly, the medial dissection is performed, starting over the anterior aspect of the vena cava, keeping any fat between the tumor and the vena cava with the tumor. The medial aspect of the dissection is an area at high risk for microscopic residual disease, given little intervening fat between tumor and vena cava. Once the adrenal vein is identified, it is ligated and divided. The tumor is then removed and marked with sutures. If adherence to or invasion of the adrenal vein or vena cava is identified, various methods can be used to obtain negative medial margins or extract tumor thrombus, including primary resection and closure if the vena cava is not narrowed greater than 50%, use of a bovine pericardial or vein patch, or resection and replacement of the vena cava with a ringed polytetrafluoroethylene graft. Rarely, venovenous or cardiopulmonary bypass is required. Clips can be placed in the surgical bed to facilitate future radiation therapy. The abdomen is then closed.

LEFT OPEN ADRENALECTOMY

An appropriate incision is again made. Once adequate exposure is obtained, the procedure begins with mobilization of the left colon by taking down the white line of Toldt; this is continued superiorly and the spleen is then released from its attachments to the level of the esophageal hiatus. The stomach, spleen, pancreas, and colon are all retracted medially if not involved by tumor in order to visualize the kidney, left adrenal gland, and aorta. The remainder of the operation is carried out in a similar manner to the contralateral side, making sure to include all the surrounding and retroperitoneal fat along with the adrenal gland. The left adrenal vein is typically identified inferomedially near the 7 or 8 o'clock position on the gland and is ligated at its insertion into the left renal vein. Careful assessment of the left adrenal vein and its junction with the left renal vein is necessary to ensure no intravenous thrombus remains. En-bloc resection of involved organs, most often the kidney, distal pancreas, and spleen, may be required.

POSTOPERATIVE CONSIDERATIONS

Patients with ACC who undergo resection are typically admitted postoperatively for anywhere from 3 to 7 days. In patients with evidence of preoperative hormone excess, serial assessment of electrolytes, volume status, and blood pressure is necessary. In those who have overt hypercortisolism, postoperative steroid supplementation is almost always required, whereas those with subclinical hypercortisolism or lack of cortisol suppression after dexamethasone suppression testing should undergo testing on postoperative day one to determine the need for steroid supplementation.[30] The total daily dose of steroids should be administered in 2 or 3 divided doses, with the larger dose in the morning to replicate the usual early morning surge of cortisol. Hydrocortisone is the preferred steroid for replacement. Prednisone is avoided, as it increases the length of time for recovery of the hypothalamic pituitary adrenal axis. Furthermore, any patient who has undergone an adrenalectomy for ACC is at risk of an Addisonian crisis and should be counseled about the need for steroid supplementation should this occur. This risk is higher in patients who have undergone bilateral adrenalectomy or unilateral adrenalectomy requiring postoperative steroid supplementation and in those taking mitotane. Because mitotane blocks cortisol production and is also an adrenolytic, patients require steroid supplementation when treated with this medication.[2,3]

STAGING AND PROGNOSIS

Multiple staging systems exist for ACC. The 2 staging systems that are most widely used are the American Joint Committee on Cancer (AJCC) 8th Edition[31] and the European Network for the Study of Adrenal Tumors (ENSAT).[32] The TNM classification for adrenal cancer was modified in the 8th Edition of the AJCC/UICC staging system to mirror the TNM classification of the ENSAT system. Additional modifications have been proposed over the past decade to further enhance the prognostic ability of these staging systems and include incorporation of age, gender, and tumor grade.[33,34] As more is known about the tumor biology of ACC, the incorporation of genomic and proteomic factors may also lead to better prognostication.[35]

There are multiple factors that influence prognosis in patients with ACC, with initial stage and tumor biology being most important.[2,3,5,8,27,33,35–39] Five-year survival for patients with ACC ranges from approximately 65% in patients with stage I disease to less than 10% in patients with stage IV disease.[1–5] Production of cortisol, high tumor grade, and increasing stage consistently predicts worse outcomes across multiple studies.[1–5] Ki-67 index is used as an alternative to mitotic rate and independently predicts recurrence, even following R0 resection.[2]

GENETIC TESTING

All patients diagnosed with ACC, as well as those with a known family history of a genetic mutation or other tumors associated with a genetic syndrome linked to adrenal cancer, should have an in depth family history taken and be referred to a genetic counselor for genetic testing.[2,8,40] Every adult patient with ACC should be offered genetic testing for Li-Fraumeni and Lynch syndromes.[2,8,40] Other hereditary syndromes associated with development of ACC include MEN-1, Beckwith–Wiedemann syndrome, familial adenomatous polyposis, neurofibromatosis type I, and Carney syndrome.[2,8,40]

ADJUVANT THERAPY

Even after complete resection, many experts will agree that adjuvant therapy is advantageous due to the high rate of local and distant recurrence following initial resection of ACC.[2] Mitotane, a derivative of the insecticide DDT, inhibits steroidogenesis and has a cytotoxic effect on cells of the adrenal cortex. It is the only medication specifically approved by the Food and Drug Administration for treatment of ACC. The usual dose is 5 to 15 g/d with target plasma concentrations of 14 to 20 mg/L.[2,41] Other cytotoxic chemotherapy regimens are not routinely used in an adjuvant manner but may be used in highly selected situations for patients at high risk for distant metastasis.[2] A new clinical trial to assess the impact of adjuvant cytotoxic chemotherapy is planned.

RADIATION THERAPY

Historically, external beam radiation therapy (XRT) was not considered beneficial for treatment of ACC. Over the past 2 decades, 2 high-volume centers have reported significant impacts on locoregional control with use of XRT in both adjuvant and palliative settings,[42,43] and forthcoming data suggest improved survival. Indications for XRT include those undergoing R1 or R2 resection. Following an R0 resection, XRT is considered in those with adverse risk factors such as high-grade disease, nodal involvement, lymphovascular invasion, and those having undergone laparoscopic resection, given the higher risk for local recurrence in some studies.[2,3,27,38,42,43] Stereotactic body radiotherapy is a more targeted alternative to conventional XRT that can be successfully used to treat small volume disease, particularly in the lungs and liver. This is well tolerated and treatment duration is much shorter (days vs weeks).

OTHER SURGICAL SITUATIONS—STAGE IV DISEASE AT PRESENTATION AND BORDERLINE RESECTABLE ADRENOCORTICAL CARCINOMA

An initial surgical approach is typically warranted for any patient who presents without evidence of metastatic disease and has an adrenal mass that appears amenable to an R0 resection based on preoperative imaging. Assessment of performance status and especially degree of debilitation due to any hormone excess is key to determining risk before offering surgical resection. Any evidence of metastatic disease should prompt discussion in a multidisciplinary setting with consideration for initial systemic treatment with chemotherapy (etoposide, doxorubicin, and cisplatin [EDP]) and mitotane rather than resection of the primary lesion.[2,22,38,44] The decision of when to offer metastasectomy at the time of initial presentation depends on many factors. If tumor response to systemic therapy is noted or at least stable without evidence of new lesions and all tumor can be resected or treated in some way with a combination of local therapies, resection may be pursued.[38] If additional metastatic lesions appear, XRT to the primary tumor may be offered, as surgical resection of the primary tumor usually does not alter survival.[3,8] Some may consider resection of the primary tumor if control of hormone excess is problematic, although control is often achievable with currently available medications, and subsequent disease progression may overcome this perceived benefit of resection relatively quickly.[45]

Locally invasive tumors without evidence of other metastatic disease, in which an R0 resection would be unlikely, may benefit from neoadjuvant therapy. Should response to mitotane and/or chemotherapy be evident, surgery may then be undertaken with an improved chance of an R0 resection. In a series from MD Anderson, patients with initially unresectable or borderline unresectable ACC who underwent neoadjuvant chemotherapy had a median disease free survival of 28 months as opposed to 13 months in patients who underwent surgery alone.[46] This approach also allows for the disease to declare itself, as those with progression of disease (primary tumor or new metastases) will likely not benefit significantly from resection.

RECURRENT DISEASE

Approximately 70% to 90% of patients with ACC will experience cancer recurrence at some point.[38,47] Most commonly, initial recurrence occurs in either the tumor bed or the lungs.[38] Survival has been found to vary based on site and extent of initial disease recurrence. Although metastases to the lungs occurred earlier, they were associated with longer survival compared with those with initial metastasis to the peritoneal cavity or metastases involving multiple organ systems.[38]

For patients found to have metastatic disease, mitotane is usually given in combination with EDP as first-line therapy. Streptozocin plus mitotane is considered second-line therapy.[48] Approximately 30% of patients will respond to mitotane- and/or cisplatin-based therapy. Given the poor long-term response of ACC with traditional chemotherapy, there has been increasing focus on providing more individualized care using targeted therapies based on actionable mutations identified using molecular testing.[2,8,22,35] Trials are ongoing.

In the past, reoperation for recurrent ACC was rarely undertaken; however, more recent work has identified some patients who will benefit from reoperation.[38,45,47] Multiple factors must be considered before proceeding with resection, including having an understanding of specific tumor characteristics (tumor grade, Ki-67 index), extent of disease to be resected, conduct of the initial resection (oncologic technique, R type—0,1,2), recurrence free interval and tempo of disease, and response to medical therapy.[38] Those with low-grade tumors often have slower disease progression compared with those with high-grade tumors, and thus survival may be prolonged with resection of recurrent disease.[2,33,38] Patients with recurrent metastatic disease are usually subjected to treatment with mitotane and EDP for 2 to 3 rounds before surgery and reimaged to determine response.[38] In those patients with response or stability, resection can be considered where all tumor can be resected or resection is necessary due to threat to a vital structure with continued growth or inability to control hormone excess. Other considerations include a patient's functional status and ability to tolerate surgery as well as consideration of tempo of disease. Reresection with evidence of new metastases on the next surveillance scan is not desirable, and instead a balance between proceeding with resection for prolonging survival and quality of life must be found.[38] Because of this, there has been a shift from formal surgical resection to utilization of various types of localized therapy to address metastatic disease in certain sites (lung, liver).[2,38,49,50] An algorithm for management of metastatic disease developed by the University of Michigan Endocrine Oncology group is shown in **Fig. 2**.[38]

HEATED INTRAOPERATIVE PERITONEAL EXTRACORPOREAL CHEMOTHERAPY FOR PERITONEAL CARCINOMATOSIS

Although heated intraoperative peritoneal extracorporeal chemotherapy (HIPEC) has been studied more extensively in the treatment of mesothelioma, ovarian, appendiceal, colorectal, and gastric malignancies, there may be a role for patients with

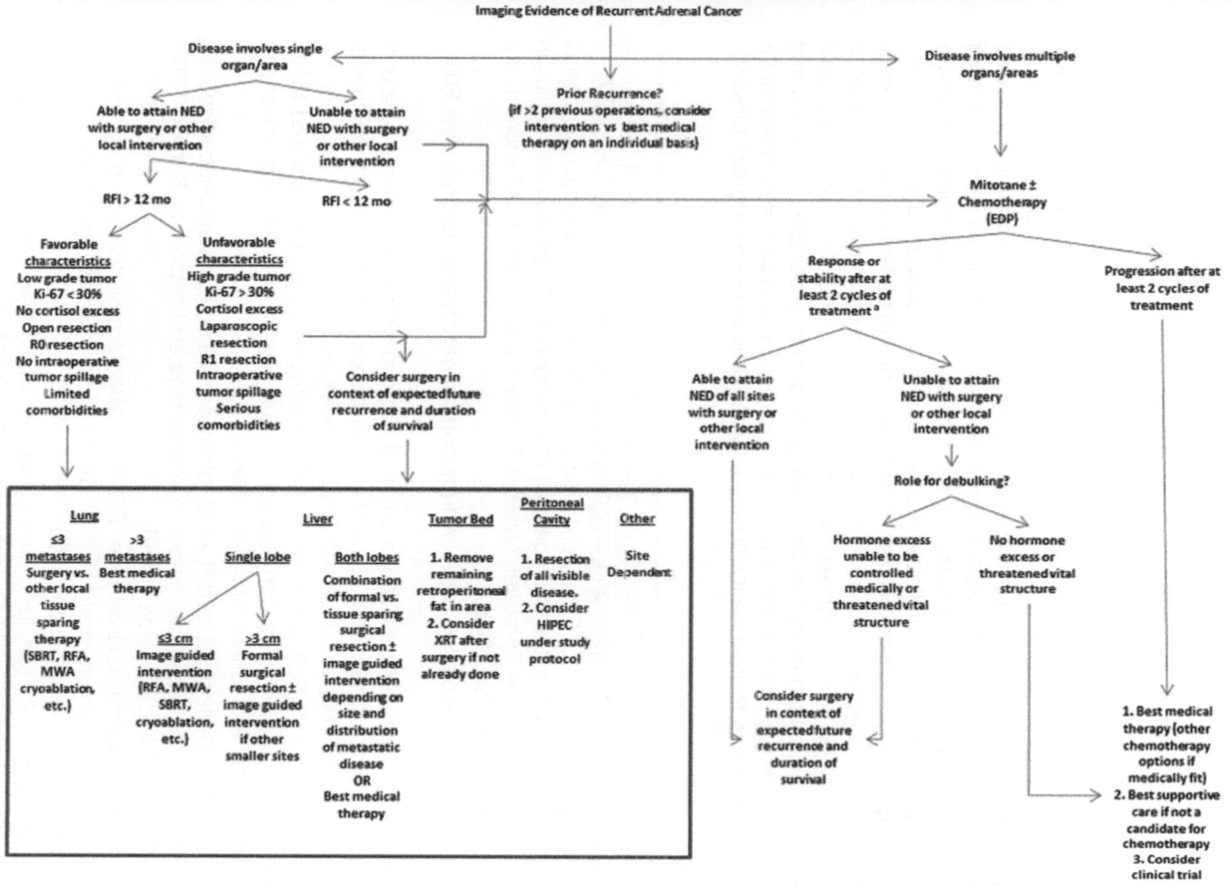

Fig. 2. University of Michigan treatment algorithm for patients with recurrent metastatic disease after primary resection of adrenocortical carcinoma with curative intent. HIPEC, hyperthermic intraperitoneal chemotherapy; MWA, microwave ablation; NED, no evidence of disease; RFA, radio-frequency ablation; RFI, recurrence-free interval; SBRT, single beam radiation therapy. [a] Chemotherapy is continued for up to 6–8 cycles until no further response is noted. (*From* Glenn JA, Else T, Hughes DT et al. Longitudinal Patterns of Recurrence in Patients with Adrenocortical Carcinoma. Surgery 2018 165(1);186–195; with permission.)

ACC.[51–53] HIPEC was previously investigated as an adjunct for the treatment of recurrent intraperitoneal ACC. Initial outcomes were not significantly changed, and the treatment itself was associated with significant morbidity and mortality. With improved understanding of the disease process and better patient selection, there may be a role for HIPEC in carefully selected patients.[52,53] Currently, new studies are underway. Chemotherapeutic agents used for HIPEC in ACC include cisplatin, carboplatin (for those with reduced renal function), mitomycin C, and oxaliplatin.[52,53]

SUMMARY

Despite being difficult to treat malignancy, advances in treatment and overall survival are being made. In large part, this is due to an increased understanding of factors identified at the time of pathologic review, including molecular profiling, which allows for selection and initiation of adjuvant treatment at an earlier time. As surgery remains the primary modality to achieve cure, it is critically important that appropriate oncologic techniques are used to minimize local and peritoneal recurrence, reserving systemic therapy to control distant disease. Careful selection of patients who may benefit from localized approaches to therapy (surgical or other intervention) can also lead to improved outcomes. With continued collaborative effort—mitotane plus traditional chemotherapy, utilization of molecular profiling to identify actionable mutations and pathways for new drug development and immunotherapies—a comprehensive multidisciplinary approach to treatment will hopefully continue to drive progress forward.

REFERENCES

1. Bilimoria KY, Shen WT, Elaraj D, et al. Adrenocortical carcinoma in the United States: treatment utilization and prognostic factors. Cancer 2008;113:3130–6.
2. Fassnacht M, Dekkers O, Else T, et al. European Society of Endocrinology Clinical Practice Guidelines on the management of adrenocortical carcinoma in adults, in collaboration with the European Network for the Study of Adrenal Tumors. Eur J Endocrinol 2018;179:G1–46.
3. Else T, Kim A, Sabolch A, et al. Adrenocortical carcinoma. Endocr Rev 2014; 35(2):282–326.
4. Nakamura Y, Yamazaki Y, Felizola SJ, et al. Adrenocortical carcinoma: review of the pathologic features, production of adrenal steroids, and molecular pathogenesis. Endocrinol Metab Clin North Am 2015;44(2):399–410.
5. Else T, Williams A, Sabolch A, et al. Adjuvant therapies and patient and tumor characteristics associated with survival of adult patients with adrenocortical carcinoma. J Clin Endocrinol Metab 2014;99(2):455–61.
6. Kendrick ML, Curlee K, Lloyd R, et al. Aldosterone-secreting adrenocortical carcinomas are associated with unique operative risks and outcomes. Surgery 2002; 132(6):1008–11 [discussion: 1012].
7. Seccia TM, Fassina A, Nussdorfer GG, et al. Aldosterone-producing adrenocortical carcinoma: an unusual cause of Conn's syndrome with an ominous clinical course. Endocr Relat Cancer 2005;12:149–59.
8. Miller BS, Else T. Personalized care of patients with adrenocortical carcinoma. A comprehensive approach. Endocr Pract 2017;23:705–15.
9. Sheps SG, Jiang NS, Klee GG, et al. Recent developments in the diagnosis and treatment of pheochromocytoma. Mayo Clin Proc 1990;65:88–95.
10. Vanderveen KA, Thompson SM, Callstrom MR, et al. Biopsy of pheochromocytomas and paragangliomas: potential for disaster. Surgery 2009;146:1158–66.

11. Caoili EM, Korobkin M, Francis IR, et al. Delayed enhanced CT of lipid-poor adrenal adenomas. AJR Am J Roentgenol 2000;175:1411–5.
12. Haider MA, Ghai S, Jhaveri K, et al. Chemical shift MR imaging of hyperattenuating (>10 HU) adrenal masses: does it still have a role? Radiology 2004;231:711–6.
13. Wong KK, Miller BS, Viglianti BL, et al. Molecular imaging in the management of adrenocortical cancer: a systematic review. Clin Nucl Med 2016;41(8):e368–82.
14. Leboulleux S, Dromain C, Bonniaud G, et al. Diagnostic and prognostic value of 18-fluorodeoxyglucose positron emission tomography in adrenocortical carcinoma: a prospective comparison with computed tomography. J Clin Endocrinol Metab 2006;91(3):920–5.
15. Miller BS, Doherty GM. Surgical management of adrenocortical tumours. Nat Rev Endocrinol 2014;10(5):282–92.
16. Sturgeon C, Shen WT, Clark OH, et al. Risk assessment in 457 adrenal cortical carcinomas: how much does tumor size predict the likelihood of malignancy? J Am Coll Surg 2006;202:423–30.
17. Fassnacht M, Arlt W, Bancos I, et al. Management of adrenal incidentalomas: European Society of Endocrinology Clinical Practice Guideline in collaboration with the European Network for the Study of Adrenal Tumors. Eur J Endocrinol 2016;175(2):G1–34.
18. Williams AR, Hammer GD, Else T. Transcutaneous biopsy of adrenocortical carcinoma is rarely helpful in diagnosis, potentially harmful, but does not affect patient outcome. Eur J Endocrinol 2014;170(6):829–35.
19. Mazzaglia PJ, Monchik JM. Limited value of adrenal biopsy in the evaluation of adrenal neoplasm: a decade of experience. Arch Surg 2009;144:465–70.
20. Delivanis DA, Erickson D, Atwell TD, et al. Procedural and clinical outcomes of percutaneous adrenal biopsy in a high-risk population for adrenal malignancy. Clin Endocrinol (Oxf) 2016;85(5):710–6.
21. Fleseriu M, Biller BM, Findling JW, et al. Mifepristone, a glucocorticoid receptor antagonist, produces clinical and metabolic benefits in patients with Cushing's syndrome. J Clin Endocrinol Metab 2012;97:2039–49.
22. Dickson PV, Kim L, Yen TWF, et al. Evaluation, staging, and surgical management for adrenocortical carcinoma: an update from the SSO Endocrine and Head and Neck Disease Site Working Group. Ann Surg Oncol 2018;25:3460–8.
23. Miller BS, Ammori JB, Gauger PG, et al. Laparoscopic resection is inappropriate in patients with known or suspected adrenocortical carcinoma. World J Surg 2010;34(6):1380–5.
24. Porpiglia F, Fiori C, Daffara F, et al. Retrospective evaluation of the outcome of open versus laparoscopic adrenalectomy for stage I & II adrenocortical cancer. Eur Urol 2010;57(5):873–8.
25. Cooper AB, Habra MA, Grubbs EG, et al. Does laparoscopic adrenalectomy jeopardize oncologic outcomes for patients with adrenocortical carcinoma? Surg Endosc 2013;26:4026–32.
26. Sgourakis G, Lanitis S, Kouloura A, et al. Laparoscopic versus open adrenalectomy for stage I/II adrenocortical carcinoma: meta-analysis of outcomes. J Invest Surg 2015;28(3):145–52.
27. Miller BS, Gauger PG, Hammer GD, et al. Resection of adrenocortical carcinoma is less complete and local recurrence occurs sooner and more often after laparoscopic adrenalectomy than after open adrenalectomy. Surgery 2012;152(6):1150–7.

28. Miller BS. Adrenalectomy: open anterior. In: Mulholland M, editor. Operative techniques in surgery, vol. 1. Philadelphia: Wolters Kluwer Health; 2015. :46:1747–54.
29. Ruffolo LI, Nessen MF, Probst CP, et al. Open adrenalectomy through a Makuuchi incision: a single institution's experience. Surgery 2018;164:1372–6.
30. Nieman LK, Biller BM, Findling JW, et al, Endocrine Society.. Treatment of Cushing's syndrome: an endocrine society clinical practice guideline. J Clin Endocrinol Metab 2015;100(8):2807–31.
31. Perrier N. Adrenal cortical carcinoma. In: Amin MB, Edge S, Greene F, et al, editors. AJCC cancer staging manual. 8th edition. New York: Springer; 2017. p. 911–8.
32. Lughezzani G, Sun M, Perrotte P, et al. The European Network for the Study of Adrenal Tumors staging system is prognostically superior to the international union against cancer-staging system: a North American validation. Eur J Cancer 2010;46(4):713–9.
33. Miller B, Gauger P, Hammer G, et al. Proposal for modification of the ENSAT staging system for adrenocortical carcinoma using tumor grade. Langenbecks Arch Surg 2010;395:955–61.
34. Asare EA, Wang TS, Winchester DP, et al. A novel staging system for adrenocortical carcinoma better predicts survival in patients with stage I/II disease. Surgery 2014;156:1378–85 [discussion: 1385–6].
35. Lippert J, Fassnacht M, Ronchi C, et al. Targeted molecular analysis in adrenocortical carcinomas: a way towards improved personalized prognostication. Endocr Abstr 2018. https://doi.org/10.1530/endoabs.56.OC11.1.
36. Luton JP, Cerdas S, Billaud L, et al. Clinical features of adrenocortical carcinoma, prognostic factors, and the effect of mitotane therapy. N Engl J Med 1990; 322(17):1195–201.
37. Terzolo M, Baudin AE, Ardito A, et al. Mitotane levels predict the outcome of patients with adrenocortical carcinoma treated adjuvantly following radical resection. Eur J Endocrinol 2013;169(3):263–70.
38. Glenn JA, Else T, Hughes DT, et al. Longitudinal patterns of recurrence in patients with adrenocortical carcinoma. Surgery 2018;165(1):186–95.
39. Gonzalez RJ, Tamm EP, Lee JE, et al. Response to mitotane predicts outcome in patients with recurrent adrenal cortical carcinoma. Surgery 2007;142:867–75 [discussion: 867–75].
40. Petr EJ, Else T. Adrenocortical carcinoma (ACC): when and why should we consider germline testing? Presse Med 2018;47:e119–25.
41. Terzolo M, Angeli A, Fassnacht M, et al. Adjuvant mitotane treatment for adrenocortical carcinoma. N Engl J Med 2007;356:2372–80.
42. Sabolch A, Else T, Griffith KA, et al. Adjuvant radiation therapy improves local control after surgical resection in patients with localized adrenocortical carcinoma. Int J Radiat Oncol Biol Phys 2015;92(2):252–9.
43. Fassnacht M, Hahner S, Polat B, et al. Efficacy of adjuvant radiotherapy of the tumor bed on local recurrence of adrenocortical carcinoma. J Clin Endocrinol Metab 2006;91:4501–4.
44. Dy BM, Strajina V, Cayo AK, et al. Surgical resection of synchronously metastatic adrenocortical cancer. Ann Surg Oncol 2015;22:146–51.
45. Dy BM, Wise KB, Richards ML, et al. Operative intervention for recurrent adrenocortical cancer. Surgery 2013;154(6):1292–9 [discussion: 1299].
46. Bednarski BK, Habra MA, Phan A, et al. Borderline resectable adrenal cortical carcinoma: a potential role for preoperative chemotherapy. World J Surg 2014; 38(6):1318–27.

47. Erdogan I, Deutschbein T, Fassnacht, et al. German Adrenocortical Carcinoma Study Group. The role of surgery in the management of recurrent adrenocortical carcinoma. J Surg Oncol 2016;114(8):971–6.
48. Fassnacht M, Terzolo M, Allolio B, et al, FIRM-ACT Study Group. Combination chemotherapy in advanced adrenocortical carcinoma. N Engl J Med 2012; 366(23):2189–97.
49. Assie G, Antoni G, Tissier F, et al. Prognostic parameters of metastatic adrenocortical carcinoma. J Clin Endocrinol Metab 2007;92:148–54.
50. Kemp CD, Ripley RT, Mathur A, et al. Pulmonary resection for metastatic adrenocortical carcinoma: The National Cancer Institute experience. Ann Thorac Surg 2011;92(4):1195–2000.
51. Dube P, Sideris L, Law C, et al. Guidelines on the use of cytoreductive surgery and hyperthermic intraperitoneal chemotherapy in patients with peritoneal surface malignancy arising from colorectal or appendiceal neoplasms. Curr Oncol 2015;22:100–12.
52. Miller BS. Surgical considerations in the treatment of adrenocortical carcinoma: 5th international ACC symposium session: who, when, and what combination? Horm Cancer 2016;7:24–8.
53. Sugarbaker PH. Peritoneal metastases from adrenal cortical carcinoma treated by cytoreductive surgery and hyperthermic intraperitoneal chemotherapy. Tumori 2016;102(6):588–92.

Surgical Approaches to the Adrenal Gland

Amin Madani, MD, PhD, FRCSC[a], James A. Lee, MD, FACS[b,*]

KEYWORDS

• Adrenalectomy • Adrenal gland • Retroperitoneum • Retroperitoneoscopic
• Laparoscopic • Minimally invasive surgery

KEY POINTS

- The adrenal gland is located in the posterior compartment of the retroperitoneum, and can be approached transabdominally or retroperitoneally through an open, laparoscopic, or retroperitoneoscopic approach.
- For laparoscopic transabdominal adrenalectomy, the sequence of steps for right and left adrenalectomy are similar, whereby the anatomy and procedure are conceptualized as reading a book.
- The book is opened by identifying and opening Gerota's fascia and read from the top-down by dissecting along the medial border of the adrenal gland from the diaphragm toward the renal hilum.
- For a retroperitoneoscopic adrenalectomy, the patient is positioned prone and access to the perirenal space is obtained from posteriorly below the ribs.
- The major landmarks are the paraspinous muscle medially, the edge of the peritoneum laterally, the contents of the perirenal space anteriorly and the ribs posteriorly.

SURGICAL ANATOMY

The adrenal glands are located in the perirenal compartment of the retroperitoneum, which also contains the kidney, perirenal/periadrenal fat, and upper ureter. This space is bordered by Gerota's fascia anteriorly and posteriorly by the posterior renal fascia, quadratus lumborum muscle, paraspinous muscle, transversus abdominis muscle, and thoracolumbar fascia. Safe dissection and access to the perirenal space for adrenalectomy is made possible by the ability to provide the appropriate retraction and identification of the avascular planes around structures in the space. Within the perirenal space, the adrenal glands are located superiorly and slightly medial to the

---

Disclosure Statement: The authors have nothing to disclose.
[a] Department of Surgery, Columbia University Irving Medical Center, 161 Fort Washington Avenue, New York, NY 10032, USA; [b] Endocrine Surgery, Columbia University Irving Medical Center, 161 Fort Washington Avenue, New York, NY 10032, USA
* Corresponding author.
E-mail address: jal74@cumc.columbia.edu

Surg Clin N Am 99 (2019) 773–791
https://doi.org/10.1016/j.suc.2019.04.013
surgical.theclinics.com

kidney. Although there is an extensive arcade of small arteries around the inferior, medial, and superior borders of the adrenal gland, the venous drainage tends to be solitary. The left adrenal vein drains into the left renal vein after converging with the inferior phrenic vein. In contrast, the right adrenal vein is short, narrow, and comes off the inferior vena cava (IVC) at a near 90°, making cannulation during adrenal venous sampling more difficult than the left side. Preoperative imaging should be obtained to determine the position of the tumor within the gland and the relationship of the adrenal/tumor to the renal hilum, kidney, and major vasculature.

CHOICE OF APPROACH

The adrenal gland can be approached either open, endoscopically, or robotically. In today's era of minimal access surgery, endoscopic adrenalectomy has become the standard of care for most adrenal tumors. Endoscopic approaches can be done either as a laparoscopic transabdominal or retroperitoneoscopic operation, both of which offer significant advantages over an open approach, including decreased hospital length of stay, postoperative pain, intraoperative blood loss, and overall 30-day post-operative complications, as well as mortality (**Table 1**). In expert hands, the need to convert to an open operation is less than 5%.[1–4] The laparoscopic transabdominal approach offers a more familiar view of the anatomy (and is easier to teach), the ability to examine the rest of the abdomen, and more working space to work with larger tumors.[5] The retroperitoneoscopic approach has a number of unique advantages over the laparoscopic transabdominal approach, including the ability to avoid the

Table 1
Summary of advantages, disadvantages, and contraindications for various approaches to adrenalectomy

	Laparoscopic Transabdominal	Retroperitoneoscopic	Open
Advantages	Ability to survey abdomen Easier to teach Larger working space for larger tumors	Less postoperative pain Improved cosmesis No need to reposition patient for bilateral adrenalectomy Shorter operative time Fewer complications	Improved exposure for locally invasive and large tumors
Disadvantages	Risk of incisional hernia Longer operative time Need to reposition patient for bilateral adrenalectomy Possible increased difficulty in patient with prior abdominal operation	Smaller workspace Potentially increased intraocular pressure for very prolonged cases	Increased morbidity Longer recovery
Contraindications	Inability to tolerate pneumoperitoneum High likelihood of malignancy (relative)[a]	Inability to tolerate prone position High likelihood of malignancy (relative)[a]	Poor performance status High perioperative risk for morbidity and mortality

[a] The likelihood of malignancy is assessed based on the size of the lesion, clinical manifestations of locally advanced disease, functionally active with sex hormone excess, and locally invasive features on imaging.

intraabdominal cavity, a more direct approach to the adrenal, obviating the need to manipulate intraabdominal structures and avoiding repositioning patients for bilateral procedures. A number of studies have shown that the retroperitoneoscopic approach has fewer complications, shorter lengths of stay, less blood loss, and faster operative times.[4–6] However, the retroperitoneoscopic approach also has the tendency to be technically more demanding owing to the smaller working space and offers surgeons a less familiar view of the anatomy. Relative contraindications to the retroperitoneoscopic approach include morbid obesity (body mass index of >45) and elevated intraocular pressure (which would be exacerbated in the prone position). Both minimally invasive approaches can be done using a robotic platform. Although robotic adrenalectomy seems to offer similar advantages to endoscopic adrenalectomy, it also comes at a much higher cost.[7]

An open approach is preferred for very large lesions and those suspicious for malignancy. Most groups suggest an open approach for lesions that are clearly adrenocortical cancers (ACC), because these lesions have a higher risk of rupture with manipulation and minimally invasive approaches may increase the risk. In particular, locally advanced tumors with invasion into adjacent organs or major vessels (such invasion into the IVC or occlusion of the left renal vein) are best approached with an open operation. However, as laparoscopic techniques and skills improve, a number of groups are approaching known ACCs using minimally invasive techniques, arguing that the enhanced visualization make it less likely that the tumor will be violated. Still, most groups also promote an open approach for tumors with a higher risk of malignancy such as clinical signs of sex hormone excess (which are strongly associated with ACC) and larger tumors. Although there is no defined size threshold, larger tumors (especially those >10 cm) have a higher risk of malignancy.[8–11]

PREOPERATIVE AND ANESTHETIC CONSIDERATIONS

The surgeon should work closely as part of a multidisciplinary team of endocrinologists, anesthesiologists, radiologists, and appropriate medical specialists to ensure that the patient undergoes the appropriate preoperative biochemical workup, anatomic localization, and perioperative medical management. Patients should also undergo cardiopulmonary and preoperative risk assessment, and optimization as warranted by the clinical scenario. Once the diagnosis is made, the preoperative preparation for patients with adrenal tumors is largely contingent on the specific pathology and is covered in detail in other sections.

Pheochromocytoma

Patients should be pharmacologically treated to counteract and/or blunt the effects of catecholamine excess. Most guidelines including the Endocrine Society Guidelines recommend alpha-blockade as the therapy of choice.[12] Typically, alpha-blockade is started at least 2 weeks before the operation and titrated until the patients begin to have symptoms (eg, nasal congestion, mild orthostasis). As the alpha-mediated vasoconstriction is released, patients should be counseled to replete their intravascular volume by increasing their salt and fluid intake. A beta-blocker may be added if the patient has persistent tachycardia, but this is often a sign that patients are not adequately resuscitated. Of note, it is critical to avoid beta-blockers before adequate alpha-blockade, because unopposed alpha-mediated vasoconstriction may precipitate a hypertensive crisis. Intraoperatively, the anesthesiologist should insure adequate intravenous access with large-bore catheters or central venous access, direct arterial blood pressure monitoring, and ready availability of short-acting vasoactive medications to treat hypertension, hypotension, and tachycardia. Close communication intraoperatively between the surgical and anesthesia team is crucial because tumor manipulation can lead to significant hemodynamic lability and instability.

Cushing's Syndrome/Disease

Patients with Cushing's and subclinical Cushing's syndrome should receive stress dose steroids before the induction of anesthesia with a gradual postoperative taper that can often last months as the contralateral gland resumes glucocorticoid production.

Hyperaldosteronism

Patients with primary hyperaldosteronism tend to have refractory hypertension, metabolic alkalosis, and hypokalemia that is difficult to control with oral supplementation. Antihypertensive agents (including aldosterone receptor antagonists) are administered to control blood pressure. To avoid unfavorable interactions with anesthetic agents, electrolyte disturbances should be also adequately treated before induction.

The use of prophylactic antibiotics is practice dependent; however, we typically administer them for patients with Cushing's syndrome and as warranted by the individual patient's clinical factors. Patients should receive deep venous thrombosis prophylaxis (either mechanical or pharmacologic) and Foley catheters, which are typically removed within a few hours after the operation as is feasible.

LAPAROSCOPIC TRANSABDOMINAL APPROACH

Patient Positioning, Port Placement, and General Principles

Laparoscopic transabdominal adrenalectomy can be done using a lateral or anterior approach, although the lateral approach is the most commonly used. During the lateral approach, gravity is used to provide passive retraction on the tissues, which helps to expose the appropriate avascular planes of dissection. In the lateral approach, the patient is placed in the lateral decubitus position with the ipsilateral adrenal facing upward (**Fig. 1**). This can be done using a beanbag or bolsters and tape to secure the patient in position, with adequate padding on all pressure points, bony prominences, and areas of potential nerve compression in the extremities. The table is flexed near

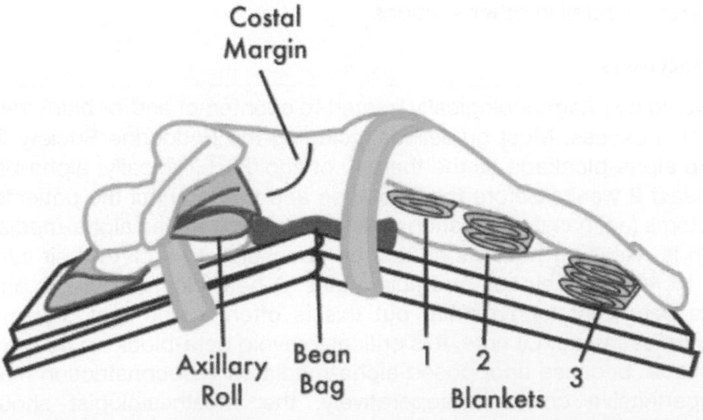

Fig. 1. Lateral decubitus position for laparoscopic transabdominal adrenalectomy. (From CollectedMed, https://collectedmed.com, with permission.)

the costal margin to maximize the distance between the iliac crest and costal margin. If the table has a kidney rest, it should be raised to further the elevation of the costal margin, thus increasing the distance between the ribs and hip even further.

Port placement is similar for both left and right approaches (**Fig. 2**). Access to the peritoneal cavity is obtained using either a Hassan or Veress needle technique 2 cm inferior to the costal margin at the midclavicular line. The Veress entry site can either be closed or used as a port site. Depending on the patient's habitus, ports are placed either subcostally or in an L-shape configuration, with the lateral port placed in the midaxillary line. For a laparoscopic transabdominal left adrenalectomy, the operation is typically done with 3 ports (1 camera and 2 working ports for the surgeon), but a fourth port can be placed medially for the assistant to help retract the spleen and pancreas, if necessary. The laparoscopic transabdominal right adrenalectomy almost always requires 4 ports (1 camera, 1 port for a liver retractor, and 2 working ports for the surgeon).

General Principles

The sequence of steps for the left and right adrenalectomies are similar and we tend to follow a technique popularized by Dr Quan Yang Duh.[13]

- *Opening the book*: The overlying structures are mobilized off the retroperitoneal space and Gerota's fascia is incised. On the right, the lateral portion of the right lobe of the liver is mobilized by incising the triangular ligament to the level of the IVC. On the left, the spleen and pancreas are mobilized free of Gerota's fascia by

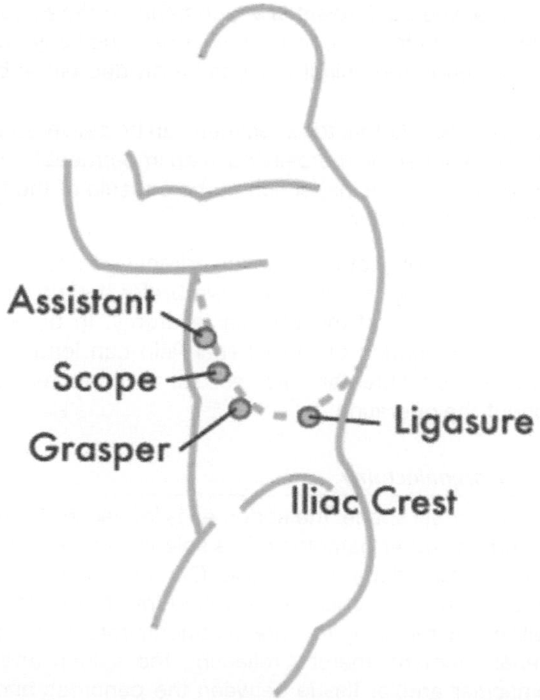

Fig. 2. Port placement for laparoscopic transabdominal adrenalectomy. (From CollectedMed, https://collectedmed.com, with permission.)

incising the lateral attachments of the spleen. Once these structures are mobilized, Gerota's fascia is exposed and divided starting at the diaphragm and moving toward the kidney. This maneuver exposes the plane (ie, the "spine of the book") between the medial aspect of the adrenal gland from the surrounding structures (ie, IVC and liver on the right, and pancreas, spleen and stomach on the left).

- *Reading from the top-down:* Once Gerota's fascia is opened widely, the plane medial to the adrenal gland is dissected starting at the superomedial border of the adrenal abutting the diaphragm and moving toward the renal hilum. During this dissection, the arcade of adrenal arteries is encountered and can be divided using either cautery or an advanced sealing device. Of note, the arterial arcade is in a layer just posterior to the level at which the adrenal vein is encountered.
- *Identifying and ligating the adrenal vein:* On the right side, the adrenal vein comes off the IVC at a right angle just inferior to the point where the IVC enters the liver. On the left side, the adrenal vein branches off the left renal vein and joins with the left inferior phrenic vein before entering the adrenal gland. As the dissection medial to the adrenal gland continues, it can be very helpful to identify the left phrenic vein and dissect along its medial border to assist in finding the adrenal vein. The adrenal vein may be ligated either using clips or an advanced sealing device. Rarely, an endoscopic stapler may be used to ligate larger veins, as may be seen in cases of large pheochromocytoma.
- *Separating the adrenal gland from the superior pole of the kidney:* Once the adrenal vein is ligated, the inferomedial and inferior border of the adrenal gland is dissected free from the top of the kidney. During this dissection, it is important to identify any superior pole renal vessels and preserve them.
- *Releasing the remaining posterolateral attachments to the abdominal wall:* Once the adrenal gland is free from the top of the kidney, the filmy attachments of the adrenal to the posterior abdominal wall can be divided either bluntly or with an energy device.
- *Delivery of the specimen:* Often, the specimen can be delivered without enlarging one of the port sites or can be morcellated in an impermeable bag. For larger tumors that would benefit from inspection of the capsule of the tumor, a port site may be enlarged for extraction.

Although some surgeons advocate ligating the adrenal vein as one of the first goals and as soon as possible during the operation, we prefer the approach described to maximize positive identification of the vascular anatomy. In particular, in cases of pheochromocytoma, early ligation of the adrenal vein can lead to congestion and proximal dilatation of small friable parasitic vessels, which increases the propensity of bleeding throughout the operation.

Left Transabdominal Adrenalectomy

Upon entry into the peritoneal space, the abdomen is inspected for any injuries owing to port placement and any other pathology. The splenic flexure of the colon is mobilized and reflected inferomedially to expose Gerota's fascia and the perirenal compartment (**Fig. 3**A). Once the colon is mobilized free of the field, the spleen and pancreas are mobilized by releasing the lateral attachments of the spleen and mobilizing the splenorenal ligament, thereby reflecting the spleen and distal pancreas medially as the avascular areolar tissue between the pancreas and Gerota's fascia is divided (see **Fig. 3**B). The medialization of the spleen should be continued until the upper portion of the greater curvature of the stomach is visualized. Once the

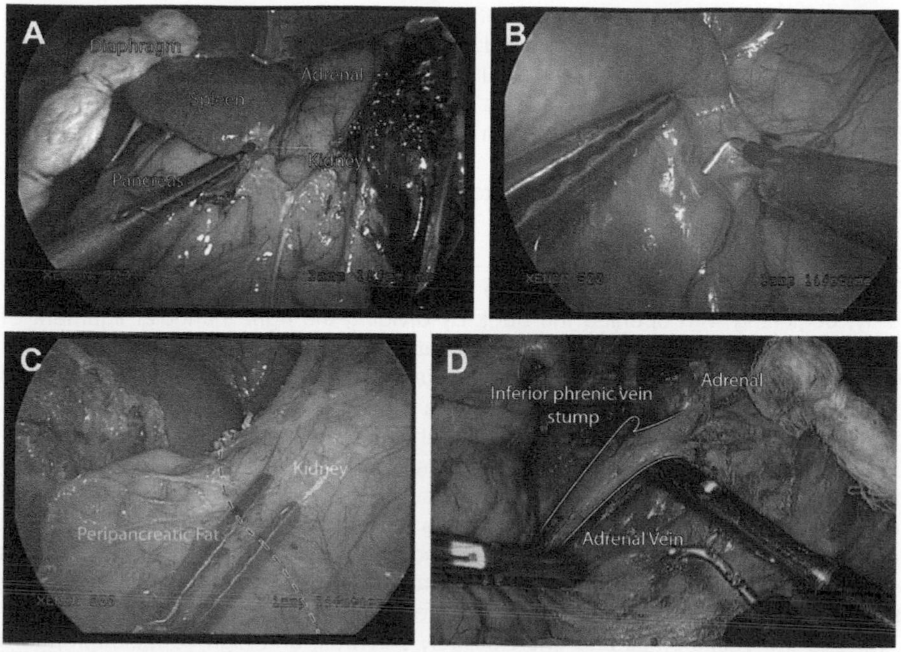

Fig. 3. During a left laparoscopic transabdominal adrenalectomy, the splenic flexure is mobilized (*A*) and lateral attachments of the spleen divided (*B*) to medialize the spleen and distal pancreas by dissecting in the avascular retropancreatic plane to expose Gerota's fascia (*C*). Once Gerota's fascia has been incised widely and the adrenal gland and periadrenal fat is exposed, the medial aspect of the adrenal gland is dissected and the left adrenal vein is exposed and skeletonized (*D*). (From CollectedMed, https://collectedmed.com, with permission.)

spleen and pancreas are mobilized off the retroperitoneum, the book is opened by entering Gerota's fascia at the superomedial border of the adrenal gland by the diaphragm and continuing the dissection toward the renal hilum. The distinct appearance of the peripancreatic fat (golden in appearance) from the perirenal fat (paler in appearance) can be used to confirm the correct plane of dissection. Care must be taken to not injure the diaphragm or stomach with energy devices during this part of the dissection. At this point, the book is read from the top down by identifying the medial border of the adrenal gland and dividing its cephalic attachments to the diaphragm and continuing along the medial border of the gland toward the renal hilum. To expose this plane adequately, inferolateral retraction is applied to the gland, and if necessary the assistant can apply countertraction on the spleen and pancreas using an instrument in a fourth port. Small arteries that are encountered in this plane are divided with an energy device as the dissection is continued inferiorly toward the renal hilum until the adrenal vein is identified and skeletonized at its confluence with the inferior phrenic vein (see **Fig. 3**C). Identification of the left adrenal vein may be facilitated by identifying the left inferior phrenic vein and dissecting along its medial border until the confluence with the left adrenal vein is encountered. The adrenal vein may be ligated with clips or an advanced energy device. The left inferior phrenic vein may also be ligated, which may be helpful with large, medially located tumors. The left adrenal gland often has a tail of tissue that extends toward the hilum of the kidney. This requires the gland to be dissected from the superior pole of the kidney at a location immediately adjacent to the capsule of the kidney by including all periadrenal fat with the specimen for an oncologically sound resection. Care should be taken at this stage to identify and protect any superior renal arteries. Finally, the remaining posterolateral attachments of the adrenal gland and its surrounding periadrenal fat are released and the specimen is extracted intact with an endoscopic retrieval bag, after ensuring hemostasis. **Table 2** summarizes all the operative steps, maneuvers, and pitfalls for laparoscopic left transabdominal adrenalectomy.

Right Transabdominal Adrenalectomy

The steps of a right adrenalectomy are generally similar to that of a left adrenalectomy, beginning with opening the book by dividing the right triangular ligament of the liver, and continuing medially approximately 1 cm away from the liver edge toward the IVC to expose and divide Gerota's fascia. It is important for the assistant to provide adequate retraction of the liver in a superomedial direction while the surgeon provides countertraction on the adrenal gland and kidney in an inferolateral direction to expose the plane adequately. The spine of the book is then opened as the dissection is meticulously carried along the superomedial edge of the adrenal gland toward the lateral edge of the IVC to mobilize the medial aspect of the adrenal gland and the surrounding periadrenal fat. Throughout this process, multiple small arteries will be encountered and can be divided with an energy device. The right adrenal vein is typically solitary and encountered just inferior to where the IVC enters the liver. Owing to the vein's small and short caliber, thin wall, and high capacitance, care must be taken in dissecting circumferentially around the right adrenal vein. Mobilization of the majority of the adrenal gland inferior to the vein may be helpful in this process. Once the medial aspect of the adrenal gland and periadrenal fat has been dissected, the remainder of the operation proceeds in a manner similar to that of a left adrenalectomy, including separating the adrenal gland from the superior pole of the kidney and renal hilum and completing the resection by taking down the posterior and lateral attachments. As on the left side, it is important to identify and preserve any superior pole renal arteries that are present. **Table 3** summarizes all the operative steps, maneuvers, and pitfalls for laparoscopic right transabdominal adrenalectomy.

RETROPERITONEOSCOPIC APPROACH

Patient Positioning

The patient is intubated on a stretcher and all venous access is placed. The patient is then placed in a modified prone position that maximizes the distance between the costal margin and iliac crest. This positioning is accomplished by transferring the patient onto noncompressible bolsters that are positioned under the hips and chest. The noncompressible bolster under the hips should be positioned at the break of the bed and an extender at the foot of the bed should be angled up to provide slight flexion at the knees (**Fig. 4**). The leg portion of the bed is then lowered to accentuate the distance between the costal margin and iliac crest. The optimal position is achieved when the space between the costal margin and iliac crest is flat and parallel to the floor. All pressure points should be padded generously, especially at the arms, knees, and shins. The patient is then prepped and draped from midchest to just above the gluteal cleft extending from the contralateral side of the spine to as low on the flank of the patient as possible. **Table 4** summarizes all the operative steps, maneuvers, and pitfalls for retroperitoneoscopic adrenalectomy.

Table 2
Summary of major operative steps for a laparoscopic transabdominal left adrenalectomy, with a list of critical maneuvers and pitfalls for each step

Step	Critical Maneuver	Pitfall
Patient positioning, port placement	Place patient in lateral decubitus position, flex the table. Place trocars subcostally or in an "L" configuration, with lateral port at the midaxillary line. Inspect peritoneal cavity and check for any injuries related to port placement.	Suboptimal positioning and port placement → inadequate exposure throughout the case Pressure sores Hyperextension of extremities Intraabdominal injury during port placement
Opening the book Mobilize splenic flexure of colon Divide the lateral attachments of spleen and medialize spleen and pancreas	Divide the gastrocolic ligament and mobilize distal transverse colon as needed. Dissect colon and mesocolon off the retropancreatic tissue and Gerota's fascia as needed. Divide the lateral attachments of the spleen 1 cm away from the spleen. Dissect in an avascular plane between the pancreas/ peripancreatic tissue (anteriorly) and Gerota's fascia (posteriorly). Open Gerota's fascia from the diaphragm toward the renal hilum. *Tip: Peripancreatic fat is golden and perirenal fat under Gerota's fascia is more pale in appearance.*	Inadequate mobilization → inadequate exposure Injury to spleen Injury to pancreas Injury to splenic artery/vein Injury to diaphragm Injury to stomach Dissecting in the wrong plane → bleeding
Reading from the top → down Mobilize the medial border of adrenal/ periadrenal fat	Divide most cephalic attachments of the adrenal gland off diaphragm/ abdominal wall. Divide superior adrenal arteries. Develop a "V-shaped" plane between peripancreatic tissue and adrenal. Expose middle adrenal arteries by retracting the adrenal laterally and divide with energy sealing device. Identify the inferior phrenic vein and dissect medial to this vessel between it and the adrenal gland. *Tip: Dissect carefully one layer at a time* *Tip: The adrenal arterial arcade is just posterior to the phrenic and adrenal vein.*	Injury to posterior stomach Injury to diaphragm Injury to inferior phrenic vein Injury to superior adrenal artery Injury to left adrenal vein Injury to left renal vein

(continued on next page)

Table 2 (*continued*)		
Step	**Critical Maneuver**	**Pitfall**
Ligating the adrenal vein	Identify/dissect/mobilize the left adrenal vein. Divide the adrenal vein with an advanced energy sealing device or clips. *Tip: The left adrenal vein can be found by tracing the inferior phrenic vein inferiorly until the confluence with the adrenal vein is encountered.*	Injury to left adrenal vein Injury to left renal vein Injury to small arteries that pass in close proximity
Freeing the adrenal gland from the renal hilum	Open Gerota's fascia immediately inferior to the adrenal gland. Retract the adrenal superolaterally. Divide the attachments between the adrenal and kidney. *Tip: Avoid grabbing the adrenal gland.*	Injury to superior renal artery → parenchymal ischemia, postoperative hypertension Inadequate oncologic margins
Removing the adrenal gland	Divide the remaining filmy attachments posteriorly and laterally. Remove the specimen using an impermeable specimen bag.	Inadequate oncologic margins Injury to the kidney

Port Positions

Appropriate port placement is critical to provide wide access to the retroperitoneal space and avoid conflicts with the hip. Three ports are used (**Fig. 5**).

- *Medial 5-mm (camera) trocar:* Immediately lateral to the paraspinous muscle, 4 to 5 cm inferior to the costovertebral angle.
- *Middle 10-mm (working) balloon tip trocar:* Midpoint between the medial and lateral ports, immediately inferior to the costal margin.
- *Lateral 5-mm (working) trocar:* As far lateral as possible (at the level of the mid-axillary line), immediately inferior to the costal margin.

The first port is placed in the middle position via a direct cut-down immediately inferior to the costal margin. Once the incision is made, the subcutaneous space is developed with a finger and Metzenbaum scissors. Once the muscle fascia is reached, the posterior pararenal space is pierced bluntly through the thoracolumbar fascia and spread with the Metzenbaum scissors to provide access for the 10-mm trocar. The motion is similar to accessing the pleural space for an open thoracostomy tube, except that the opening is made inferior to the rib. Access to the correct space is confirmed by feeling the smooth internal surface of the ribs. Blunt finger dissection medially and laterally clears an opening for the medial and lateral ports. The lateral port is placed directly into the space immediately inferior to the costal margin with a finger in the space guiding it appropriately. The medial port is then placed at approximately a 30° to 45° angle so that the tip enters the space just below the costal margin under direct guidance onto a finger in the retroperitoneal space. Finally, the 10-mm balloon tip trocar is placed and inflated into position.

Table 3
Summary of major operative steps for a laparoscopic transabdominal right adrenalectomy, with a list of critical maneuvers and pitfalls for each step

Step	Critical Maneuver	Pitfall
Patient positioning, port placement	Place patient in lateral decubitus position, flex the table. Place trocars subcostally or in an "L" configuration, with lateral port at the midaxillary line. Inspect the peritoneal cavity and check for any injuries related to port placement.	Suboptimal positioning and port placement → inadequate exposure throughout the case Pressure sores Hyperextension of extremities Intraabdominal injury during port placement
Opening the book Dividing the right triangular ligament and peritoneum overlying adrenal	Divide the triangular ligament from lateral to medial. Retract liver superomedially. Open Gerota's fascia from the superolateral margin of the adrenal toward the IVC 1 cm away from liver edge. Use the left hand to provide inferolateral retraction to the adrenal and superior pole of the kidney, while assistant applies superomedial rotation of the liver. Continue opening Gerota's fascia toward the renal hilum 1 cm from lateral edge of IVC. *Tip: Dissect carefully 1 layer at a time and carefully identify hepatic veins and IVC.*	Inadequate mobilization → inadequate exposure Injury to hepatic veins, IVC, right adrenal vein, or other small veins draining directly into IVC Injury to liver capsule
Reading from the top → down Mobilize medial aspect of adrenal gland	Divide most cephalic attachments of the adrenal gland off diaphragm/ abdominal wall. Divide superior adrenal arteries. Develop a "V-shaped" plane between the adrenal and liver/IVC. Expose and divide middle adrenal arteries by retracting the adrenal laterally. *Tip: The right adrenal vein is typically very short and comes off the IVC just inferior to where the IVC enters the liver at roughly a right angle and enters the adrenal on the anterior surface of the gland.* *Tip: Although the majority of patients have a single adrenal vein, there may be multiple veins.*	Injury to hepatic veins, IVC, right adrenal vein, or other small veins draining directly into IVC

(*continued on next page*)

Table 3
(*continued*)

Step	Critical Maneuver	Pitfall
Ligating the adrenal vein	Identify/dissect/mobilize adrenal vein. Divide the adrenal vein with an advanced energy sealing device or clips. *Tip: Mobilization of the majority of the adrenal gland inferior to the vein can be helpful.*	Injury to right adrenal vein or IVC
Freeing the adrenal gland from the renal hilum	Open Gerota's fascia immediately inferior to the adrenal gland. Retract the adrenal superolaterally. Divide the attachments between the adrenal and kidney. *Tip: Avoid grabbing the adrenal gland.*	Injury to superior renal artery of kidney → parenchymal ischemia, postoperative hypertension Inadequate oncologic margins
Removing the adrenal gland	Divide the remaining filmy attachments posteriorly and laterally. Remove the specimen using an impermeable specimen bag.	Inadequate oncologic margins Injury to the kidney

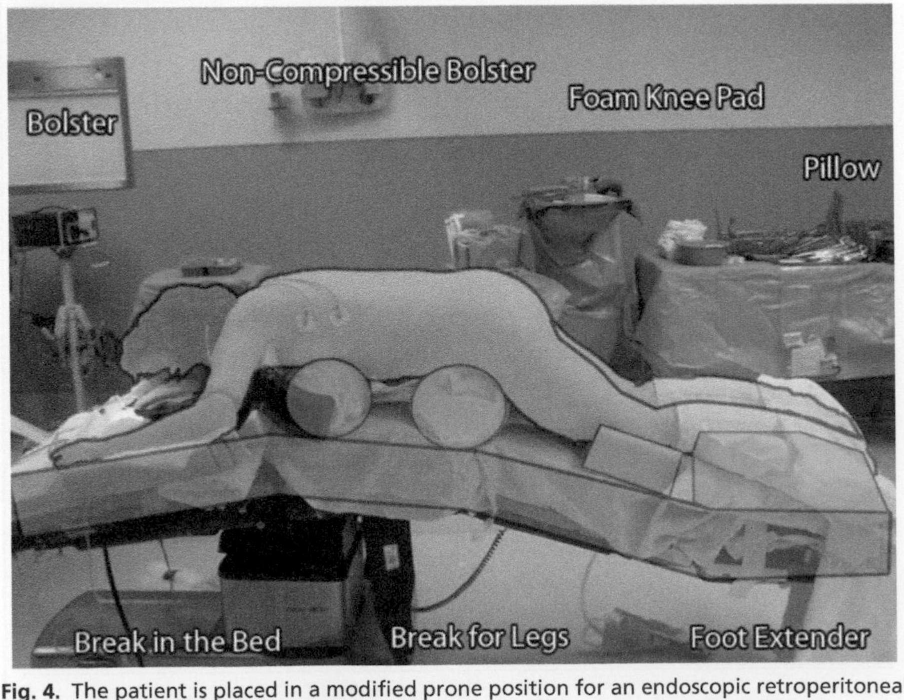

Fig. 4. The patient is placed in a modified prone position for an endoscopic retroperitoneal adrenalectomy. (From CollectedMed, https://collectedmed.com, with permission.)

Table 4
Summary of major operative steps during retroperitoneoscopic adrenalectomy, with a list of critical maneuvers and pitfalls for each step

Step	Critical Maneuver	Pitfall
Patient positioning		Suboptimal positioning → inadequate exposure Suboptimal ergonomics
Port placement	Make a 1.0- to 1.5-cm incision for middle port and enter the retroperitoneal space bluntly through the fascia below the costal margin. Place a medial 5-mm port, 4–5 cm inferior to costal margin, immediately lateral to paraspinous muscle, at a 30°–45° angle so that the tip enters just inferior to the costovertebral angle under direct palpation. Place a lateral 5-mm port as lateral as possible just inferior to the costal margin under direct palpation. Insert a 10-mm balloon port into the middle port site. Insufflate to 20–25 mm Hg.	Ports placed inadequately → limited working space for use of instruments Higher insufflation pressures may lead to subcutaneous emphysema and less commonly increased partial pressure of carbon dioxide levels
Entering Gerota's fascia	Divide Gerota's fascia widely from side to side. Bluntly divide the filmy posterior attachments of the kidney, adrenal, perirenal, and periadrenal fat to let gravity autoretract the adrenal toward the table.	Inadvertently opening the peritoneum will cause the peritoneal space to bulge into the retroperitoneal space, decreasing the working space Dissecting in the wrong space (posterior pararenal space)
Separating the superior pole of the kidney from the adrenal gland	Identify the superior pole of the kidney. Once the superior pole of the kidney is identified, the plane between the kidney and adrenal is accentuated by placing the retracting instrument on the anterior surface of the kidney and retracting inferomedially. The plane between the kidney and adrenal is dissected from lateral to medial with a combination of blunt and sharp dissection progressively rotating the kidney inferiorly and medially. *Tip: On the left side, the upper pole of the kidney should also be mobilized along the medial side toward the renal hilum to facilitate identification of the tongue of adrenal tissue that runs toward the hilum.*	Injury to adrenal vein Injury to renal vein Injury to superior pole artery of kidney → parenchymal ischemia, postoperative hypertension

(continued on next page)

Table 4 (continued)		
Step	**Critical Maneuver**	**Pitfall**
Identifying and ligating the adrenal vein	Retract the adrenal laterally and dissect the medial border. On the right, this plane is between the adrenal and IVC. On the left, this plane is between the adrenal and inferior phrenic vein. Divide the adrenal arterial arcade, which lies in the layer just posterior to the venous layer. Identify and dissect the adrenal vein circumferentially. Divide the adrenal vein with an advanced energy sealing device or clips. *Tip: The right adrenal vein is short and comes off the IVC at a right angle just inferior to the where the IVC enters the liver.* *Tip: The left adrenal vein enters the gland at the inferomedial aspect of the gland and branches off a common trunk with the inferior phrenic vein.* *Tip: The adrenal veins enter the adrenal on the anterior surface of the gland, which is toward the table in this view.*	Injury to adrenal vein Left: injury to left renal vein, inferior phrenic vein Right: injury to IVC Injury to small feeding arteries that pass in close proximity
Removing the adrenal gland	Dissect adrenal gland and its surrounding fat off the remaining attachments to the paraspinous muscle and peritoneum. Extract specimen using an impermeable specimen bag. Reduce insufflation pressure (10–15 mm Hg) to identify bleeding.	Inadequate oncologic margins Not identifying bleeding vessels that were masked by tamponade effect of high insufflation pressures → postoperative hemorrhage

General Principles and Dissection

The major landmarks for this operation consist of the paraspinous muscle medially, the edge of the peritoneum laterally, the contents of the perirenal space (kidney, adrenal gland, perirenal fat) anteriorly, and the ribs posteriorly (**Fig. 6**). A high insufflation pressure (approximately 25 mm Hg) provides adequate visualization and tamponades any small bleeding vessels. Hypercarbia and crepitus may develop requiring brief periods of desufflation or lower insufflation pressures.

Entry into Gerota's fascia (posterior renal fascia)

After port placement, a 30° camera is inserted into the middle port with the camera stem facing toward the table to obtain an upward (posterior) angled view. An advanced energy sealing device is placed in the lateral port and Gerota's fascia is entered and opened widely from the paraspinous muscle to the peritoneum. The tissue surrounding the medial port is cleared away and the camera is then inserted into

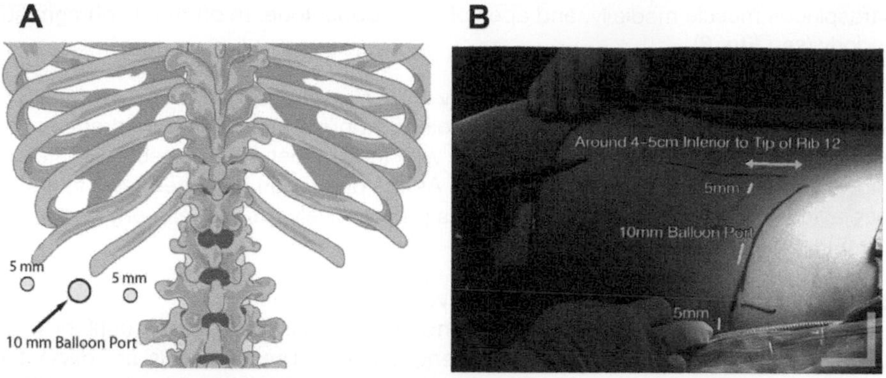

Fig. 5. Port positions for a left (*A*) and right (*B*) retroperitoneoscopic adrenalectomy. (From CollectedMed, https://collectedmed.com, with permission.)

the medial port (stem facing upward for a downward view). The advanced energy sealing device is placed in the dominant hand and an atraumatic grasper such as a fenestrated bowel grasper is placed in the nondominant hand and used as a retractor. The posterior attachments of the perinephric and periadrenal fat are swept down (anteriorly) bluntly using gravity as an aid, bringing into view the peritoneum laterally,

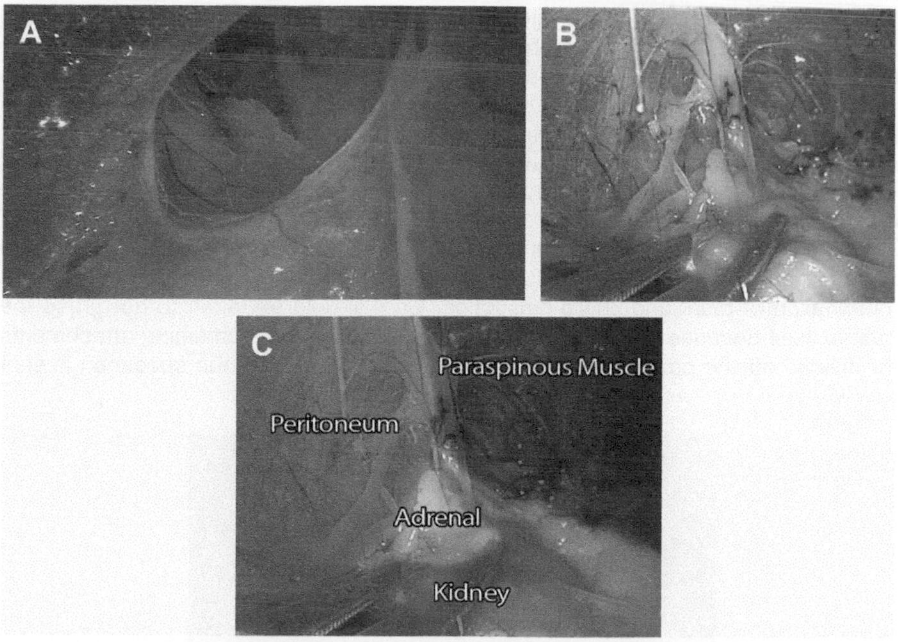

Fig. 6. Gerota's fascia is entered (*A*) and opened widely from the paraspinous muscle to the peritoneum. The posterior attachments of the perinephric and periadrenal fat are swept down (anteriorly) while keeping the dissection anterior to Gerota's fascia, bringing into view the peritoneum laterally, paraspinous muscle medially and apex of the retroperitoneum off the diaphragm superiorly (*B*, *C*). The images are from a left retroperitoneoscopic adrenalectomy. (From CollectedMed, https://collectedmed.com, with permission.)

paraspinous muscle medially, and apex of the retroperitoneum off the diaphragm superiorly (see **Fig. 6**).

Separating the superior pole of the kidney from the adrenal gland

After identifying the kidney, the superior pole is mobilized from the periadrenal fat by placing inferomedial traction on the kidney with the grasper. This dissection is started on the anterolateral surface of the kidney. As the dissection is carried from lateral to medial toward the renal hilum, the kidney is progressively rotated inferiorly and medially (**Fig. 7**).

Identification and division of the adrenal vein

The medial attachments of the adrenal gland are then dissected bluntly until the layer containing the adrenal arterial arcade is encountered. These vessels are dissected and divided using an advanced energy sealing device. On the right side, the IVC is identified and the gland can be dissected from inferior to superior along the medial border of the adrenal using a combination of blunt and sharp dissection. The right adrenal vein is encountered on the anterior surface of the adrenal gland just below where the IVC enters the liver. Once the adrenal vein is dissected circumferentially, we ligate the vein using the advanced energy sealing device or clips. On the left side, the inferior phrenic vein is identified and the adrenal gland is dissected free from its medial border using a combination of blunt and sharp dissection and is traced toward the renal hilum to identify the take-off of the left adrenal vein (**Fig. 8**). As with the right adrenal vein, the left adrenal vein enters the anterior surface of the adrenal gland. As mentioned, the left adrenal gland often has a tongue of tissue that extends inferiorly toward the renal vein, which should be dissected carefully and completely. Once the adrenal vein is ready to be divided, we grasp the adrenal vein at its insertion point into the adrenal with the atraumatic grasper and divide the adrenal vein with an advanced energy sealing device or clips. Using the stump of the vein on the specimen side as a handle, we can then manipulate the gland and surrounding fat to facilitate the rest of the dissection.

Specimen extraction and closure

Once the adrenal vein and arteries are divided, the adrenal gland should be held in place almost exclusively by filmy areolar tissue, which may be dissected using a combination of blunt and sharp dissection. Care should be taken to not grasp the adrenal itself because the gland can be easily ruptured. The remaining attachments are divided off the paraspinous muscle and peritoneum, and the specimen is sent

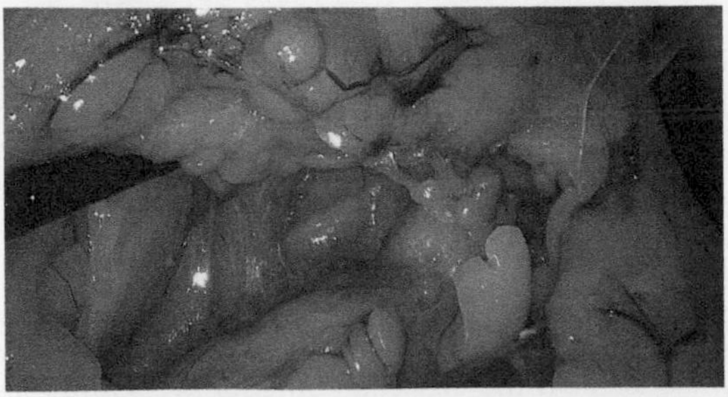

Fig. 7. During a left retroperitoneoscopic adrenalectomy, the dissection is started on the lateral surface of the kidney and carried medially toward the renal hilum, while the kidney is progressively rotated inferiorly and medially.

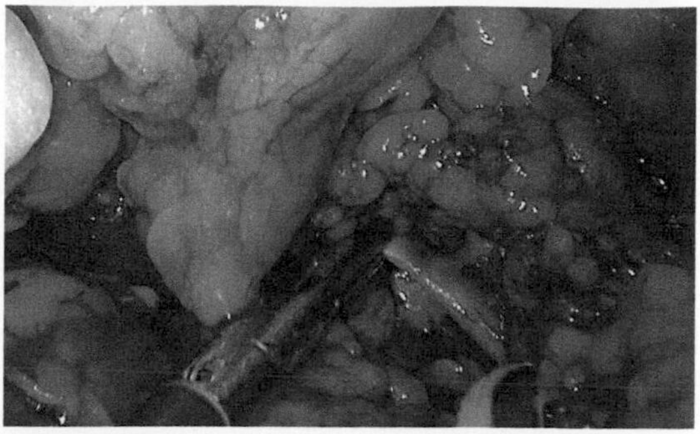

Fig. 8. The adrenal gland is dissected free from its medial border using a combination of blunt and sharp dissection to identify the left adrenal vein up to its takeoff (in this case, the inferior phrenic vein on the left).

off to pathology using an endoscopic retrieval bag. The dissection bed is reassessed carefully under a lower insufflation pressure (10–15 mm Hg) to identify any bleeding vessels, and the port sites are closed in a standard fashion. If the middle port needs to be expanded for specimen extraction, we reapproximate the muscle with a figure-of-8 absorbable stitch. Otherwise, it is not necessary to close this port site because port site hernias are exceedingly rare in the retroperitoneoscopic approach.

OPEN APPROACH

Because most open cases tend to be planned for ACC, it is essential to adhere to basic oncologic principles, such as avoiding any dissection that could lead to tumor fracture and tumor cell seeding. In some cases, concomitant resection of adjacent organs, such as a kidney, liver, colon, spleen, or pancreas, or in rare cases, a vascular reconstruction of the IVC, may be required. Good preoperative imaging is imperative to guide the operation. In cases of ACC, vascular imaging with a contrast study, intravascular ultrasound examination, or magnetic resonance venogram may be helpful to determine if tumor thrombus is present. To minimize the risk of locoregional recurrence and to achieve an appropriate resection, it is imperative to choose an incision that will achieve optimal exposure.

Choice of Incision

There are 4 common surgical approaches for open adrenalectomy: upper midline incision, subcostal incision, modified Makuuchi ("J") incision and a thoracoabdominal incision. Several factors should be taken into consideration when deciding the optimal incision:

- Size of tumor and need for any concomitant resection (eg, nephrectomy, nonanatomic or anatomic hepatectomy), or vascular reconstruction;
- Location of mass and direction of invasion; and
- Existing position of the patient during conversion from a laparoscopic procedure.

A posterior approach can also be undertaken with the patient in prone position, using a curvilinear incision that begins paramedian and extends laterally. This approach requires removal of the 12th rib to widely expose the retroperitoneal space. The remainder of the operation proceeds in a manner similar to an endoscopic retroperitoneal adrenalectomy.

Open Right Adrenalectomy

A right subcostal or modified Makuuchi incision is typically done in most settings and provides adequate exposure for a safe dissection. For an open right adrenalectomy, the right lobe of the liver needs to be completely mobilized by dividing the triangular ligament, while rotating the liver superomedially to expose the infrahepatic and retrohepatic IVC as well as the retrocaval collateral vessels. In addition, the duodenum and pancreas may need to be Kocherized and the hepatic flexure of the colon may also need to be mobilized.

For very large tumors, or if there is evidence of hepatic involvement, diaphragmatic involvement, or tumor thrombus, a thoracoabdominal incision may be necessary. In cases where a right hepatectomy is planned, another option is to perform a liver resection using a transabdominal approach before actually mobilizing the right liver, using the so-called hanging maneuver. This maneuver requires extrahepatic inflow control (right hepatic artery and right portal vein) followed by transection of the liver parenchyma down to the level of the IVC and division of the right hepatic vein. For cases where the tumor invades into the liver but not into the diaphragm, this technique avoids a thoracotomy and the remainder of the mass is dissected off the IVC and suprarenal fossa, as described elsewhere in this article.

Securing the right adrenal vein can be challenging for locally advanced ACCs that extend into the IVC. After mobilizing the right liver, colon, duodenum, and pancreas and exposing the IVC, the adrenal vein is exposed and assessed for any potential tumor thrombus extending to the IVC.

Open Left Adrenalectomy

Typically, this operation is done either through a left subcostal or a left-sided "J" incision. A midline laparotomy can be done, but this approach tends to have less robust exposure. It is quite uncommon to require a thoracoabdominal incision to achieve the necessary exposure for an open left adrenalectomy and these are typically reserved for very aggressive and locally advanced tumors. Another important consideration for open left adrenalectomies for ACC is the potential for tumor invasion into the left renal vein requiring a nephrectomy, as well as the removal of any tumor thrombus extending into the IVC.

POSTOPERATIVE CARE

Most patients undergoing an uneventful minimally invasive adrenalectomy can be discharged on postoperative day 1 after immediate resumption of a diet and early mobilization.

Pheochromocytoma

Patients should be monitored for any hemodynamic fluctuations or instability, especially hypotension, and treated accordingly with fluid resuscitation with or without short-acting vasoactive agents. Most patients have an uneventful postoperative course and do not require an intensive care unit setting.

Cushing's Syndrome/Disease

As discussed elsewhere in this article, in addition to receiving perioperative intravenous steroids, these patients require a slow and gradual steroid taper, often over a periods of months. They should also be closely monitored in the postoperative period for any signs and symptoms of an Addisonian crisis (acute adrenal insufficiency).

Hyperaldosteronism

Aldosterone receptor antagonists and potassium supplementation should be stopped after surgery, whereas other antihypertensive medications can be either reduced or stopped. Serum potassium and aldosterone levels should be checked on postoperative day 1 and serum potassium levels should be checked weekly for 4 weeks for hyperkalemia, which may indicate mineralocorticoid deficiency.

REFERENCES

1. Elfenbein DM, Scarborough JE, Speicher PJ, et al. Comparison of laparoscopic versus open adrenalectomy: results from American College of Surgeons-National Surgery Quality Improvement Project. J Surg Res 2013;184(1):216–20.
2. Shen WT, Kebebew E, Clark OH, et al. Reasons for conversion from laparoscopic to open or hand-assisted adrenalectomy: review of 261 laparoscopic adrenalectomies from 1993 to 2003. World J Surg 2004;28(11):1176–9.
3. Turrentine FE, Stukenborg GJ, Hanks JB, et al. Elective laparoscopic adrenalectomy outcomes in 1099 ACS NSQIP patients: identifying candidates for early discharge. Am Surg 2015;81(5):507–14.
4. Walz MK, Alesina PF, Wenger FA, et al. Posterior retroperitoneoscopic adrenalectomy–results of 560 procedures in 520 patients. Surgery 2006;140(6):943–8 [discussion: 8–50].
5. Lee CR, Walz MK, Park S, et al. A comparative study of the transperitoneal and posterior retroperitoneal approaches for laparoscopic adrenalectomy for adrenal tumors. Ann Surg Oncol 2012;19(8):2629–34.
6. Epelboym I, Digesu CS, Johnston MG, et al. Expanding the indications for laparoscopic retroperitoneal adrenalectomy: experience with 81 resections. J Surg Res 2014;187(2):496–501.
7. Samreen S, Fluck M, Hunsinger M, et al. Laparoscopic versus robotic adrenalectomy: a review of the national inpatient sample. J Robot Surg 2019;13(1):69–75.
8. Autorino R, Bove P, De Sio M, et al. Open versus laparoscopic adrenalectomy for adrenocortical carcinoma: a meta-analysis of surgical and oncological outcomes. Ann Surg Oncol 2016;23(4):1195–202.
9. Brix D, Allolio B, Fenske W, et al. Laparoscopic versus open adrenalectomy for adrenocortical carcinoma: surgical and oncologic outcome in 152 patients. Eur Urol 2010;58(4):609–15.
10. Donatini G, Caiazzo R, Do Cao C, et al. Long-term survival after adrenalectomy for stage I/II adrenocortical carcinoma (ACC): a retrospective comparative cohort study of laparoscopic versus open approach. Ann Surg Oncol 2014;21(1): 284–91.
11. Kebebew E, Siperstein AE, Clark OH, et al. Results of laparoscopic adrenalectomy for suspected and unsuspected malignant adrenal neoplasms. Arch Surg 2002;137(8):948–51 [discussion: 52–3].
12. Lenders JW, Duh QY, Eisenhofer G, et al. Endocrine S. Pheochromocytoma and paraganglioma: an endocrine society clinical practice guideline. J Clin Endocrinol Metab 2014;99(6):1915–42.
13. Yeh M, Livhits M, Duh Q. The adrenal glands. In: Townsend C Jr, Beauchamp R, Evers B, et al, editors. Sabiston textbook of surgery. 20th edition. Philadelphia: Elsevier; 2017. p. 963–95.

Evaluation and Management of Neuroendocrine Tumors of the Pancreas

Aaron T. Scott, MD[a], James R. Howe, MD[a,b,*]

KEYWORDS

• Pancreas • Neuroendocrine tumor • PNET • Surgery

KEY POINTS

- Pancreatic neuroendocrine tumors arise from islet cells or their precursors and may cause symptoms from mass effect or hormone production.
- The standard treatment for localized pancreatic neuroendocrine tumors is pancreatico-duodenectomy or distal pancreatectomy, but enucleation or observation may be considered for small tumors.
- Approximately 60% of pancreatic neuroendocrine tumors will present with metastases, most commonly to the liver.
- The treatment for metastatic pancreatic neuroendocrine tumors is multimodal and includes primary resection, surgical debulking, liver-directed therapy, and a variety of systemic treatments.
- Pancreatic neuroendocrine tumors carry a significantly more favorable prognosis when compared with pancreatic adenocarcinoma.

INTRODUCTION

Neuroendocrine tumors (NETs) are a diverse group of neoplasms arising from cells in the diffuse neuroendocrine system. At least 17 different types of neuroendocrine cells are found in the pancreas and gastrointestinal tract.[1] In the pancreas, they are located in the islets of Langerhans, which were first described by their namesake in 1869.[2] There are 5 well-defined pancreatic islet cell types that produce biologically active peptides including insulin, glucagon, somatostatin, pancreatic polypeptide, and

---

Disclosure Statement: The authors have no conflicts of interest to disclose.
This work was supported by the T32 grant CA148062-0 (A.T. Scott) and SPORE grant P50 CA174521-01 (J.R. Howe).

[a] Department of Surgery, University of Iowa Carver College of Medicine, Iowa City, IA, USA;
[b] Division of Surgical Oncology and Endocrine Surgery, University of Iowa Hospitals and Clinics, 200 Hawkins Drive, 4644 JCP, Iowa City, IA 52242, USA
* Corresponding author.
E-mail address: james-howe@uiowa.edu

Surg Clin N Am 99 (2019) 793–814
https://doi.org/10.1016/j.suc.2019.04.014

ghrelin.[3] Pancreatic NETs (PNETs) are also capable of hormone production and are believed to arise from islet cells or, more likely, their precursors.[1,4] Tumors that overproduce hormones may be associated with distinct clinical syndromes and are referred to as functional; those that do not secrete hormones, secrete them in minimal quantities, or secrete peptides that do not result in an obvious syndrome (eg, pancreatic polypeptide) are termed nonfunctional. PNETS may produce multiple hormones[5] and are referred to by the name of the hormone whose effects dominate the clinical picture appended with "-oma," as in insulinoma or gastrinoma.

HISTORY

The first report of a PNET was by Albert Nicholls, who described an adenoma arising from the islets of Langerhans in 1902.[6] The term *karzinoide* (carcinoid) was introduced in 1907 by Siegfried Oberndorfer to describe small tumors of the distal ileum resembling carcinoma, but with less malignant potential.[7] Although the term originally referred specifically to ileal tumors, over the next half century the definition would be expanded until nearly any NET could be referred to as a carcinoid, regardless of its primary site.[8] In 1924, Seale Harris described several patients with symptoms of hypoglycemia, which the authors attributed to hypersecretion of insulin by the pancreas.[9] Convincing evidence of insulinoma was first presented by Wilder and colleagues in 1927, who reported a patient with recurrent hypoglycemic episodes who was found at exploratory surgery to have an unresectable distal pancreatic mass. Autopsy of the same patient revealed nodal and liver metastases, and the tumor cells were noted to bear a "striking" resemblance to islets of Langerhans. Further evidence that the tumor was an insulinoma was provided when the effect of tumor extract injected in rabbits mimicked that of insulin.[10] Two years after this report, Roscoe Graham enucleated a 1.5-cm insulinoma from the pancreas of a patient suffering from recurrent hypoglycemic episodes, successfully curing her disease.[11] In the decades after the initial reports of hyperinsulinism and insulinoma, syndromes associated with oversecretion of various other peptides by islet cell tumors were described, although the responsible hormone was not always correctly identified until later: serotonin in 1931, glucagon in 1942, adrenocorticotropic hormone in 1950, gastrin in 1955, vasoactive intestinal peptide in 1958, parathyroid hormone-related peptide in 1973, somatostatin in 1977, growth hormone-releasing factor (GRF) in 1978, neurotensin in 1981, and cholecystokinin in 2013.[12–23]

EPIDEMIOLOGY

PNETs have an approximate incidence of 0.5 per 100,000 persons per year and account for fewer than 10% of all NETs.[24,25] The mean age at diagnosis is 57 to 58 years, and the peak incidence is in the seventh decade.[26–29] At least 70% of these tumors are nonfunctional, and the most common functional PNETs are insulinomas, followed by gastrinomas.[29–32] Together, these 3 subtypes account for the large majority of PNETs. The incidence of other tumors, such as VIPomas, glucagonomas, and somatostatinomas, is not well-defined, but they are significantly rarer.[31,32] Most PNETs are malignant, and upwards of 60% of patients will have metastatic disease at the time of diagnosis.[1,26,27] Insulinomas, which are benign in 90% of cases, are the exception to this rule; as a consequence, their incidence is frequently underestimated in population-based studies, which use data from cancer registries, such as the Surveillance, Epidemiology, and End Results database.[24,29,31,32] The majority of PNETs are sporadic, but as many as 10% to 20% are associated with inherited cancer syndromes such as multiple endocrine neoplasia type 1, Von Hippel-Lindau syndrome

(VHL), tuberous sclerosis complex, neurofibromatosis type 1, or glucagon cell hyperplasia and neoplasia.[32–37] Of these, multiple endocrine neoplasia type 1 is the most frequently associated with PNETs.

Despite the high frequency of metastases, the prognosis of patients with PNETs is favorable, particularly when compared with pancreatic adenocarcinoma. The median overall survival for patients in the Surveillance, Epidemiology, and End Results database diagnosed with PNETs between 1973 and 2012 was 3.6 years. However, over this time period there has been significant improvement in survival, particularly for patients with advanced stage disease.[24,26] The median overall survival for patients with metastatic PNETs is now 5 years, and for patients with surgically resected, nonmetastatic tumors the 20-year disease specific survival is just over 50%.[24,38]

PRESENTATION

The presentation of PNETs varies considerably. When present, the symptoms of nonfunctional tumors are generally nonspecific and related to tumor mass effect, but these tumors are increasingly being detected incidentally on imaging before developing symptoms.[39,40] In contrast, functional tumors are frequently associated with dramatic hormonal syndromes, leading to an earlier diagnosis and improved prognosis.[28] The clinical presentations of PNET subtypes are summarized in **Table 1**.[18,29–32,41–46] Despite the stark differences in presentation, the diagnostic workup and treatment of functional and nonfunctional tumors are largely similar.[1,5,45] Although the majority of PNETs occur sporadically, they may also arise in association with several hereditary cancer syndromes, the characteristics of which are shown in **Table 2**.[33,34,36,47–52]

DIAGNOSIS

The diagnosis of PNET ultimately depends on immunohistochemical examination of tumor tissue for confirmation; however, serum markers and imaging also play a critical role in the workup of these tumors. The diagnostic sequence varies from patient to patient, depending on the presentation; those who present with hormonal symptoms may initially undergo blood testing, whereas nonfunctional tumors are frequently discovered incidentally on imaging. Regardless of whether biochemical testing precedes imaging or vice versa, patients with PNETs will usually undergo both as part of their diagnostic workup.[45,53–55]

Biochemical

Laboratory testing involves the use of both biomarkers that are common to most PNETs as well as specific hormones that are secreted by functional PNETs and responsible for the associated syndromes. Chromogranin A (CgA) is an acidic glycoprotein that is found in the secretory granules of all neuroendocrine cells and is among the most widely studied biomarkers for NETs. Serum CgA is elevated in patients with PNETs and is correlated with both disease burden and survival.[56,57] A recent metaanalysis on CgA for the diagnosis of NETs reported that the pooled sensitivity and specificity were 73% and 95%, respectively; however, these values vary depending on the specific assay and diagnostic thresholds used.[58] Moreover, clinicians should be aware that elevated CgA may be associated with hypertension, renal dysfunction, treatment with proton pump inhibitors, and a variety of other benign and malignant diseases unrelated to NETs.[59] Pancreastatin, a protein derived from CgA, is another potential biomarker. Although pancreastatin is less sensitive for the diagnosis of NETs than CgA, it is also less susceptible to nonspecific elevation and has been shown to

Table 1
Clinical presentation of various PNET subtypes

Tumor	Hormone	Symptoms
Nonfunctional PNET	Varies (pancreatic polypeptide, chromogranin A, others in small quantities)	Asymptomatic, abdominal/back pain, nausea/vomiting, pancreatitis, obstructive jaundice
Insulinoma	Insulin	Hypoglycemic symptoms (tremor, palpitations, anxiety, hunger, cognitive impairment, seizure, coma), fasting hypoglycemia, rapid correction with glucose (Whipple's triad)
Gastrinoma	Gastrin	Severe, medically refractory peptic ulcer disease, gastroesophageal reflux, diarrhea (Zollinger-Ellison syndrome)
VIPoma	Vasoactive intestinal peptide (VIP)	Watery diarrhea, hypokalemia, achlorhydria (WDHA syndrome, pancreatic cholera or Verner Morrison syndrome)
Glucagonoma	Glucagon	Necrolytic migratory erythema, weight loss, diabetes mellitus, diarrhea, venous thrombosis
Somatostatinoma	Somatostatin	Diabetes, gallstones, steatorrhea, weight loss
Pancreatic carcinoid	Serotonin, tachykinins	Flushing, diarrhea, bronchospasm, valvular heart disease (carcinoid syndrome)
ACTHoma	Adrenocorticotropic hormone (ACTH)	Obesity, facial plethora, round face (moon facies), hirsutism, hypertension, bruising, fatigue, depression, dorsal fat pad, glucose intolerance, stria, proximal weakness, menstrual irregularities, decreased fertility (Cushing's syndrome)
GRFoma	Growth hormone-releasing factor (GRF or GHRF)	Coarse facial features, enlarged hands and feet, macroglossia, deepening voice, skin thickening, sleep apnea, arthritis, cardiovascular disease, insulin resistance, fatigue, weakness (acromegaly)
PTHrPoma	Parathyroid hormone-related protein (PTHrP)	Nephrolithiasis, weakness, bone pain, nausea, constipation, polyuria, depression (hypercalcemia)

Data from Refs.[18,29–32,41–46]

correlate with survival in surgical patients.[56,57,60] Other biomarkers that are variably elevated in patients with PNETs include neuron-specific enolase, chromogranin B, and pancreatic polypeptide, although none of these are as widely validated as CgA.[56,57] Given the limitations of the available biomarkers, a 51-gene, polymerase chain reaction-based assay (NETest) has recently been developed for the diagnosis and surveillance of NETs. The NETest has superior sensitivity and specificity (94% and 96%, respectively) for PNETs when compared with CgA; however, the test is significantly more expensive than serum testing for other makers.[61]

Biochemical testing for functional PNETs is directed by symptoms of hormone excess (see **Table 1**). Insulinomas present with inappropriately high insulin levels in the setting of hypoglycemia, characterized by Whipple's triad: hypoglycemic symptoms, low plasma glucose, and resolution of symptoms with the administration of glucose. The diagnosis should be confirmed by measurement of elevated insulin,

Table 2
Characteristics of hereditary cancer syndromes associated with PNETs

Syndrome	Gene	Inheritance	Incidence of PNETs	Other Characteristics
Multiple endocrine neoplasia type 1	*MEN1*	Autosomal dominant	20%–70% symptomatic PNET, nonfunctional most common followed by gastrinoma, nearly 100% develop multiple pancreatic microadenomas	Parathyroid hyperplasia (95%–100%), pituitary tumors (30%–50%), angiofibromas (85%), adrenal adenoma (30%–40%), gastric NETs (10%–35%)
Von Hippel-Lindau syndrome	*VHL*	Autosomal dominant	10%–20%, almost all nonfunctional	Retinal and CNS hemangioblastoma (60%–80%), renal cell carcinoma (25%–70%), pheochromocytoma (10%–20%), pancreatic cysts (35%–80%), epididymal cystadenoma (25%–60%)
Neurofibromatosis type 1	*NF1*	Autosomal dominant	0%–10%, characteristically ampullary/duodenal somatostatinomas	Café-au-lait macules (99%), neurofibromas (99%), skin fold freckling (85%), Lisch nodules (95%), optic pathway glioma (15%), learning problems (60%) skeletal abnormalities, pheochromocytomas, malignant peripheral nerve sheath tumors
Tuberous sclerosis complex	*TSC1, TSC2*	Autosomal dominant	Rare, may be functional or nonfunctional	Variable presentation: hamartomas affecting brain, skin, kidneys, and eyes; classically seizures, developmental delay, and angiofibromas
Glucagon cell hyperplasia and neoplasia (Mahvash syndrome)	*GCCR*	Autosomal recessive	100%, microglucagonomas and macroglucagonomas	Background of glucagon cell hyperplasia

Abbreviation: CNS, central nervous system.
Data from Refs.[33,34,36,47–52]

proinsulin and C-peptide during a hypoglycemic episode, which is often induced by a supervised 72-hour fast. In patients with refractory peptic ulcer disease, the presence of a gastrinoma may be confirmed by serum gastrin greater than 10 times the upper limit of normal in the setting of gastric pH 2 or less, or moderately elevated gastrin with a positive secretin or glucagon stimulation test. Proton pump inhibitors should be discontinued for 1 to 2 weeks before measurement of the fasting serum gastrin, during which time acid suppression may be maintained with histamine type 2 blockers. Biochemical testing can help support the diagnosis for other functional PNETs, but given their rarity, there are no universally accepted diagnostic thresholds.[46,56,57]

Imaging

Imaging studies play a vital role in the diagnosis and workup of PNETs. Computed tomography (CT) is the most commonly used modality, and it has several favorable characteristics when compared with other studies: it is quick, widely available, and provides excellent anatomic definition of the pancreas, and of lymph node or liver metastases (**Figs. 1** and **2**). The mean sensitivity of CT for PNETs is 82%.[62,63] MRI has a similar mean sensitivity of 79% for primary PNETs, but is significantly more sensitive than CT for the detection of liver metastases, particularly when hepatocyte specific contrast agents are used (eg, Eovist).[63–65] Because of this, MRI is primarily used to evaluate liver tumor burden, particularly in patients for whom hepatic debulking is being considered.[53,54]

Somatostatin receptors are expressed by 80% to 100% of PNETs, with the exception of insulinomas for which the rate of expression is 50% to 70%.[66] Functional imaging techniques include indium-111 somatostatin receptor scintigraphy (^{111}In-SRS, octreoscan) and gallium-68 positron emission tomography (^{68}Ga-PET, Netspot), both of which use radiolabeled somatostatin analogs (SSAs) to localize NETs (see

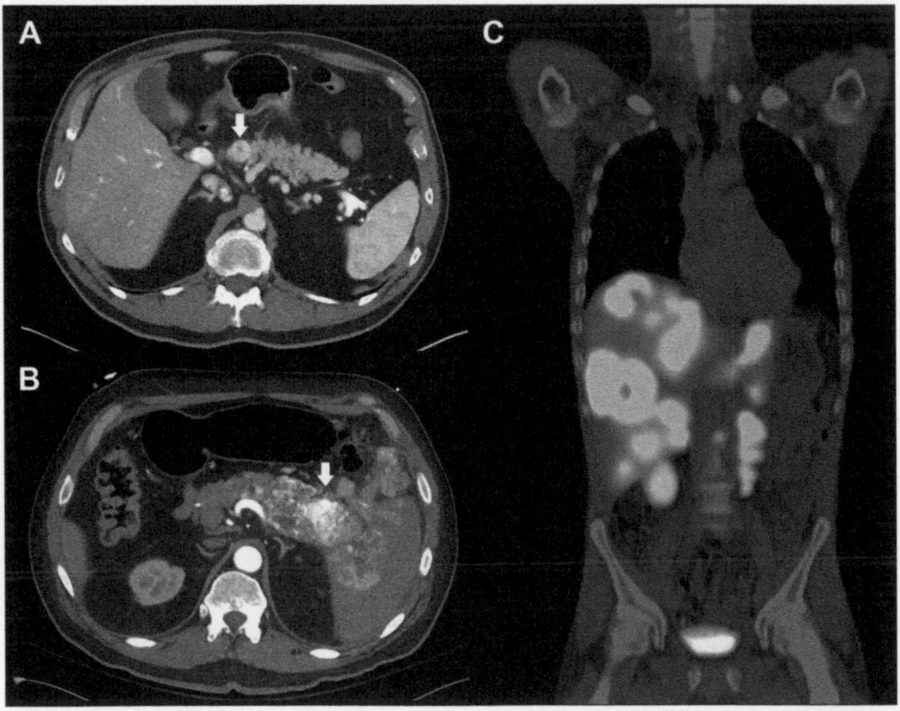

Fig. 1. (*A*) Arterial phase CT showing a well-circumscribed, enhancing PNET (*arrow*). (*B*) Arterial phase CT showing an enhancing PNET (*arrow*), which is directly invading the spleen and peritoneal cavity. (*C*) ^{68}Ga-PET allows the entire body to be imaged in a single study. In this patient, who had previously undergone primary PNET resection, extensive metastases are seen in the liver, paraaortic lymph nodes, and left supraclavicular lymph nodes.

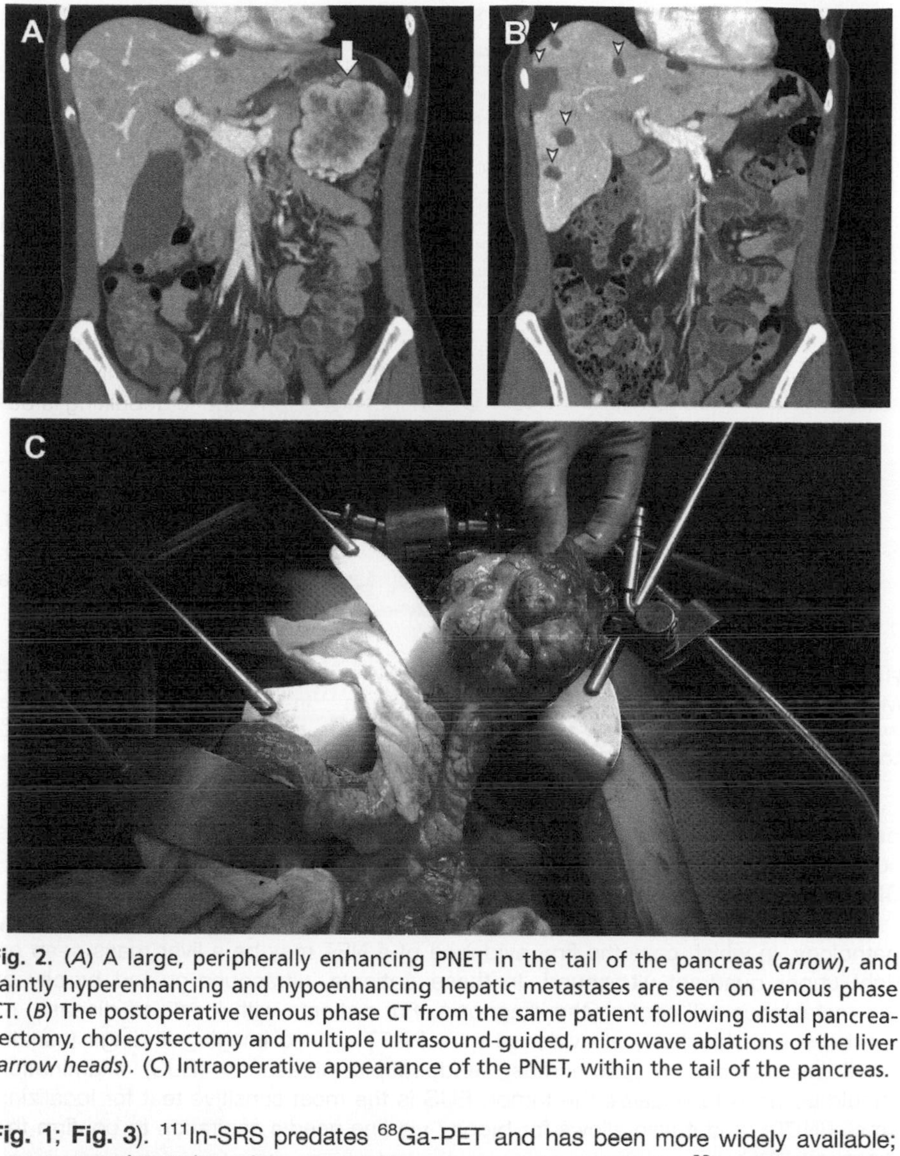

Fig. 2. (*A*) A large, peripherally enhancing PNET in the tail of the pancreas (*arrow*), and faintly hyperenhancing and hypoenhancing hepatic metastases are seen on venous phase CT. (*B*) The postoperative venous phase CT from the same patient following distal pancreatectomy, cholecystectomy and multiple ultrasound-guided, microwave ablations of the liver (*arrow heads*). (*C*) Intraoperative appearance of the PNET, within the tail of the pancreas.

Fig. 1; **Fig. 3**). ^{111}In-SRS predates ^{68}Ga-PET and has been more widely available; however, owing to its quicker acquisition and superior sensitivity, ^{68}Ga-PET is rapidly becoming the functional imaging modality of choice.[62,63] A recent metaanalysis found the pooled sensitivity and specificity of ^{68}Ga-PET for the diagnosis of NETs were 93% and 91%, respectively.[67] Somatostatin receptor–based imaging will often clearly show distant metastases that are not apparent on conventional imaging, and is very useful for evaluating the entire body in a single scan, or for equivocal lesions on CT or MRI. Although the spatial resolution of ^{68}Ga-PET is superior to that of ^{111}In-SRS, the noncontrasted CT scan, which accompanies it does not provide adequate anatomic definition for surgical planning, and a contrast enhanced CT and/or MRI is still required for this purpose. Finally, while fluorodeoxyglucose with PET (FDG-PET) is widely used to image other malignancies, well-differentiated PNETs are comparatively slow growing and frequently do not show avid glucose uptake. FDG-PET may

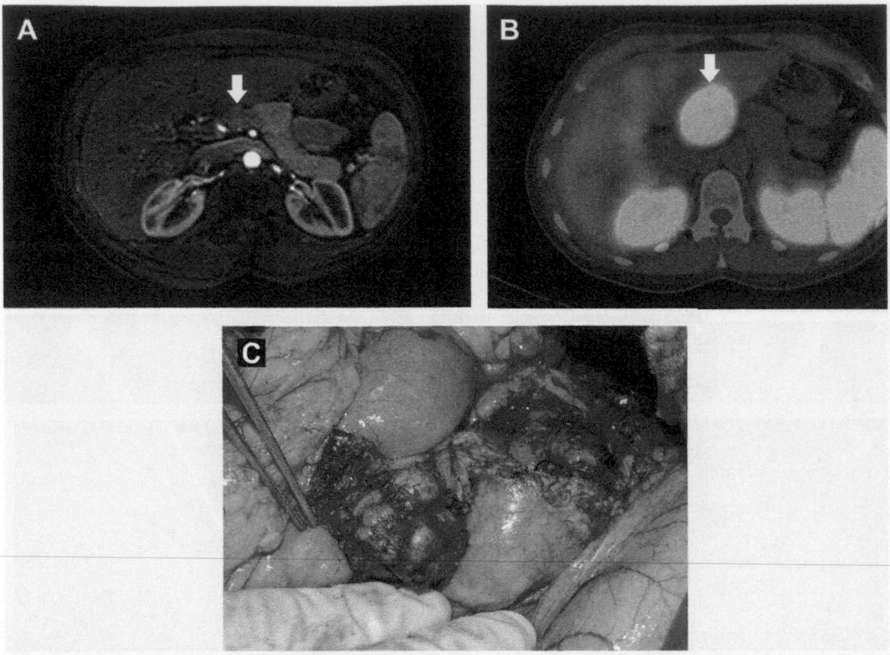

Fig. 3. (*A*) Hypoenhancing pancreatic neck mass shown on contrast enhanced, T1 weighted MRI (*arrow*). (*B*) The same mass shows intense uptake on ^{111}In-SRS (*arrow*). (*C*) The mass was well-encapsulated and not near the pancreatic duct; thus, enucleation and lymphadenectomy were performed.

be used for imaging poorly differentiated tumors, which are also less likely to express somatostatin receptors, and thus less likely to show up well on ^{68}Ga-PET or ^{111}In-SRS.[68]

Patients who present with liver metastases can have symptoms mimicking biliary pathology, in which case the first evidence of a NET may be a liver mass seen on right upper quadrant ultrasound. In these patients, ultrasound-guided biopsy of the metastases will confirm the diagnosis. For patients with localized disease, or for those with biochemical evidence of a PNET but no imaging findings (usually small insulinomas or gastrinomas), endoscopic ultrasound (EUS) examination should be used to visualize the tumor. EUS is the most sensitive test for localizing small PNETs, and it also allows for biopsy via fine needle aspiration to confirm the diagnosis.[69–71]

Pathology

PNETs are definitively diagnosed by immunohistochemistry and histologic examination of the tumor.[45,72,73] Tissue may be obtained via EUS examination and fine needle aspiration of the pancreatic tumor, by percutaneous core needle biopsy of a liver metastasis, or by surgical resection, although every effort should be made to obtain a tissue diagnosis before operation. Immunohistochemical examination of the tumor should include staining for general NET markers, commonly chromogranin and synaptophysin, as well as markers for the site of origin, which is particularly important for NET liver metastases of unknown origin. First-line immunohistochemistry markers for this purpose include PAX6 (paired box 6), PAX8 (paired box 8), ISL1 (islet 1),

CDX2 (caudal type homeobox 2), and TTF1 (thyroid transcription factor 1). Of these, PAX6, PAX8, and ISL1 serve as pancreatic markers, and CDX2 positivity suggests a small bowel NET and TTF1 indicates a lung NET.[72,73] Once the neuroendocrine nature of the tumor has been established, the tumor should be graded by the Ki-67 index (proliferative index) and mitotic rate according to 2017 World Health Organization classification (**Table 3**).[35] Due to the limited amount of material returned by FNA, biopsies obtained using this technique may be more prone to sampling error, and tend to underestimate tumor grade.[71,74] PNETs are staged according to the 8th edition of the AJCC Cancer Staging Manual (seen here), or the ENETS system, which is largely similar.[75] A study comparing validity of these two staging systems found them to be equally valid, and that a model which employed the Ki-67 index as a continuous variable was more prognostic than either.[76]

MANAGEMENT

The treatment of PNETs is a multidisciplinary effort, incorporating surgery, SSAs, targeted therapy, and cytotoxic chemotherapy. A number of recent trials have significantly expanded the therapeutic options, and guidelines for treatment continue to evolve.

Surgery

Surgery is the mainstay of treatment for PNETs.[31,45,53–55] For patients with localized disease, resection is frequently curative, and even those with distant metastases may derive significant benefit in terms of both symptom control and survival from surgical debulking.[77,78] The surgical approach to PNETs depends on the size and location of the tumor, functional status, and presence or absence of distant metastases. Resection of PNETs may be accomplished by pancreaticoduodenectomy (Whipple procedure) or distal pancreatectomy; however, the high morbidity associated with major pancreatic resection combined with the indolent growth of well-differentiated PNETs has led to the adoption of more conservative strategies for small tumors, including enucleation or careful observation.[79]

Localized Disease

For patients with PNETs confined to the pancreas and regional lymph nodes, treatment options include distal pancreatectomy, pancreaticoduodenectomy, central

Table 3
2017 World Health Organization classification of PNETs

Classification/Grade	Ki-67 Proliferative Index	Mitotic Index (per 10 HPF)
Well-differentiated NET		
Grade 1	<3%	<2
Grade 2	3%–20%	2–20
Grade 3	>20%	>20
Poorly differentiated NEC		
Grade 3	>20%	>20

Abbreviation: HPF, high-power field.
Data from Lloyd RV, Osamura RY, Klöppel G, Rosai J. WHO classification of tumours of endocrine organs. 4th Edition ed. Lyon, France: International Agency for Research on Cancer; 2017.

pancreatectomy, enucleation, or observation. All PNETs larger than 2 cm and functional tumors, irrespective of size, should be resected.[31,45,53–55] Incidentally discovered PNETs less than 2 cm in size generally exhibit benign behavior,[80] and the increasingly frequent diagnosis of small, nonfunctional PNETs has heightened the controversy over how these tumors should be managed. Single-institutional studies have shown that a nonoperative approach to PNETs smaller than 2 cm is feasible and safe: with an average follow-up of 3 to 4 years, no patients under observation developed metastases and there was no disease-specific mortality.[81,82] The risks of observation must be balanced against the complication rate for patients undergoing resection of PNETs, which is roughly 30%, and as high as 45% in patients undergoing pancreaticoduodenectomy or total pancreatectomy.[83] In an effort to avoid these complications, close observation rather than resection may be considered for well-differentiated PNETs less than 2 cm, particularly those confirmed to be low grade by biopsy.[46,54] However, recommendations for conservative management should be interpreted with caution: reviews of the Surveillance, Epidemiology, and End Results and National Cancer Data Base databases have found that nearly 30% of PNETs less than 2 cm had nodal involvement, clearly demonstrating the malignant potential of these tumors, and studies supporting the safety of observation had relatively short follow-up.[81,82,84,85] Additionally, a metaanalysis of studies comparing resection with nonsurgical management found that surgery was associated with a significant overall survival benefit, even for PNETs less than 2 cm.[79]

When the decision to resect is made, enucleation can be considered for tumors that are well-circumscribed, small, well-differentiated, not in close proximity to the pancreatic duct, and without evidence of nodal or distant metastases (see **Fig. 3**).[45,54,55] The primary advantage of enucleation versus standard pancreatic resection is that the former is associated with a lower rate of postoperative pancreatic insufficiency,[55] although this advantage may primarily apply only to pancreatic head masses.[86] Additionally, pancreatic enucleation is associated with a similar rate of overall complications, and a higher rate of postoperative pancreatic fistula when compared with standard resection.[79,86] Small tumors located in the pancreatic body that are too close to the duct to allow for enucleation may be resected via central pancreatectomy.[31,55]

Formal pancreatic resection should be performed for tumors that are larger than 2 to 3 cm, abutting the pancreatic duct, intermediate or high grade, or suspicious for lymph node involvement.[31,54,55] Pancreaticoduodenectomy is performed for tumors of the pancreatic head, and tumors in the body or tail are resected via distal pancreatectomy, with or without splenic preservation. Regional lymphadenectomy should be performed as a matter of course with pancreatic resection, because more than 50% of tumors larger than 2 cm will have nodal metastases.[46,54,84,87] Recurrence is common even after R0 resection and is significantly more likely in patients with nodal metastases.[46,87]

Although several factors, including tumor size greater than 3 to 4 cm, lymph node involvement, tumor vascularity as assessed by CT, and Ki-67 index greater than 5%, are associated with an increased likelihood of recurrence,[87–89] the optimal frequency and duration of follow-up has not been conclusively established. Surveillance should include imaging with CT scans or MRI and monitoring of serum markers, particularly if these were elevated preoperatively. Follow-up is initially at 3 to 6 months, and then every 6 to 12 months in the absence of recurrence, but this schedule may be more frequent for high-grade tumors. Given the risk of late recurrence, surveillance should be continued for at least 7 years after resection. ^{68}Ga-PET may be used to evaluate equivocal evidence of disease recurrence.[53,55]

Metastatic Disease

Although patients with distant metastases have generally passed the point at which curative resection may be hoped for, surgery continues to play a central role in their treatment.[45,54,55,77,78,90–92] The liver is the overwhelmingly favored site of metastasis for PNETs, accounting for roughly 80% of all metastases, but metastases to the bone, distant lymph nodes, and peritoneal cavity (by direct invasion) are also frequent.[93] Significant hepatic replacement by tumor is common, and, among patients with metastatic disease, liver failure is the most common cause of death. In contrast with surgery for metastatic adenocarcinoma, the importance of margin status is deemphasized, and there is a proportionally greater emphasis on preservation of normal hepatic parenchyma. There seems to be minimal benefit associated with R0/R1 resection compared with R2, and even when R0 margins are achieved, eventual disease recurrence is nearly universal.[90,91] Numerous surgical series have shown that cytoreductive surgery improves survival and symptomatic control, and historically this has been attempted when 90% cytoreduction was deemed feasible. Although a significant majority of patients will be considered unresectable at this threshold, recent studies have shown similar results may be achieved using a lower cutoff of 70% debulking. To achieve adequate cytoreduction in patients with numerous, bilobar liver metastases, parenchyma-sparing techniques including enucleation and intraoperative, ultrasound-guided ablation are used (see **Fig. 2**), with similar results compared with formal hepatectomy.[77,78,92]

Cytoreductive surgery is largely accepted as a standard treatment for PNET liver metastases,[45,54,55] but precise indications and contraindications for surgery continue to be defined. Broadly, patients should be considered for debulking if they have well-differentiated, grade 1 or 2, metastatic PNETs with less than 50% hepatic replacement (preferably <25%) with a surgically amenable distribution (ie, not miliary), normal or near-normal liver function, and no evidence of carcinoid heart disease or other major comorbidities. Extrahepatic metastases should not be considered a contraindication to hepatic debulking, and peritoneal tumor deposits may be resected concurrently.[77,92] For patients with extensive liver involvement who are ineligible for hepatic debulking, but are otherwise well-suited for surgery and have no evidence of extrahepatic disease, liver transplantation seems to offer improved survival.[94,95] However, the potential benefits of transplant must be carefully weighed against the scarcity of available grafts and the prospect of lifelong immunosuppression. Moreover, the indications for transplant, as defined by the Milan NET criteria,[95] are very similar to those for hepatic debulking, further complicating patient selection.

Primary tumor resection should be considered in patients with metastatic disease to avoid obstructive complications from the pancreatic mass and further metastatic seeding. In most cases, this procedure may be performed simultaneously; the primary exception is for pancreaticoduodenectomy and hepatic ablation, which should be performed in a staged fashion to avoid the theoretic risk of hepatic abscess formation. Even in the case of unresectable metastatic disease, there may be a survival advantage associated with resection of the primary tumor,[96] although studies showing a benefit may be prone to selection bias.

Patients with metastatic PNETs are usually treated long-term with SSAs such as octreotide long-acting-repeatable or lanreotide. The incidence of gallstones in these patients is roughly 50%, significantly higher than in the general population. Because the rate of symptomatic biliary disease remains low, prophylactic cholecystectomy is not recommended as a separate operation. However, the risk of developing complications from gallstones is sufficiently increased to warrant cholecystectomy for patients undergoing primary resection or hepatic cytoreduction, particularly because laparoscopic cholecystectomy may be more difficult after liver surgery.[97]

Patients with distant metastases should be assumed to have residual tumor following surgery and should undergo routine biochemical and radiographic surveillance.[53,55,90] Patients should be seen in 3 to 6 months after surgery, and then every 6 to 12 months thereafter. Rapid progression or high-grade disease warrants more frequent surveillance.[53,55]

Surgical Approach

In general, PNETs are approached via laparotomy to facilitate adequate inspection of the abdomen and debulking of nodal or distant metastases. However, for patients with small localized tumors, distal pancreatectomy or enucleation may be performed laparoscopically with similar outcomes.[54,55,98] The role of laparoscopy for metastatic disease is significantly more limited. For patients with PNETs and liver-dominant disease, laparoscopic hepatic ablation offers a less invasive alternative to open surgery, with equivalent rates of symptomatic improvement, significantly less morbidity, and a much shorter hospital course.[99]

Hereditary Syndromes

Many of the principles of management are common between sporadic and inherited PNETs, but there are some special considerations for patients with hereditary syndromes such as MEN-1 and VHL. The surgical management of MEN-1 is covered in Colleen M. Kiernan and Elizabeth G. Grubbs' article, "Surgical Management of MEN-1 and MEN-2," in this issue, and this effort will not be duplicated here. The most common pancreatic manifestations of VHL are multiple cysts or serous cystadenomas; however, PNETs are also seen in approximately 10% to 20% of these patients.[48,52,55,100] PNETs associated with VHL are frequently multiple and usually nonfunctional. They are also significantly more likely to be benign than sporadic tumors, and have longer recurrence-free survival after resection.[52,100] The risk of progression for PNETs less than 1.5 cm in patients with VHL seems to be very low, and this observation, coupled with the high incidence of multifocal tumors, has led to recommendations against routine resection of asymptomatic PNETs smaller than 1.5 cm.[100] Tumors greater than 3 cm in size, with a doubling time of less than 500 days or exon 3 mutations are significantly more likely to metastasize, and, therefore, these factors are indications for resection in patients with VHL.[101]

Liver-Directed Therapy

For patients with PNET liver metastases, percutaneous ablation and hepatic artery embolization (HAE) are less invasive options for hepatic cytoreduction compared with surgery. Percutaneous ablation of liver metastases may be performed using radiofrequency ablation, microwave ablation, or cryoablation.[45,54,55,102,103] A direct comparison of each modality for the treatment of PNET liver metastases is difficult owing to the limited data in the literature, but extrapolation from the treatment of hepatocellular cancer suggests that outcomes are similar.[104,105] Microwave ablation has several theoretic advantages over radiofrequency ablation, including faster ablation time and higher intertumoral temperature, and may be superior for larger lesions.[104,106] Reported rates of symptomatic improvement and complete ablation are both greater than 90%.[103,106] Percutaneous ablation is a reasonable option for the treatment of 1 or only a few metastases, particularly in patients who are not candidates for surgical resection.[45]

HAE takes advantage of the fact that liver metastases are preferentially supplied by the hepatic artery, in contrast with the normal liver parenchyma, which receives much of its blood supply from the portal vein. A catheter is introduced into the hepatic artery and used to deliver therapy locally to the metastatic lesions rather than systemically. Bland HAE is performed using polyvinyl alcohol particles, which occlude blood flow to the metastases, inducing hypoxic necrosis. Chemotherapy or radioactive microspheres may also be delivered via the catheter (chemoembolization and radioembolization, respectively), but at this time no one method has been shown to be definitively superior.[107] Patients are admitted after embolization for the management of a constellation of symptoms referred to as postembolization syndrome. This self-limited syndrome is characterized by fever, abdominal pain, nausea, and vomiting and occurs in up to 90% of patients after the procedure.[108] HAE is indicated for patients with liver-dominant disease and a patent portal vein who are not candidates for operative hepatic debulking.[45,54,55]

Medical Therapy

For patients with localized PNETs, resection is often curative, and no further treatment is needed in the absence of recurrence. For patients with metastases, a number of systemic therapies are available for disease control and symptom palliation. Streptozocin was one of the first agents to show activity against PNETs, but significant side effects and the more recent introduction of less toxic therapies have limited its use.[109,110] The antiproliferative properties of SSAs were demonstrated by the CLARINET trial and, owing to their favorable side effect profile and inhibition of hormone secretion, long-acting SSAs are considered first-line therapy for metastatic PNETs.[45,54,55,111,112] The tyrosine kinase inhibitor sunitinib and the mammalian target of rapamycin inhibitor everolimus are second-line treatments that are generally well-tolerated and are associated with modest improvements in progression-free survival.[113,114] Although previous chemotherapeutic regimens have provided only moderate survival benefits and substantial toxicity, the combination of capecitabine and temozolomide (CAPTEM) has been introduced as a promising new regimen with high objective response rates, improved survival, and superior tolerability.[115,116] Finally, peptide receptor radionuclide therapy was recently shown to significantly increase progression-free survival in patients with metastatic NETs in the NETTER-1 trial. Although this trial enrolled only patients with midgut NETs, other nonrandomized trials have shown similar results in NETs arising from other sites, and peptide receptor radionuclide therapy was recently approved by the US Food and Drug Administration for the treatment of all NETs.[117] A summary of selected randomized, controlled trials for the treatment of PNETs are presented in **Table 4**.

High-Grade Pancreatic Neuroendocrine Tumors

Until recently, all high-grade PNETs, defined by a Ki-67 index of greater than 20%, were classified as neuroendocrine carcinoma (NEC); as of the latest World Health Organization classifications, they are now divided into high-grade well-differentiated NETs and poorly differentiated NEC (see **Table 3**).[35] NEC may be further subdivided into small cell and large cell types, but it is unclear how this classification may affect prognosis or treatment.[118,119] With a median survival of 5 to 21 months, these tumors are significantly rarer and more aggressive than well-differentiated, grade 1 and 2 PNETs, and their management is distinct in several respects.[118–120] High-grade PNETs are more metabolically active and less likely to express somatostatin receptors. Thus, they are more likely to be detected by FDG-PET and less likely to show uptake on somatostatin receptor based imaging when compared with low-grade

Table 4
Selected randomized controlled trials for the treatment of PNETs

Trial	Year	Enrollment	Patients Enrolled	Intervention	Comparator	Progression Free Survival	Response Rate
Moertel et al	1980	Unresectable, metastatic PNETs	84	STZ 500 mg/m^2 + FU 400 mg/m^2 daily × 5 d, q6w	STZ 500 mg/m^2 daily × 5 d, q6w	Not reported	63% vs 36% ($P < .01$)
Raymond et al	2011	Well-differentiated, progressive, unresectable PNETs	171	Sunitinib 37.5 mg/daily	Placebo	11.4 vs 5.5 mo ($P < .001$)	9.3% vs 0% ($P = .007$)
RADIANT-3	2011	Low or intermediate-grade, unresectable, progressive PNETs	410	Everolimus 10 mg/daily	Placebo	11.0 vs 4.6 mo ($P < .001$)	5% vs 2% ($P < .001$)
CLARINET	2014	Nonfunctioning enteropancreatic NETs or gastrinoma, SSR+, unresectable, Ki-67 <10%, 96% stable disease	204 (45% PNETs)	Lanreotide 120 mg q28d	Placebo	65.1% vs 33.0% at 24 mo ($P < .001$)	Not reported
NETTER-1	2017	Well-differentiated, unresectable, progressive midgut NETs, SSR+, Ki-67 <20%	229	177Lu-Dotatate peptide receptor radionuclide therapy 7.4 GBq q8w + octreotide LAR 30 mg q4w	Octreotide LAR 60 mg q4w	65.2% vs 10.8% at 20 mo ($P < .001$)	18% vs 3% ($P < .001$)
E2211	2018	Low or intermediate-grade, unresectable, progressive PNETs	144	CAP 750 mg/m^2 BID × 14 d + TMZ 200 mg/m^2 daily × 5 d	TMZ 200 mg/m^2 daily × 5 d	22.7 vs 14.4 mo ($P = .023$)	Not reported

Abbreviations: CAP, capecitabine; FU, follow-up; LAR, long-acting-repeatable; STZ, streptozocin; TMZ, temozolomide.
Data from Refs.[53,109,112–114,117]

tumors.[68] On immunohistochemical examination, high-grade tumors are less likely to stain positively for chromogranin, and the typical markers used to assign a site of origin cannot be reliably applied.[72,118,119]

Surgical resection should be considered for localized, high-grade PNETs and should involve formal oncologic resection (pancreaticoduodenectomy or distal pancreatectomy with lymphadenectomy) rather than enucleation.[53,54,118] Patients with metastases derive minimal benefit from cytoreduction, and should not be considered for debulking surgery.[78] Adjuvant chemotherapy and follow-up every 3 months after resection is recommended owing to the high risk of recurrence.[53,118] Standard first-line chemotherapy for high-grade PNETs consists of cisplatin or carboplatin plus etoposide or irinotecan.[53,54,110,118] A number of other agents have been suggested as second-line therapy, but none are well-validated.[53,54,110,118] Among high-grade PNETs, those with a Ki-67 index between 20% and 55% were less likely to respond to platinum-based chemotherapy, but were associated with better survival than those with a Ki-67 index of greater than 55%.[119] This finding may reflect the difference between well-differentiated, high-grade PNETs, which typically have Ki-67 indices closer to 20%, and poorly differentiated NECs, which typically have much higher Ki-67 indices. SSAs, everolimus, and sunitinib play a limited role in the treatment of high-grade PNETs.

SUMMARY

PNETs are rare malignancies characterized by indolent growth and a propensity to metastasize. The heterogeneity of PNETs is striking: they may present with debilitating hormonal syndromes, diffuse liver metastases, or as asymptomatic, incidentally discovered masses. Similarly, their prognosis runs the gamut from extremely favorable, as is the case with the majority of insulinomas, to dismal for poorly differentiated NEC. Once a PNET is suspected, the diagnostic workup should consist of biochemical testing for NET markers and thorough imaging, which may include CT scans, MRI, EUS examination, and ^{68}Ga-PET. The diagnosis is confirmed by verifying immunohistochemistry positivity for NET markers, at which point the tumor is graded according to the World Health Organization classification. Pancreatic tumors, which are low grade, nonfunctional, stable in size and smaller than 2 cm, may be safely observed, whereas those that do not meet these criteria are indicated for resection. Standard resections include pancreaticoduodenectomy for head masses and central or distal pancreatectomy for body and tail masses. Enucleation is an option for selected tumors smaller than 3 cm that are not abutting the pancreatic duct. Patients with well-differentiated, metastatic PNETs should be considered for surgical debulking, with or without concurrent primary resection, to improve survival and for symptom control. Other options for hepatic cytoreduction include percutaneous ablation, HAE, and liver transplantation in highly selected patients. A wide variety of systemic therapies are now available for the treatment of metastatic disease including SSAs, everolimus, sunitinib, peptide receptor radionuclide therapy and CAPTEM. High-grade PNETs carry a grave prognosis and are treated primarily with platinum-based chemotherapy. Formal oncologic resection may be considered for localized disease, but does not play a role in the treatment of metastatic, high-grade tumors.

REFERENCES

1. Schimmack S, Svejda B, Lawrence B, et al. The diversity and commonalities of gastroenteropancreatic neuroendocrine tumors. Langenbecks Arch Surg 2011; 396(3):273–98.

2. Langerhans P. Beiträge zur mikroskopischen Anatomie der Bauchspeicheldrüse. Berlin: Buchdruckerei von Gustav Lange; 1869.
3. Da Silva Xavier G. The cells of the islets of Langerhans. J Clin Med 2018;7(3):54.
4. Vortmeyer AO, Huang S, Lubensky I, et al. Non-islet origin of pancreatic islet cell tumors. J Clin Endocrinol Metab 2004;89(4):1934–8.
5. Modlin IM, Moss SF, Gustafsson BI, et al. The archaic distinction between functioning and nonfunctioning neuroendocrine neoplasms is no longer clinically relevant. Langenbecks Arch Surg 2011;396(8):1145–56.
6. Nicholls AG. Simple adenoma of the pancreas arising from an Island of Langerhans. J Med Res 1902;8(2):385–95.
7. Oberndorfer S. Karzinoide Tumoren des Dünndarms. Frankf Z Pathol 1907;1:425–32.
8. Williams ED, Sandler M. The classification of carcinoid tumours. Lancet 1963;1(7275):238–9.
9. Harris S. Hyperinsulinism and dysinsulinism. J Am Med Assoc 1924;83(10):729–33.
10. Wilder RM, Allan FN, Power MH, et al. Carcinoma of the islands of the pancreas: hyperinsulinism and hypoglycemia. J Am Med Assoc 1927;89(5):348–55.
11. Howland G, Campbell WR, Maltby EJ, et al. Dysinsulinism: convulsions and coma due to islet cell tumor of the pancreas, with operation and cure. J Am Med Assoc 1929;93(9):674–9.
12. Arnett JH, Long CF. A case of congenital stenosis of the pulmonary valve, with late onset of cyanosis: death from carcinoma of the pancreas. Am J Med Sci 1931;182:212.
13. Peart WS, Porter KA, Robertson JI, et al. Carcinoid syndrome due to pancreatic-duct neoplasm secreting 5-hydroxytryptophan and 5-hydroxytryptamine. Lancet 1963;1(7275):239–43.
14. Becker S, Kahn D, Rothman S. Cutaneous manifestations of internal malignant tumors. Archives of Dermatology and Syphilology 1942;45(6):1069–80.
15. Del Castillo EB, Trucco E, Manzuoli J. [Cushing's disease and cancer of the pancreas]. Presse Med 1950;58(43):783–5.
16. Balls KF, Nicholson JTL, Goodman HL, et al. Functioning islet-cell carcinoma of the pancreas with Cushing's syndrome. J Clin Endocrinol Metab 1959;19(9):1134–43.
17. Zollinger RM, Ellison EH. Primary peptic ulcerations of the jejunum associated with islet cell tumors of the pancreas. Ann Surg 1955;142(4):709–23.
18. Verner JV, Morrison AB. Islet cell tumor and a syndrome of refractory watery diarrhea and hypokalemia. Am J Med 1958;25(3):374–80.
19. DeWys WD, Stoll R, Au WY, et al. Effects of streptozotocin on an islet cell carcinoma with hypercalcemia. Am J Med 1973;55(5):671–6.
20. Larsson LI, Hirsch MA, Holst JJ, et al. Pancreatic somatostatinoma. Clinical features and physiological implications. Lancet 1977;1(8013):666–8.
21. Caplan RH, Koob L, Abellera RM, et al. Cure of acromegaly by operative removal of an islet cell tumor of the pancreas. Am J Med 1978;64(5):874–82.
22. Feurle GE, Helmstaedter V, Tischbirek K, et al. A multihormonal tumor of the pancreas producing neurotensin. Dig Dis Sci 1981;26(12):1125–33.
23. Rehfeld JF, Federspiel B, Bardram L. A neuroendocrine tumor syndrome from cholecystokinin secretion. N Engl J Med 2013;368(12):1165–6.
24. Dasari A, Shen C, Halperin D, et al. Trends in the incidence, prevalence, and survival outcomes in patients with neuroendocrine tumors in the United States. JAMA Oncol 2017;3(10):1335–42.

25. Lawrence B, Gustafsson BI, Chan A, et al. The epidemiology of gastroentero-pancreatic neuroendocrine tumors. Endocrinol Metab Clin North Am 2011;40(1):1–18, vii.
26. Yao JC, Hassan M, Phan A, et al. One hundred years after "carcinoid": epidemiology of and prognostic factors for neuroendocrine tumors in 35,825 cases in the United States. J Clin Oncol 2008;26(18):3063–72.
27. Hallet J, Law CH, Cukier M, et al. Exploring the rising incidence of neuroendocrine tumors: a population-based analysis of epidemiology, metastatic presentation, and outcomes. Cancer 2015;121(4):589–97.
28. Halfdanarson TR, Rabe KG, Rubin J, et al. Pancreatic neuroendocrine tumors (PNETs): incidence, prognosis and recent trend toward improved survival. Ann Oncol 2008;19(10):1727–33.
29. Yao JC, Eisner MP, Leary C, et al. Population-based study of islet cell carcinoma. Ann Surg Oncol 2007;14(12):3492–500.
30. Fottner C, Ferrata M, Weber MM. Hormone secreting gastro-entero-pancreatic neuroendocrine neoplasias (GEP-NEN): when to consider, how to diagnose? Rev Endocr Metab Disord 2017;18(4):393–410.
31. Kuo JH, Lee JA, Chabot JA. Nonfunctional pancreatic neuroendocrine tumors. Surg Clin North Am 2014;94(3):689–708.
32. Halfdanarson TR, Rubin J, Farnell MB, et al. Pancreatic endocrine neoplasms: epidemiology and prognosis of pancreatic endocrine tumors. Endocr Relat Cancer 2008;15(2):409–27.
33. de Wilde RF, Edil BH, Hruban RH, et al. Well-differentiated pancreatic neuroendocrine tumors: from genetics to therapy. Nat Rev Gastroenterol Hepatol 2012;9(4):199–208.
34. Jensen RT, Berna MJ, Bingham DB, et al. Inherited pancreatic endocrine tumor syndromes: advances in molecular pathogenesis, diagnosis, management, and controversies. Cancer 2008;113(7 Suppl):1807–43.
35. Lloyd RV, Osamura RY, Klöppel G, et al. WHO classification of tumours of endocrine organs. 4th Edition. Lyon (France): International Agency for Research on Cancer; 2017.
36. Sipos B, Sperveslage J, Anlauf M, et al. Glucagon cell hyperplasia and neoplasia with and without glucagon receptor mutations. J Clin Endocrinol Metab 2015;100(5):E783–8.
37. Niina Y, Fujimori N, Nakamura T, et al. The current strategy for managing pancreatic neuroendocrine tumors in multiple endocrine neoplasia type 1. Gut Liver 2012;6(3):287–94.
38. Chi W, Warner RRP, Chan DL, et al. Long-term outcomes of gastroenteropancreatic neuroendocrine tumors. Pancreas 2018;47(3):321–5.
39. Birnbaum DJ, Gaujoux S, Cherif R, et al. Sporadic nonfunctioning pancreatic neuroendocrine tumors: prognostic significance of incidental diagnosis. Surgery 2014;155(1):13–21.
40. Vagefi PA, Razo O, Deshpande V, et al. Evolving patterns in the detection and outcomes of pancreatic neuroendocrine neoplasms: the Massachusetts General Hospital experience from 1977 to 2005. Arch Surg 2007;142(4):347–54.
41. Oberg K, Eriksson B. Endocrine tumours of the pancreas. Best Pract Res Clin Gastroenterol 2005;19(5):753–81.
42. Li J, Luo G, Fu D, et al. Preoperative diagnosis of nonfunctioning pancreatic neuroendocrine tumors. Med Oncol 2011;28(4):1027–31.
43. Whipple AO, Frantz VK. Adenoma of islet cells with hyperinsulinism: a review. Ann Surg 1935;101(6):1299–335.

44. Ito T, Igarashi H, Jensen RT. Pancreatic neuroendocrine tumors: clinical features, diagnosis and medical treatment: advances. Best Pract Res Clin Gastroenterol 2012;26(6):737–53.
45. Kulke MH, Anthony LB, Bushnell DL, et al. NANETS treatment guidelines: well-differentiated neuroendocrine tumors of the stomach and pancreas. Pancreas 2010;39(6):735–52.
46. Falconi M, Eriksson B, Kaltsas G, et al. ENETS consensus guidelines update for the management of patients with functional pancreatic neuroendocrine tumors and non-functional pancreatic neuroendocrine tumors. Neuroendocrinology 2016;103(2):153–71.
47. Thakker RV, Newey PJ, Walls GV, et al. Clinical practice guidelines for multiple endocrine neoplasia type 1 (MEN1). J Clin Endocrinol Metab 2012;97(9):2990–3011.
48. Maher ER, Neumann HP, Richard S. von Hippel-Lindau disease: a clinical and scientific review. Eur J Hum Genet 2011;19(6):617–23.
49. Ferner RE, Huson SM, Thomas N, et al. Guidelines for the diagnosis and management of individuals with neurofibromatosis 1. J Med Genet 2007;44(2):81–8.
50. Larson AM, Hedgire SS, Deshpande V, et al. Pancreatic neuroendocrine tumors in patients with tuberous sclerosis complex. Clin Genet 2012;82(6):558–63.
51. Staley BA, Vail EA, Thiele EA. Tuberous sclerosis complex: diagnostic challenges, presenting symptoms, and commonly missed signs. Pediatrics 2011;127(1):e117–25.
52. Erlic Z, Ploeckinger U, Cascon A, et al. Systematic comparison of sporadic and syndromic pancreatic islet cell tumors. Endocr Relat Cancer 2010;17(4):875–83.
53. Kunz PL, Reidy-Lagunes D, Anthony LB, et al. Consensus guidelines for the management and treatment of neuroendocrine tumors. Pancreas 2013;42(4):557–77.
54. Singh S, Dey C, Kennecke H, et al. Consensus recommendations for the diagnosis and management of pancreatic neuroendocrine tumors: guidelines from a Canadian National Expert Group. Ann Surg Oncol 2015;22(8):2685–99.
55. Falconi M, Bartsch DK, Eriksson B, et al. ENETS consensus guidelines for the management of patients with digestive neuroendocrine neoplasms of the digestive system: well-differentiated pancreatic non-functioning tumors. Neuroendocrinology 2012;95(2):120–34.
56. Vinik AI, Chaya C. Clinical presentation and diagnosis of neuroendocrine tumors. Hematol Oncol Clin North Am 2016;30(1):21–48.
57. Hofland J, Zandee WT, de Herder WW. Role of biomarker tests for diagnosis of neuroendocrine tumours. Nat Rev Endocrinol 2018;14(11):656–69.
58. Yang X, Yang Y, Li Z, et al. Diagnostic value of circulating chromogranin a for neuroendocrine tumors: a systematic review and meta-analysis. PLoS One 2015;10(4):e0124884.
59. Marotta V, Zatelli MC, Sciammarella C, et al. Chromogranin A as circulating marker for diagnosis and management of neuroendocrine neoplasms: more flaws than fame. Endocr Relat Cancer 2018;25(1):R11–29.
60. Sherman SK, Maxwell JE, O'Dorisio MS, et al. Pancreastatin predicts survival in neuroendocrine tumors. Ann Surg Oncol 2014;21(9):2971–80.
61. Modlin IM, Kidd M, Bodei L, et al. The clinical utility of a novel blood-based multi-transcriptome assay for the diagnosis of neuroendocrine tumors of the gastrointestinal tract. Am J Gastroenterol 2015;110(8):1223–32.
62. Maxwell JE, Howe JR. Imaging in neuroendocrine tumors: an update for the clinician. Int J Endocr Oncol 2015;2(2):159–68.

63. Sundin A, Arnold R, Baudin E, et al. ENETS consensus guidelines for the standards of care in neuroendocrine tumors: radiological, nuclear medicine & hybrid imaging. Neuroendocrinology 2017;105(3):212–44.
64. Dromain C, de Baere T, Lumbroso J, et al. Detection of liver metastases from endocrine tumors: a prospective comparison of somatostatin receptor scintigraphy, computed tomography, and magnetic resonance imaging. J Clin Oncol 2005;23(1):70–8.
65. Tirumani SH, Jagannathan JP, Braschi-Amirfarzan M, et al. Value of hepatocellular phase imaging after intravenous gadoxetate disodium for assessing hepatic metastases from gastroenteropancreatic neuroendocrine tumors: comparison with other MRI pulse sequences and with extracellular agent. Abdom Radiol (NY) 2018;43(9):2329–39.
66. Reubi JC. Somatostatin and other Peptide receptors as tools for tumor diagnosis and treatment. Neuroendocrinology 2004;80(Suppl 1):51–6.
67. Treglia G, Castaldi P, Rindi G, et al. Diagnostic performance of Gallium-68 somatostatin receptor PET and PET/CT in patients with thoracic and gastroenteropancreatic neuroendocrine tumours: a meta-analysis. Endocrine 2012;42(1):80–7.
68. Squires MH 3rd, Volkan Adsay N, Schuster DM, et al. Octreoscan versus FDG-PET for neuroendocrine tumor staging: a biological approach. Ann Surg Oncol 2015;22(7):2295–301.
69. Puli SR, Kalva N, Bechtold ML, et al. Diagnostic accuracy of endoscopic ultrasound in pancreatic neuroendocrine tumors: a systematic review and meta analysis. World J Gastroenterol 2013;19(23):3678–84.
70. Rosch T, Lightdale CJ, Botet JF, et al. Localization of pancreatic endocrine tumors by endoscopic ultrasonography. N Engl J Med 1992;326(26):1721–6.
71. Zilli A, Arcidiacono PG, Conte D, et al. Clinical impact of endoscopic ultrasonography on the management of neuroendocrine tumors: lights and shadows. Dig Liver Dis 2018;50(1):6–14.
72. Bellizzi AM. Assigning site of origin in metastatic neuroendocrine neoplasms: a clinically significant application of diagnostic immunohistochemistry. Adv Anat Pathol 2013;20(5):285–314.
73. Klimstra DS, Modlin IR, Adsay NV, et al. Pathology reporting of neuroendocrine tumors: application of the Delphic consensus process to the development of a minimum pathology data set. Am J Surg Pathol 2010;34(3):300–13.
74. Weynand B, Borbath I, Bernard V, et al. Pancreatic neuroendocrine tumour grading on endoscopic ultrasound-guided fine needle aspiration: high reproducibility and inter-observer agreement of the Ki-67 labelling index. Cytopathology 2014;25(6):389–95.
75. Amin MB, Edge S, Greene F, et al, editors. AJCC cancer staging manual. 8th edition. New York: Springer International Publishing; 2017.
76. Ellison TA, Wolfgang CL, Shi C, et al. A single institution's 26-year experience with nonfunctional pancreatic neuroendocrine tumors: a validation of current staging systems and a new prognostic nomogram. Ann Surg 2014;259(2):204–12.
77. Morgan RE, Pommier SJ, Pommier RF. Expanded criteria for debulking of liver metastasis also apply to pancreatic neuroendocrine tumors. Surgery 2018;163(1):218–25.
78. Scott AT, Breheny PJ, Keck KJ, et al. Effective cytoreduction can be achieved in patients with numerous neuroendocrine tumor liver metastases (NETLMs). Surgery 2019;165(1):166–75.

79. Finkelstein P, Sharma R, Picado O, et al. Pancreatic neuroendocrine tumors (panNETs): analysis of overall survival of nonsurgical management versus surgical resection. J Gastrointest Surg 2017;21(5):855–66.
80. Bettini R, Partelli S, Boninsegna L, et al. Tumor size correlates with malignancy in nonfunctioning pancreatic endocrine tumor. Surgery 2011;150(1):75–82.
81. Lee LC, Grant CS, Salomao DR, et al. Small, nonfunctioning, asymptomatic pancreatic neuroendocrine tumors (PNETs): role for nonoperative management. Surgery 2012;152(6):965–74.
82. Gaujoux S, Partelli S, Maire F, et al. Observational study of natural history of small sporadic nonfunctioning pancreatic neuroendocrine tumors. J Clin Endocrinol Metab 2013;98(12):4784–9.
83. Smith JK, Ng SC, Hill JS, et al. Complications after pancreatectomy for neuroendocrine tumors: a national study. J Surg Res 2010;163(1):63–8.
84. Jutric Z, Grendar J, Hoen HM, et al. Regional metastatic behavior of nonfunctional pancreatic neuroendocrine tumors: impact of lymph node positivity on survival. Pancreas 2017;46(7):898–903.
85. Kuo EJ, Salem RR. Population-level analysis of pancreatic neuroendocrine tumors 2 cm or less in size. Ann Surg Oncol 2013;20(9):2815–21.
86. Jilesen AP, van Eijck CH, Busch OR, et al. Postoperative outcomes of enucleation and standard resections in patients with a pancreatic neuroendocrine tumor. World J Surg 2016;40(3):715–28.
87. Hashim YM, Trinkaus KM, Linehan DC, et al. Regional lymphadenectomy is indicated in the surgical treatment of pancreatic neuroendocrine tumors (PNETs). Ann Surg 2014;259(2):197–203.
88. Yamamoto Y, Okamura Y, Uemura S, et al. Vascularity and tumor size are significant predictors for recurrence after resection of a pancreatic neuroendocrine tumor. Ann Surg Oncol 2017;24(8):2363–70.
89. Genc CG, Falconi M, Partelli S, et al. Recurrence of pancreatic neuroendocrine tumors and survival predicted by Ki67. Ann Surg Oncol 2018;25(8):2467–74.
90. Mayo SC, de Jong MC, Pulitano C, et al. Surgical management of hepatic neuroendocrine tumor metastasis: results from an international multi-institutional analysis. Ann Surg Oncol 2010;17(12):3129–36.
91. Sarmiento JM, Heywood G, Rubin J, et al. Surgical treatment of neuroendocrine metastases to the liver: a plea for resection to increase survival. J Am Coll Surg 2003;197(1):29–37.
92. Maxwell JE, Sherman SK, O'Dorisio TM, et al. Liver-directed surgery of neuroendocrine metastases: what is the optimal strategy? Surgery 2016;159(1):320–33.
93. Riihimaki M, Hemminki A, Sundquist K, et al. The epidemiology of metastases in neuroendocrine tumors. Int J Cancer 2016;139(12):2679–86.
94. Moris D, Tsilimigras DI, Ntanasis-Stathopoulos I, et al. Liver transplantation in patients with liver metastases from neuroendocrine tumors: a systematic review. Surgery 2017;162(3):525–36.
95. Mazzaferro V, Pulvirenti A, Coppa J. Neuroendocrine tumors metastatic to the liver: how to select patients for liver transplantation? J Hepatol 2007;47(4):460–6.
96. Almond LM, Hodson J, Ford SJ, et al. Role of palliative resection of the primary tumour in advanced pancreatic and small intestinal neuroendocrine tumours: a systematic review and meta-analysis. Eur J Surg Oncol 2017;43(10):1808–15.
97. Trendle MC, Moertel CG, Kvols LK. Incidence and morbidity of cholelithiasis in patients receiving chronic octreotide for metastatic carcinoid and malignant islet cell tumors. Cancer 1997;79(4):830–4.

98. Fernandez-Cruz L, Blanco L, Cosa R, et al. Is laparoscopic resection adequate in patients with neuroendocrine pancreatic tumors? World J Surg 2008;32(5):904–17.
99. Mazzaglia PJ, Berber E, Milas M, et al. Laparoscopic radiofrequency ablation of neuroendocrine liver metastases: a 10-year experience evaluating predictors of survival. Surgery 2007;142(1):10–9.
100. de Mestier L, Gaujoux S, Cros J, et al. Long-term prognosis of resected pancreatic neuroendocrine tumors in von Hippel-Lindau disease is favorable and not influenced by small tumors left in place. Ann Surg 2015;262(2):384–8.
101. Blansfield JA, Choyke L, Morita SY, et al. Clinical, genetic and radiographic analysis of 108 patients with von Hippel-Lindau disease (VHL) manifested by pancreatic neuroendocrine neoplasms (PNETs). Surgery 2007;142(6):814–8 [discussion: 818.e1-2].
102. Lewis MA, Hobday TJ. Treatment of neuroendocrine tumor liver metastases. Int J Hepatol 2012;2012:973946.
103. Mohan H, Nicholson P, Winter DC, et al. Radiofrequency ablation for neuroendocrine liver metastases: a systematic review. J Vasc Interv Radiol 2015;26(7):935–42.e1.
104. Facciorusso A, Di Maso M, Muscatiello N. Microwave ablation versus radiofrequency ablation for the treatment of hepatocellular carcinoma: a systematic review and meta-analysis. Int J Hyperthermia 2016;32(3):339–44.
105. Mahnken AH, Konig AM, Figiel JH. Current technique and application of percutaneous cryotherapy. Rofo 2018;190(9):836–46.
106. Groeschl RT, Pilgrim CH, Hanna EM, et al. Microwave ablation for hepatic malignancies: a multiinstitutional analysis. Ann Surg 2014;259(6):1195–200.
107. Kennedy AS. Hepatic-directed therapies in patients with neuroendocrine tumors. Hematol Oncol Clin North Am 2016;30(1):193–207.
108. Leung DA, Goin JE, Sickles C, et al. Determinants of postembolization syndrome after hepatic chemoembolization. J Vasc Interv Radiol 2001;12(3):321–6.
109. Moertel CG, Hanley JA, Johnson LA. Streptozocin alone compared with streptozocin plus fluorouracil in the treatment of advanced islet-cell carcinoma. N Engl J Med 1980;303(21):1189–94.
110. Garcia-Carbonero R, Rinke A, Valle JW, et al. ENETS consensus guidelines for the standards of care in neuroendocrine neoplasms. systemic therapy 2: chemotherapy. Neuroendocrinology 2017;105(3):281–94.
111. Rinke A, Muller HH, Schade-Brittinger C, et al. Placebo-controlled, double-blind, prospective, randomized study on the effect of octreotide LAR in the control of tumor growth in patients with metastatic neuroendocrine midgut tumors: a report from the PROMID Study Group. J Clin Oncol 2009;27(28):4656–63.
112. Caplin ME, Pavel M, Cwikla JB, et al. Lanreotide in metastatic enteropancreatic neuroendocrine tumors. N Engl J Med 2014;371(3):224–33.
113. Raymond E, Dahan L, Raoul JL, et al. Sunitinib malate for the treatment of pancreatic neuroendocrine tumors. N Engl J Med 2011;364(6):501–13.
114. Yao JC, Shah MH, Ito T, et al. Everolimus for advanced pancreatic neuroendocrine tumors. N Engl J Med 2011;364(6):514–23.
115. Ramirez RA, Beyer DT, Chauhan A, et al. The role of capecitabine/temozolomide in metastatic neuroendocrine tumors. Oncologist 2016;21(6):671–5.
116. Kunz PL, Catalano PJ, Nimeiri H, et al. A randomized study of temozolomide or temozolomide and capecitabine in patients with advanced pancreatic neuroendocrine tumors: a trial of the ECOG-ACRIN Cancer Research Group (E2211) [Abstract]. J Clin Oncol 2018;36(15_suppl):4004.

117. Strosberg J, El-Haddad G, Wolin E, et al. Phase 3 trial of (177)Lu-Dotatate for Midgut neuroendocrine tumors. N Engl J Med 2017;376(2):125–35.
118. Ilett EE, Langer SW, Olsen IH, et al. Neuroendocrine carcinomas of the gastroenteropancreatic system: a comprehensive review. Diagnostics (Basel) 2015; 5(2):119–76.
119. Sorbye H, Welin S, Langer SW, et al. Predictive and prognostic factors for treatment and survival in 305 patients with advanced gastrointestinal neuroendocrine carcinoma (WHO G3): the NORDIC NEC study. Ann Oncol 2013;24(1): 152–60.
120. Strosberg JR, Cheema A, Weber J, et al. Prognostic validity of a novel American Joint Committee on Cancer Staging Classification for pancreatic neuroendocrine tumors. J Clin Oncol 2011;29(22):3044–9.

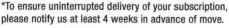

Printed and bound by CPI Group (UK) Ltd, Croydon, CR0 4YY

Printed and bound by CPI Group (UK) Ltd, Croydon, CR0 4YY
03/10/2024
01040408-0006